Genetics of Epilepsy and Genetic Epilepsies

Fondazione Pierfranco e Luisa Mariani
Viale Bianca Maria 28
20129 Milan, Italy

Telephone: +39 02 795458
Fax: +39 02 76009582
Publications coordinator: Valeria Basilico
e-mail: publications@fondazione-mariani.org
www.fondazione-mariani.org

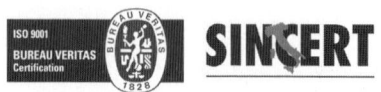

Spinal Cord Injuries: Advances in Rehabilitation

Spinal Cord Injuries: Advances in Rehabilitation

Editors

Mohit Arora
Ashley Craig

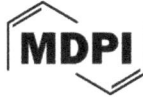

Basel • Beijing • Wuhan • Barcelona • Belgrade • Novi Sad • Cluj • Manchester

Editors

Mohit Arora
John Walsh Centre for
Rehabilitation Research
Northern Sydney Local Health
District
St Leonards, NSW
Australia

Ashley Craig
John Walsh Centre for
Rehabilitation Research
Northern Sydney Local Health
District
St Leonards, NSW
Australia

Editorial Office
MDPI AG
Grosspeteranlage 5
4052 Basel, Switzerland

This is a reprint of articles from the Special Issue published online in the open access journal *Journal of Clinical Medicine* (ISSN 2077-0383) (available at: https://www.mdpi.com/journal/jcm/special_issues/J1BH0XBOK7).

For citation purposes, cite each article independently as indicated on the article page online and as indicated below:

Lastname, A.A.; Lastname, B.B. Article Title. *Journal Name* **Year**, *Volume Number*, Page Range.

ISBN 978-3-7258-2139-6 (Hbk)
ISBN 978-3-7258-2140-2 (PDF)
doi.org/10.3390/books978-3-7258-2140-2

© 2024 by the authors. Articles in this book are Open Access and distributed under the Creative Commons Attribution (CC BY) license. The book as a whole is distributed by MDPI under the terms and conditions of the Creative Commons Attribution-NonCommercial-NoDerivs (CC BY-NC-ND) license.

Contents

About the Editors vii

Preface ix

Mohit Arora and Ashley R. Craig
Special Issue—Spinal Cord Injuries: Advances in Rehabilitation
Reprinted from: *J. Clin. Med.* **2024**, *13*, 1782, doi:10.3390/jcm13061782 1

Yuna Kim, Myungeun Lim, Seo Young Kim, Tae Uk Kim, Seong Jae Lee, Soo-Kyung Bok, et al.
Integrated Machine Learning Approach for the Early Prediction of Pressure Ulcers in Spinal Cord Injury Patients
Reprinted from: *J. Clin. Med.* **2024**, *13*, 990, doi:10.3390/jcm13040990 5

Anamaria Gherle, Carmen Delia Nistor-Cseppento, Diana-Carina Iovanovici, Iulia Ruxandra Cevei, Mariana Lidia Cevei, Danche Vasileva, et al.
Secondary Sarcopenia and Spinal Cord Injury: Clinical Associations and Health Outcomes
Reprinted from: *J. Clin. Med.* **2024**, *13*, 885, doi:10.3390/jcm13030885 23

Mohit Arora, Ilaria Pozzato, Candice McBain, Yvonne Tran, Danielle Sandalic, Daniel Myles, et al.
Cognitive Reserve and Its Association with Cognitive and Mental Health Status following an Acute Spinal Cord Injury
Reprinted from: *J. Clin. Med.* **2023**, *12*, 4258, doi:10.3390/jcm12134258 38

Jane Duff, Rebecca Ellis, Sally Kaiser and Lucy C Grant
Psychological Screening, Standards and Spinal Cord Injury: Introducing Change in NHS England Commissioned Services
Reprinted from: *J. Clin. Med.* **2023**, *12*, 7667, doi:10.3390/jcm12247667 50

Julia Tijsse Klasen, Tijn van Diemen, Nelleke G. Langerak and Ilse J. W. van Nes
Effects of Adaptations in an Interdisciplinary Follow-Up Clinic for People with Spinal Cord Injury in the Chronic Phase: A Prospective Cohort Study
Reprinted from: *J. Clin. Med.* **2023**, *12*, 7572, doi:10.3390/jcm12247572 75

Jacob Schoffl, Mohit Arora, Ilaria Pozzato, Candice McBain, Dianah Rodrigues, Elham Vafa, et al.
Heart Rate Variability Biofeedback in Adults with a Spinal Cord Injury: A Laboratory Framework and Case Series
Reprinted from: *J. Clin. Med.* **2023**, *12*, 7664, doi:10.3390/jcm12247664 88

Camila Quel de Oliveira, Anita Bundy, James W. Middleton, Kathryn Refshauge, Kris Rogers and Glen M. Davis
Activity-Based Therapy for Mobility, Function and Quality of Life after Spinal Cord Injuries—A Mixed-Methods Case Series
Reprinted from: *J. Clin. Med.* **2023**, *12*, 7588, doi:10.3390/jcm12247588 105

Monzurul Alam, Yan To Ling, Md Akhlasur Rahman, Arnold Yu Lok Wong, Hui Zhong, V. Reggie Edgerton and Yong-Ping Zheng
Restoration of Over-Ground Walking via Non-Invasive Neuromodulation Therapy: A Single-Case Study
Reprinted from: *J. Clin. Med.* **2023**, *12*, 7362, doi:10.3390/jcm12237362 122

Dewa Putu Wisnu Wardhana, Sri Maliawan, Tjokorda Gde Bagus Mahadewa, Rohadi Muhammad Rosyidi and Sinta Wiranata
The Impact of Machine Learning and Robot-Assisted Gait Training on Spinal Cord Injury: A Systematic Review and Meta-Analysis
Reprinted from: *J. Clin. Med.* **2023**, *12*, 7230, doi:10.3390/jcm12237230 . . . . **135**

Alicja Widuch-Spodyniuk, Beata Tarnacka, Bogumił Korczyński and Justyna Wiśniowska
Impact of Robotic-Assisted Gait Therapy on Depression and Anxiety Symptoms in Patients with Subacute Spinal Cord Injuries (SCIs)—A Prospective Clinical Study
Reprinted from: *J. Clin. Med.* **2023**, *12*, 7153, doi:10.3390/jcm12227153 . . . . **152**

Sylvia M. Gustin, Mark Bolding, William Willoughby, Monima Anam, Corey Shum, Deanna Rumble, et al.
Cortical Mechanisms Underlying Immersive Interactive Virtual Walking Treatment for Amelioration of Neuropathic Pain after Spinal Cord Injury: Findings from a Preliminary Investigation of Thalamic Inhibitory Function
Reprinted from: *J. Clin. Med.* **2023**, *12*, 5743, doi:10.3390/jcm12175743 . . . . **171**

Amy J. Starosta, Katherine S. Wright, Charles H. Bombardier, Faran Kahlia, Jason Barber, Michelle C. Accardi-Ravid, et al.
A Case Study of Hypnosis Enhanced Cognitive Therapy for Pain in a Ventilator Dependent Patient during Inpatient Rehabilitation for Spinal Cord Injury
Reprinted from: *J. Clin. Med.* **2023**, *12*, 4539, doi:10.3390/jcm12134539 . . . . **184**

Soshi Samejima, Claire Shackleton, Raza N. Malik, Kawami Cao, Anibal Bohorquez, Tom E. Nightingale, et al.
Spinal Cord Stimulation Prevents Autonomic Dysreflexia in Individuals with Spinal Cord Injury: A Case Series
Reprinted from: *J. Clin. Med.* **2023**, *12*, 2897, doi:10.3390/jcm12082897 . . . . **198**

About the Editors

Mohit Arora

Dr. Arora is a Senior Lecturer within the Faculty of Medicine and Health at The University of Sydney. He also serves as a Senior Research Fellow at the John Walsh Centre for Rehabilitation Research, situated in the Kolling Institute of Northern Sydney Local Health District. With a dedicated research career spanning over 15 years, Dr. Arora has significantly contributed to the field through more than 70 journal articles and book chapters, highlighting his expertise and dedication to advancing spinal cord injury knowledge and treatment. His successful acquisition of over AUD 6 million in research funding underscores his capacity to spearhead impactful studies. Dr. Arora's research ambitiously navigates through development of educational resources for people with spinal cord injury utilising co-design approaches, secondary health conditions after spinal cord injury including cognitive impairments, determinants of psychosocial health, and the integration of technology (such as VR and AI) in spinal cord injury rehabilitation. His proficiency extends to clinical trials, systematic reviews, and cohort studies, alongside methodological pursuits in survival analysis, cost-effectiveness, and cost-utility analyses. His academic excellence was recognised in 2012 with the Prime Minister's Australia Asia Post Graduate Endeavour Research Award, facilitating his PhD studies at the University of Sydney. In 2021, his contributions were further acknowledged when he was invited by the Australian Government's Department of Home Affairs to apply for the Global Talent Visa Program. Additionally, Dr. Arora lends his expertise as an editorial member of several peer-reviewed scientific journals.

Ashley Craig

Dr. Craig is the Professor of Rehabilitation Studies in the Faculty of Medicine and Health, The University of Sydney. He is also a Senior Researcher in the John Walsh Centre for Rehabilitation Research, Kolling Institute, Royal North Shore Hospital. Professor Craig has been involved in spinal cord injury research for over 30 years and has published over 350 journal papers, books, and book chapters. He has won over AUD 40 million in research funding. His research is focused on better understanding the process and dynamics involved in adjusting to the impairment associated with injury, including mental health, fatigue, pain, sleep, quality of life, and physiological factors like autonomic nervous system function and brain activity. He is also a senior clinical psychologist and does one day a week in a clinical setting treating adults with injury, pain, and mental health conditions. He was awarded an honorary doctorate from South West University for his contribution to neurological research in 2004.

Preface

Welcome to this Special Issue, a collection that not only shines a light on the profound challenges posed by spinal cord injuries but also indicates a hope through groundbreaking advancements in rehabilitation. As Guest Editors, we are honoured to present a compilation of research that is at the forefront of innovation in the field, offering new avenues for enhancing the quality of life and life expectancy of those affected by spinal cord injury, a life-altering and devastating condition.

Spinal cord injury can disrupt every facet of bodily function, and therefore, it demands a multifaceted approach to rehabilitation. The journey towards optimal physical and psychological adjustments is complex and ongoing. It is with this understanding that the current Special Issue seeks to contribute to the body of knowledge, presenting research that is both innovative and pragmatic. The breadth of topics covered is expansive, from examining the role of cognitive reserve in mitigating cognitive impairment to the potential of electrical stimulation for improving mobility and managing autonomic dysreflexia. The included articles also delve into the use of machine learning for the early prediction of pressure ulcers and robot-assisted gait training, activity-based therapy, and the application of hypnosis-enhanced cognitive behaviour therapy for pain management. Every article in this Speciasl Issue offers insights into cutting-edge interventions.

We would like to extend our heartfelt gratitude to all the contributing authors and the dedicated team at MDPI for their invaluable efforts. Their expertise, commitment, and hard work have been instrumental in bringing this Special Issue to fruition. It is through their collective contributions that we are able to offer this significant resource to the SCI community. It is our hope that this Special Issue will not only inform and inspire but also pave the way for significant advancements in the care and rehabilitation of individuals with spinal cord injuries. These contributions stand as testament to the relentless pursuit of improvement in the lives of those affected, showcasing the innovative spirit of researchers and practitioners in the field. We invite you to explore these articles that form a significant contribution to the evolving field of spinal cord injury rehabilitation.

Mohit Arora and Ashley Craig
Editors

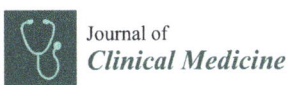

Editorial

Special Issue—Spinal Cord Injuries: Advances in Rehabilitation

Mohit Arora [1,2] **and Ashley R. Craig** [1,2,*]

1. Faculty of Medicine and Health, The University of Sydney, Sydney, NSW 2000, Australia; mohit.arora@sydney.edu.au
2. John Walsh Centre for Rehabilitation Research, Kolling Institute, Northern Sydney Local Health District, St Leonards, NSW 2065, Australia
* Correspondence: a.craig@sydney.edu.au

Spinal cord injury (SCI) is a severe, neurological disorder resulting from traumatic injury (such as a motor vehicle crash or fall) or non-traumatic injury associated with disease (such as cancer or infection) that results in impaired voluntary motor control and sensory function, usually leading to lifelong severe disability [1–4]. Secondary health conditions are common, compounding dysfunction and lowering quality of life [2,3], with prevalent conditions including autonomic nervous system dysfunction, cardiovascular disorder, cognitive impairment, bladder and bowel infection, skin disorders, sleep disorders, chronic pain and mental health disorder [2–4]. Consequently, people with SCI are vulnerable to experiencing barriers to achieving adjustment, such as inadequate resilience and coping skills to deal with the disability and any secondary health conditions [3–6]. Furthermore, social participation and social mobility can be impeded, family and social networks diminished and employment opportunities greatly lessened [4,6–10]. In such a complex and severe injury and coupled with the need for improved rehabilitation treatments and strategies, advances are required across the whole spectrum of SCI assessment and interventions that target the disability and secondary conditions.

SCI rehabilitation has been defined as a goal-oriented process constructed to optimize recovery of residual physical function, with the objective of gaining the highest possible level of personal adjustment, autonomy and independence [4,11]. To address the multiple challenges a person with SCI faces, it is crucial that the multidisciplinary health team (MDT) involved in SCI rehabilitation strategically collaborate to assist the person with SCI in attaining optimal recovery [4]. Additionally, the MDT must also work closely with social, educational and vocational services to achieve rehabilitation goals [11]. Evidence suggests that SCI rehabilitation resulted in improved management of secondary conditions as well as increased life expectancy in people with SCI [12]. However, the occurrence of disorders associated with SCI remains very high [4–6], and life expectancy is still well below that of the general population [13].

Given the above, it is critical that advances in SCI rehabilitation continue to occur to ensure optimal physical and psychological adjustment to SCI and that quality of life and life expectancy continue to improve. Arguably, one vital strategy for achieving this is through the appropriate communication of innovative research that features advances in SCI rehabilitation. With this in mind, researchers exploring strategies designed to promote innovation in SCI rehabilitation were invited throughout 2023 to submit their research to a Special Issue titled Advances in SCI Rehabilitation. We were extremely pleased with the response.

Thirteen high-quality papers written by highly experienced and internationally renowned researchers were accepted for publication in the Special Issue, covering the following topics:

(i) Innovative rehabilitation approaches to secondary conditions (Contribution 1: prediction of pressure ulcers after SCI; Contribution 2: investigation into sarcopenia after

Citation: Arora, M.; Craig, A.R. Special Issue—Spinal Cord Injuries: Advances in Rehabilitation. *J. Clin. Med.* **2024**, *13*, 1782. https://doi.org/10.3390/jcm13061782

Received: 12 March 2024
Accepted: 18 March 2024
Published: 20 March 2024

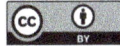

Copyright: © 2024 by the authors. Licensee MDPI, Basel, Switzerland. This article is an open access article distributed under the terms and conditions of the Creative Commons Attribution (CC BY) license (https:// creativecommons.org/licenses/by/ 4.0/).

SCI the involuntary loss of skeletal muscle mass and strength and Contribution 3: a prospective study on the association between cognitive impairment after SCI and cognitive reserve before SCI).

(ii) Improvements in national approaches to screening and follow-up strategies (Contribution 4: evidence concerning national change in England in, among other things, screening for mental health, and Contribution 5: investigating changes to follow-up processes after SCI rehabilitation in the Netherlands).

(iii) Research into novel treatments that could provide essential advances in SCI rehabilitation (Contribution 6: a case study and laboratory framework on the possible beneficial effects of heart rate variability biofeedback and paced breathing after SCI; Contribution 7: evidence for the benefits of activity-based therapy for mobility and life quality after SCI; Contribution 8: research investigating restoration of walking after SCI using neuromodulation therapy; Contribution 9: a systematic review and meta-analysis on benefits of robot-assisted gait training after SCI; Contribution 10: a prospective study on the effects of robot-assisted gait therapy on mental health after SCI; Contribution 11: preliminary research on the beneficial effects of virtual reality (walking) for neuropathic pain after SCI; Contribution 12: a case study presenting evidence for beneficial effects of Hypnosis Enhanced Cognitive Therapy for pain after SCI and Contribution 13: a case study on the beneficial effects of spinal cord stimulation on autonomic dysreflexia after SCI.

These thirteen papers offer exciting SCI advances in rehabilitation. They all deal with a very complex disorder that results in debilitating life-long injury and impairment. These papers provide preliminary evidence that could deliver novel solutions to significant gaps in our understanding of the management of SCI. To highlight just a few.

Autonomic dysreflexia (AD) is a severe and potentially life-threatening syndrome after SCI involving abnormal reaction of the autonomic nervous system to sensory stimuli that provoke a sympathetic nervous system reflex. This then results in vasoconstriction that leads to dangerously increased blood pressure [14]. Treatments for AD are limited, and preliminary research with three individuals with SCI using epidural spinal cord stimulation at the level of the lumbosacral spinal cord showed great promise, reducing vascular sympathetic nervous system activation when provoked [14]. This type of therapy, therefore, has the potential to be used to reduce the risk of AD. Electrical stimulation was also used to restore standing and walking in individuals with SCI [15]. The case study results presented in the Special Issue [16] were based on an individual with chronic tetraplegia. This person received multiple weeks of stimulation training (e.g., standing, sitting up, treadmill walking and active cycling). The results were promising. The participant showed significant improvement in lower-limb volitional movements and, after the study, was to walk short distances with aids [16].

Chronic pain is a prevalent secondary condition after SCI, and treatments are limited and problematic, such as the overuse of opioid medications [17]. While pain management strategies like cognitive behavior therapies are known to be effective [18], these strategies are limited for individuals with SCI who are ventilator-dependent. Novel research that employed hypnotic cognitive therapy that relies less on verbal interaction showed promise for relieving pain symptoms in an individual with SCI [19].

The studies reported in this Special Issue are certainly cutting-edge and, importantly, informed by evidence-based groundbreaking research. They will, therefore, form the basis of future research that investigates critical gaps in our knowledge about SCI rehabilitation and play a pivotal foundation for transformative advances in SCI rehabilitation. The advances reported in this Special Issue will then hopefully be followed by a translation of findings into SCI rehabilitation programs around the world with the ultimate goal of enhancing the quality of life for people living with SCI worldwide.

Conflicts of Interest: The authors declare no conflict of interest.

List of Contributions:

1. Kim, Y.; Lim, M.; Kim, S.Y.; Kim, T.U.; Lee, S.J.; Bok, S.K.; Park, S.; Han, Y.; Jung, H.Y.; Hyun, J.K. Integrated Machine Learning Approach for the Early Prediction of Pressure Ulcers in Spinal Cord Injury Patients. *J. Clin. Med.* **2024**, *13*, 990.
2. Gherle, A.; Nistor-Cseppento, C.D.; Iovanovici, D.C.; Cevei, I.R.; Cevei, M.L.; Vasileva, D.; Deac, S.; Stoicanescu, D. Secondary Sarcopenia and Spinal Cord Injury: Clinical Associations and Health Outcomes. *J. Clin. Med.* **2024**, *13*, 885.
3. Arora, M.; Pozzato, I.; McBain, C.; Tran, Y.; Sandalic, D.; Myles, D.; Middleton, J.W.; Craig, A. Cognitive Reserve and Its Association with Cognitive and Mental Health Status following an Acute Spinal Cord Injury. *J. Clin. Med.* **2023**, *12*, 4258.
4. Duff, J.; Ellis, R.; Kaiser, S.; Grant, L.C. Psychological Screening, Standards and Spinal Cord Injury: Introducing Change in NHS England Commissioned Services. *J. Clin. Med.* **2023**, *12*, 7667.
5. Tijsse Klasen, J.; van Diemen, T.; Langerak, N.G.; van Nes, I.J. Effects of Adaptations in an Interdisciplinary Follow-Up Clinic for People with Spinal Cord Injury in the Chronic Phase: A Prospective Cohort Study. *J. Clin. Med.* **2023**, *12*, 7572.
6. Schoffl, J.; Arora, M.; Pozzato, I.; McBain, C.; Rodrigues, D.; Vafa, E.; Middleton, J.; Davis, G.M.; Gustin, S.M.; Bourke, J.; et al. Heart Rate Variability Biofeedback in Adults with a Spinal Cord Injury: A Laboratory Framework and Case Series. *J. Clin. Med.* **2023**, *12*, 7664.
7. Quel de Oliveira, C.; Bundy, A.; Middleton, J.W.; Refshauge, K.; Rogers, K.; Davis, G.M. Activity-Based Therapy for Mobility, Function and Quality of Life after Spinal Cord Injuries—A Mixed-Methods Case Series. *J. Clin. Med.* **2023**, *12*, 7588.
8. Alam, M.; Ling, Y.T.; Rahman, M.A.; Wong, A.Y.; Zhong, H.; Edgerton, V.R.; Zheng, Y.P. Restoration of Over-Ground Walking via Non-Invasive Neuromodulation Therapy: A Single-Case Study. *J. Clin. Med.* **2023**, *12*, 7362.
9. Wardhana, D.P.; Maliawan, S.; Mahadewa, T.G.; Rosyidi, R.M.; Wiranata, S. The Impact of Machine Learning and Robot-Assisted Gait Training on Spinal Cord Injury: A Systematic Review and Meta-Analysis. *J. Clin. Med.* **2023**, *12*, 7230.
10. Widuch-Spodyniuk, A.; Tarnacka, B.; Korczyński, B.; Wiśniowska, J. Impact of Robotic-Assisted Gait Therapy on Depression and Anxiety Symptoms in Patients with Subacute Spinal Cord Injuries (SCIs)—A Prospective Clinical Study. *J. Clin. Med.* **2023**, *12*, 7153.
11. Gustin, S.M.; Bolding, M.; Willoughby, W.; Anam, M.; Shum, C.; Rumble, D.; Mark, V.W.; Mitchell, L.; Cowan, R.E.; Richardson, E.; et al. Cortical Mechanisms Underlying Immersive Interactive Virtual Walking Treatment for Amelioration of Neuropathic Pain after Spinal Cord Injury: Findings from a Preliminary Investigation of Thalamic Inhibitory Function. *J. Clin. Med.* **2023**, *12*, 5743.
12. Starosta, A.J.; Wright, K.S.; Bombardier, C.H.; Kahlia, F.; Barber, J.; Accardi-Ravid, M.C.; Wiechman, S.A.; Crane, D.A.; Jensen, M.P. A Case Study of Hypnosis Enhanced Cognitive Therapy for Pain in a Ventilator Dependent Patient during Inpatient Rehabilitation for Spinal Cord Injury. *J. Clin. Med.* **2023**, *12*, 4539.
13. Samejima, S.; Shackleton, C.; Malik, R.N.; Cao, K.; Bohorquez, A.; Nightingale, T.E.; Sachdeva, R.; Krassioukov, A.V. Spinal Cord Stimulation Prevents Autonomic Dysreflexia in Individuals with Spinal Cord Injury: A Case Series. *J. Clin. Med.* **2023**, *12*, 2897.

References

1. David, G.; Mohammadi, S.; Martin, A.R.; Cohen-Adad, J.; Weiskopf, N.; Thompson, A.; Freund, P. Traumatic and nontraumatic spinal cord injury: Pathological insights from neuroimaging. *Nat. Rev. Neurol.* **2019**, *15*, 718–731. [CrossRef] [PubMed]
2. Adriaansen, J.J.; Post, M.W.; de Groot, S.; van Asbeck, F.W.; Stolwijk-Swuste, J.M.; Tepper, M.; Lindeman, E. Secondary health conditions in persons with spinal cord injury: A longitudinal study from one to five years post-discharge. *J. Rehabil. Med.* **2013**, *45*, 1016–1022. [CrossRef] [PubMed]
3. Geyh, S.; Ballert, C.; Sinnott, A.; Charlifue, S.; Catz, A.; D'Andrea Greve, J.M.; Post, M.W. Quality of life after spinal cord injury: A comparison across six countries. *Spinal Cord* **2013**, *51*, 322–326. [CrossRef] [PubMed]
4. Craig, A.; Tran, Y.; Arora, M.; Pozzato, I.; Middleton, J.W. Investigating Dynamics of the Spinal Cord Injury Adjustment Model: Mediation Model Analysis. *J. Clin. Med.* **2022**, *11*, 4557. [CrossRef] [PubMed]
5. Chevalier, Z.; Kennedy, P.; Sherlock, O. Spinal cord injury, coping and psychological adjustment: A literature review. *Spinal Cord* **2009**, *47*, 778–782. [CrossRef] [PubMed]
6. Krause, J.S. Changes in adjustment after spinal cord injury: A 20-year longitudinal study. *Rehabil. Psychol.* **1998**, *43*, 41–55. [CrossRef]

7. Kennedy, P.; Lude, P.; Taylor, N. Quality of life, social participation, appraisals and coping post spinal cord injury: A review of four community samples. *Spinal Cord* **2006**, *44*, 95–105. [CrossRef] [PubMed]
8. Tsai, I.; Graves, D.E.; Chan, W.; Darkoh, C.; Lee, M.S.; Pompeii, L.A. Environmental barriers and social participation in individuals with spinal cord injury. *Rehabil. Psychol.* **2017**, *62*, 36–44. [CrossRef] [PubMed]
9. Zürcher, C.; Tough, H.; Fekete, C.; SwiSCI Study Group. Mental health in individuals with spinal cord injury: The role of socioeconomic conditions and social relationships. *PLoS ONE* **2019**, *14*, e0206069. [CrossRef] [PubMed]
10. Murphy, G.C.; Middleton, J.; Quirk, R.; De Wolf, A.; Cameron, I.D. Predicting employment status at 2 years' postdischarge from spinal cord injury rehabilitation. *Rehabil. Psychol.* **2011**, *56*, 251–256. [CrossRef] [PubMed]
11. World Health Organisation. *A Glossary of Terms for Community Health Care and Services for Older Personnel*; World Health Organisation Centre for Development, Ageing and Health Technical Report; World Health Organisation: Geneva, Switzerland, 2004; Volume 5.
12. Middleton, J.W.; Dayton, A.; Walsh, J.; Rutkowski, S.B.; Leong, G.; Duong, S. Life expectancy after spinal cord injury: A 50-year study. *Spinal Cord* **2012**, *50*, 803–811. [CrossRef]
13. Savic, G.; DeVivo, M.J.; Frankel, H.L.; Jamous, M.A.; Soni, B.M.; Charlifue, S. Long-term survival after traumatic spinal cord injury: A 70-year British study. *Spinal Cord* **2017**, *55*, 651–658. [CrossRef] [PubMed]
14. Samejima, S.; Shackleton, C.; Malik, R.N.; Cao, K.; Bohorquez, A.; Nightingale, T.E.; Sachdeva, R.; Krassioukov, A.V. Spinal Cord Stimulation Prevents Autonomic Dysreflexia in Individuals with Spinal Cord Injury: A Case Series. *J. Clin. Med.* **2023**, *12*, 2897. [CrossRef] [PubMed]
15. Sayenko, D.G.; Rath, M.; Ferguson, A.R.; Burdick, J.W.; Havton, L.A.; Edgerton, V.R.; Gerasimenko, Y.P. Self-assisted standing enabled by non-invasive spinal stimulation after spinal cord injury. *J. Neurotrauma* **2019**, *36*, 1435–1450. [CrossRef] [PubMed]
16. Alam, M.; Ling, Y.T.; Rahman, M.A.; Wong, A.Y.; Zhong, H.; Edgerton, V.R.; Zheng, Y.P. Restoration of Over-Ground Walking via Non-Invasive Neuromodulation Therapy: A Single-Case Study. *J. Clin. Med.* **2023**, *12*, 7362. [CrossRef] [PubMed]
17. Siddall, P.J.; Loeser, J.D. Pain following spinal cord injury. *Spinal Cord* **2001**, *39*, 63–73. [CrossRef] [PubMed]
18. Heutink, M.; Post, M.; Overdulve, C.; Pfennings, L.; van de Vis, W.; Vrijens, N.; Lindeman, E. Which pain coping strategies and cognitions are associated with outcomes of a cognitive behavioral intervention for neuropathic pain after spinal cord injury? *Top. Spinal Cord Inj. Rehabil.* **2013**, *19*, 330–340. [CrossRef] [PubMed]
19. Starosta, A.J.; Wright, K.S.; Bombardier, C.H.; Kahlia, F.; Barber, J.; Accardi-Ravid, M.C.; Wiechman, S.A.; Crane, D.A.; Jensen, M.P. A Case Study of Hypnosis Enhanced Cognitive Therapy for Pain in a Ventilator Dependent Patient during Inpatient Rehabilitation for Spinal Cord Injury. *J. Clin. Med.* **2023**, *12*, 4539. [CrossRef] [PubMed]

Disclaimer/Publisher's Note: The statements, opinions and data contained in all publications are solely those of the individual author(s) and contributor(s) and not of MDPI and/or the editor(s). MDPI and/or the editor(s) disclaim responsibility for any injury to people or property resulting from any ideas, methods, instructions or products referred to in the content.

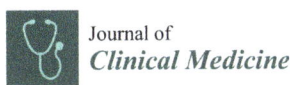

Article

Integrated Machine Learning Approach for the Early Prediction of Pressure Ulcers in Spinal Cord Injury Patients

Yuna Kim [1,†], Myungeun Lim [2,†], Seo Young Kim [1], Tae Uk Kim [1], Seong Jae Lee [1], Soo-Kyung Bok [3], Soojun Park [2], Youngwoong Han [2], Ho-Youl Jung [2,*] and Jung Keun Hyun [1,4,5,*]

1. Department of Rehabilitation Medicine, College of Medicine, Dankook University, Cheonan 31116, Republic of Korea; kimyuna727@dkuh.co.kr (Y.K.); syoungrm@dkuh.co.kr (S.Y.K.); magnarbor@dankook.ac.kr (T.U.K.); rmlee@dankook.ac.kr (S.J.L.)
2. Digital Biomedical Research Division, Electronics and Telecommunications Research Institute, Daejeon 34129, Republic of Korea; melim@etri.re.kr (M.L.); psj@etri.re.kr (S.P.); hanhero@etri.re.kr (Y.H.)
3. Department of Rehabilitation Medicine, College of Medicine, Chungnam National University, Daejeon 35015, Republic of Korea; skbok@cnuh.co.kr
4. Department of Nanobiomedical Science and BK21 NBM Global Research Center for Regenerative Medicine, Dankook University, Cheonan 31116, Republic of Korea
5. Institute of Tissue Regeneration Engineering, Dankook University, Cheonan 31116, Republic of Korea
* Correspondence: hoyoul.jung@etri.re.kr (H.-Y.J.); rhhyun@dankook.ac.kr (J.K.H.); Tel.: +82-42-860-1502 (H.-Y.J.); +82-41-550-6480 (J.K.H.)
† These authors contributed equally to this work.

Abstract: (1) Background: Pressure ulcers (PUs) substantially impact the quality of life of spinal cord injury (SCI) patients and require prompt intervention. This study used machine learning (ML) techniques to develop advanced predictive models for the occurrence of PUs in patients with SCI. (2) Methods: By analyzing the medical records of 539 patients with SCI, we observed a 35% incidence of PUs during hospitalization. Our analysis included 139 variables, including baseline characteristics, neurological status (International Standards for Neurological Classification of Spinal Cord Injury [ISNCSCI]), functional ability (Korean version of the Modified Barthel Index [K-MBI] and Functional Independence Measure [FIM]), and laboratory data. We used a variety of ML methods—a graph neural network (GNN), a deep neural network (DNN), a linear support vector machine (SVM_linear), a support vector machine with radial basis function kernel (SVM_RBF), K-nearest neighbors (KNN), a random forest (RF), and logistic regression (LR)—focusing on an integrative analysis of laboratory, neurological, and functional data. (3) Results: The SVM_linear algorithm using these composite data showed superior predictive ability (area under the receiver operating characteristic curve (AUC) = 0.904, accuracy = 0.944), as demonstrated by a 5-fold cross-validation. The critical discriminators of PU development were identified based on limb functional status and laboratory markers of inflammation. External validation highlighted the challenges of model generalization and provided a direction for future research. (4) Conclusions: Our study highlights the importance of a comprehensive, multidimensional data approach for the effective prediction of PUs in patients with SCI, especially in the acute and subacute phases. The proposed ML models show potential for the early detection and prevention of PUs, thus contributing substantially to improving patient care in clinical settings.

Keywords: spinal cord injury; pressure ulcer; machine learning; prediction model; laboratory test

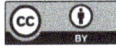

1. Introduction

Spinal cord injury (SCI) results primarily from traumatic events and can cause considerable sensory and motor impairments and complications [1]. Among the myriad challenges that patients with SCI encounter, pressure ulcers (PUs) are notable; previous studies revealed that over 20% of SCI individuals develop PUs, with significant implications for morbidity, mortality, and quality of life, especially in developing countries [2,3].

Untreated PUs have a significant impact on patient well-being and place a high financial burden on healthcare systems. These ulcers exacerbate physical and emotional distress and reduce patients' quality of life [4]. Economically, the treatment of PUs is costly, with the U.S. healthcare system spending approximately USD 26.8 billion annually [5].

These PUs typically occur over bony prominences due to prolonged pressure, and key sites for PUs include the sacrum, heels, and ischial tuberosities, with complications ranging from infections to delayed rehabilitation, underscoring the need for early prediction and intervention [6]. Prevention is crucial in the management of pressure ulcers, especially for individuals at higher risk such as those with spinal cord injuries, and regular repositioning, careful skin inspection, and the use of pressure-relieving devices are key strategies [7]. The prediction and early identification of pressure ulcers are vital, as early-stage ulcers can often be managed more easily and heal faster compared to advanced ulcers, thus highlighting the importance of innovative prediction and intervention strategies in healthcare [8]. The severity of SCI varies, with more severe cases, such as complete tetraplegia, showing a higher PU risk due to an extensive loss of sensory and motor functions [9]. This increased risk is attributed to prolonged immobility and areas prone to sores, like the sacrum and heels [10]. The management and prediction of PUs in patients with SCI have advanced through the use of traditional clinical assessments and monitoring tools [11]. While the Braden Scale, Norton Scale, and Spinal Cord Injury Pressure Ulcer Scale (SCIPUS) are commonly used in clinical settings, their predictive accuracy varies considerably among individual patients with SCI, as highlighted in previous studies [12,13]. The Braden Scale evaluates factors like sensory perception and moisture, the Norton Scale focuses on physical condition and activity, and the Spinal Cord Injury Pressure Ulcer Scale is tailored specifically to patients with SCI, considering aspects like spasticity and sweating [12]. In previous studies, the Braden Scale has demonstrated the highest overall accuracy, whereas the Norton Scale has exhibited greater specificity [12,14]. However, another study reported that functional assessments, such as the Functional Independence Measure (FIM), outperformed both the SCIPUS and Braden Scales in terms of accuracy [15]. This variability highlights the need for more individualized and effective assessment tools for pressure ulcer risk assessment in this patient population. Molecular markers, including proinflammatory cytokines like interleukin (IL)-1α, show promise in early pressure ulcer detection, though their clinical application remains exploratory [16,17]. The challenges encompass enhancing predictive accuracy and ensuring that methods are cost-effective, accessible, and universally applicable. Tackling the challenges of pressure ulcer management requires a combination of clinical expertise and cutting-edge technologies, including alternative support surfaces and wireless patient monitoring systems. These technologies are integral for risk identification, effective repositioning, and microclimate control, thereby emphasizing the need for a patient-centric care approach [18].

In recent years, machine learning (ML) has become a significant factor in healthcare, particularly in areas such as diagnosis, prognosis, and personalized treatment [19]. ML uses algorithms, ranging from simple decision trees to sophisticated deep learning models, to uncover complex patterns and correlations, leveraging increased computational power and extensive healthcare datasets [20]. For instance, decision trees use a tree-like structure to represent decisions and their potential outcomes, which makes them highly interpretable and adaptable to different data types [21]. On the other hand, deep learning models employ layered neural networks to analyze data in a complex manner, making them particularly effective at identifying subtle patterns in large datasets [22]. Advanced algorithms are currently being utilized in spinal cord injury (SCI) care to predict neurological and functional recovery through the analysis of medical records and imaging data [22,23]. Machine learning techniques, including these algorithms, are being explored for patients with SCI to identify risk factors for pressure ulcers (PUs) [24]. This addresses the challenge of limited clinical integration due to previously undefined risk factors.

The primary goal of our study is to establish optimal prediction models by comprehensively integrating clinical, physical, and biological parameters, with a focus on improving the accuracy of prognostic predictions for pressure ulcers during the acute and subacute phases of hospitalization in patients with SCI. The secondary goal is to translate these models into practical tools for clinical application to enable the early intervention and effective prevention of pressure ulcers, thereby significantly improving patient outcomes during their hospital stay.

2. Subjects and Methods

2.1. Ethics and Study Design

This retrospective observational study was approved by the institutional review board (IRB) of Dankook University Hospital (IRB No. 2021-05-021) and was conducted in accordance with the ethical guidelines of the 1975 Declaration of Helsinki. We reviewed the medical records of 1117 patients with SCI from Dankook University Hospital (DKUH) and Chungnam National University Hospital (CNUH) in South Korea. Patients were included if they underwent surgical or conservative treatment for traumatic or nontraumatic SCI with confirmed spinal cord signal changes by spinal magnetic resonance imaging (MRI) as demonstrated in previous studies [25,26] from May 1996 to May 2021. The clinical data during the initial hospitalization period for SCI were collected by three researchers, who were specifically assigned to ensure impartiality and minimize bias. These researchers were not involved in the statistical analysis or development of the ML model due to a separation of roles that was implemented to maintain the objectivity and integrity of both the data collection and analysis phases. The clinical parameters included baseline characteristics, such as sex, age, height, weight, alcohol consumption, smoking status, and medical history; subscale and total score of the International Standards for Neurological Classification of Spinal Cord Injury (ISNCSCI), the Korean version of the modified Barthel Index (K-MBI), and Functional Independence Measure (FIM), which were initially assessed during the initial hospitalization period for SCI. We obtained all the laboratory data from the laboratory medicine department of each hospital. The laboratory parameters included complete blood count (CBC), electrolytes, lipid battery, glucose, albumin, protein, C-reactive protein (CRP), the erythrocyte sedimentation rate (ESR), procalcitonin, blood urea nitrogen (BUN), creatinine, aspartate transaminase (AST), alanine transaminase (ALT), and total bilirubin. The patients with SCI who experienced PUs at least once during the hospitalization period were classified into the PU group, while the patients who never experienced PUs were classified into the non-PU group. For the PU group, we extracted only clinical and laboratory data from 3 days to 60 days before the onset of PU.

2.2. Machine Learning Analysis

In this study, the recursive feature elimination (RFE) technique was used for feature selection. In the RFE method, a given machine learning algorithm is trained on the initial set of baseline features, after which the importance of each feature is computed. The least important feature is then iteratively eliminated at each step. This elimination process is repeated until the optimal set of features that contributes significantly to the model remains. The linear support vector machine (SVM_linear) classifier was selected as the training algorithm. The selection process was implemented using the RFE with a cross-validation (RFECV) module provided by the scikit-learn library [27], which ensures robust feature selection by considering the cross-validation performance during the elimination process.

We utilized various machine learning methods, combining advanced deep learning with traditional techniques. We employed the graph neural network–graph convolutional network (GNN-GCN) and deep neural network (DNN), which are complex artificial neural networks. GNN-GCN analyzes data structured in graphs, while DNN processes data through interconnected layers [28]. Traditional methods used for classification include linear support vector machine (SVM_linear) and support vector machine with a radial basis function kernel (SVM_RBF) for decision boundary-based classification, K-nearest neighbors (KNN) for proximity-based classification, random forest (RF) as an ensemble of decision trees to improve prediction accuracy, and logistic regression (LR) for binary outcome probabilities.

The GNN-GCN model was trained using a graph matrix computed by Euclidean distances between input data, while the other models were trained directly on input data. The GNN-GCN and DNN models were implemented using PyTorch 1.10 [29], and the other ML methods were implemented using scikit-learn 0.24.

Fivefold cross-validation was performed to evaluate the model performance. The dataset was randomized and divided into five partitions, one of which was used for testing and the other for training. To ensure balanced case–control ratios in each partition, a stratified K-fold cross-validation method was used. Cross-validation was repeated five times to ensure a robust and reliable evaluation. Model performance was evaluated by accuracy, area under the receiver operating characteristic curve (AUC), and F1-score.

To improve the interpretability of the problem, we performed additional analyses on the decision tree. The decision tree was trained with entropy as the partitioning criterion. The graph shows the use of features for prediction and the corresponding criteria.

2.3. Statistics

All the laboratory, neurological, and functional data were compared between the two hospitals using PASW 20.0 (IBM Corp., New York, NY, USA). The Shapiro–Wilk test was used to assess the normality of the distribution of all the numerical data from each group. The chi-squared test was used for categorial parameters, and the independent t test was used for continuous parameters to compare the differences between the two groups. $p < 0.05$ indicated statistical significance.

3. Results

3.1. Flow of the Machine Learning Algorithm

Figure 1 outlines the flow of our machine learning algorithm. Clinical data, sourced from the two participating hospitals, were collected during several preprocessing stages. This involved imputation using the KNN method and subsequent filtering of missing values (NaN). Data from patients with a feature coverage exceeding 80% were subjected to imputation, while those with a feature coverage less than 70% were discarded during the NaN filtering stage. For the PU cohort, data were further curated to capture only the interval, spanning 3 days prior to PU onset, up to 60 days before its incidence. Concurrently, laboratory data pertaining to the PU group were processed through date filtering and imputed using mean values. The processed clinical and laboratory datasets were subsequently combined and applied to feature selection. Using these consolidated data, seven distinct machine learning models were developed. The efficacy of the combinations was determined through a 5-fold cross-validation procedure, with performance metrics presented in terms of accuracy, AUC, and F1-score.

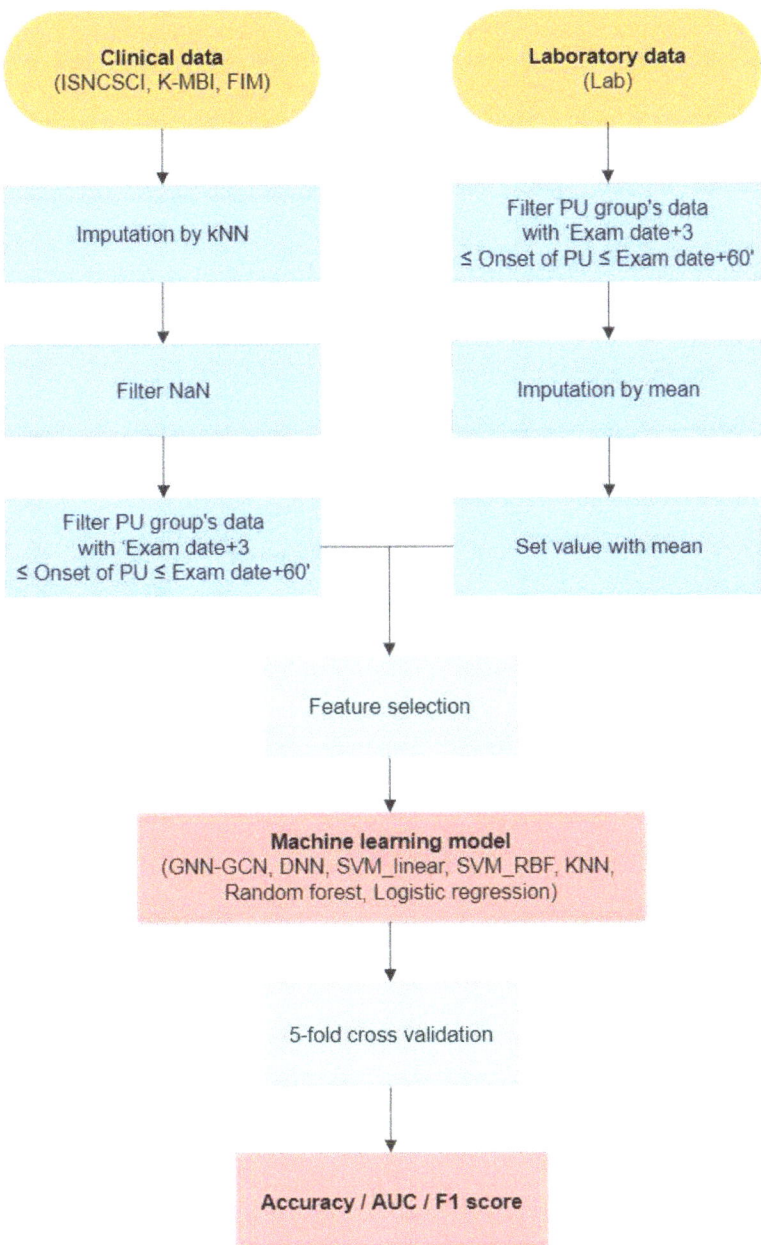

Figure 1. Flow of the machine learning process.

3.2. Data Characteristics and Dataset Selection for Each Hospital

Table 1 presents the baseline characteristics of patients from Dankook University Hospital (DKUH) and Chonnam National University Hospital (CNUH), categorized by the presence or absence of pressure ulcers. While DKUH focused on the formulation and refinement of machine learning algorithms, CNUH was utilized exclusively for external validation. Notably, patients with pressure ulcers exhibited longer hospital stays across both institutions. For our machine learning models, we utilized parameters from the ISNCSCI, K-MBI, FIM, and 20 laboratory indicators. A detailed analysis revealed significant differences in certain metrics. Within the ISNCSCI, total motor scores, especially for the right and left lower extremities, showed marked disparities. Sensory scores, both light touch and pinprick, varied notably between groups. According to the K-MBI metrics, distinctions were evident in toileting, stair climbing, dressing, and ambulation, among others. The FIM highlighted differences in bladder and bowel controls. Finally, laboratory results revealed contrasting hemoglobin levels, hematocrit levels, and platelet counts between the groups.

Table 1. Baseline characteristics of patients with and without pressure ulcers at DKUH and CNUH.

Parameters	DKUH (n = 238)			CNUH (n = 385)		
	Non-PU (n = 199)	PU (n = 39)	p Value	Non-PU (n = 362)	PU (n = 23)	p Value
Baseline characteristics						
Sex (male)	158 (79.4%)	31 (79.5%)	0.99	247 (68.2%)	19 (82.6%)	0.148
Age	54.22 ± 14.26	48.95 ± 17.02	0.042 *	58.51 ± 15.62	57.00 ± 17.91	0.657
Height	166.85 ± 7.71	167.85 ± 7.51	0.867	165.00 ± 9.06	166.55 ± 9.54	0.495
Weight	65.18 ± 10.59	65.17 ± 11.66	0.996	64.55 ± 12.38	63.41 ± 9.89	0.680
Alcohol consumption	99 (50.0%)	26 (66.7%)	0.057	103 (28.6%)	6 (26.1%)	0.795
Smoking status	73 (36.9%)	16 (41.0%)	0.624	97 (27.0%)	5 (21.7%)	0.579
Diabetes mellitus	37 (18.7%)	8 (20.5%)	0.79	67 (18.5%)	4 (17.4%)	0.893
Hypertension	60 (30.3%)	13 (33.3%)	0.708	130 (35.9%)	8 (34.8%)	0.913
Neurologic disease	34 (17.1%)	4 (10.5%)	0.313	16 (4.4%)	0 (0.0%)	0.303
Cardiovascular disease	2 (1.0%)	3 (7.7%)	0.008 *	38 (10.5%)	0 (0.0%)	0.102
Pulmonary disease	9 (4.5%)	4 (10.3%)	0.15	25 (6.9%)	2 (8.7%)	0.745
Clinical parameters						
Hospital days	53.49 ± 31.87	96.72 ± 67.15	0.000 *	68.15 ± 42.92	118.17 ± 81.66	0.008 *
Braden scale	15.48 ± 3.62	13.69 ± 2.45	0.000 *	Null	Null	Null
Traumatic injury	158 (79.8%)	33 (84.6%)	0.487	199 (55.0%)	16 (69.6%)	0.172
Mechanism of injury						
Traffic accident	67 (37.8%)	14 (40.0%)		59 (30.1%)	5 (31.3%)	
Falls	58 (32.6%)	12 (34.3%)		48 (24.5%)	8 (50.0%)	
Hit by falling objects	12 (6.7%)	4 (11.4%)	0.581	7 (3.6%)	0 (0.0%)	0.183
Sports	0 (0%)	0 (0%)		2 (1.0%)	0 (0.0%)	
Others	41 (23.0%)	5 (14.3%)		80 (40.8%)	3 (18.8%)	
Combined injury	42 (21.1%)	13 (33.3%)	0.098	56 (15.5%)	6 (26.1%)	0.179
Number of operations	1.13 ± 0.741	1.51 ± 1.048	0.035 *	0.82 ± 1.01	0.61 ± 0.84	0.333
Total time of operations (min)	229.58 ± 146.85	256.77 ± 164.36	0.301	269.18 ± 176.42	245.67 ± 85.33	0.692
GCS total	14.69 ± 0.92	14.06 ± 2.76	0.212	14.00 ± 2.68	12.00 ± 1.41	0.337
GCS Eye	3.83 ± 0.44	3.63 ± 0.942	0.236	3.75 ± 0.87	4.00 ± 0.00	0.700
GCS Motor	5.93 ± 0.30	5.66 ± 0.90	0.098	5.83 ± 0.58	6.00 ± 0.00	0.700
GCS Verbal	4.92 ± 0.64	4.78 ± 1.52	0.605	4.50 ± 1.17	2.00 ± 1.41	0.018 *
ISNCSCI						
ASIA impairment scale (AIS)						
A	12 (6.3%)	14 (36.8%)		23 (7.6%)	7 (31.8%)	
B	9 (4.8%)	5 (13.2%)		8 (2.6%)	4 (18.2%)	
C	27 (14.3%)	12 (31.6%)	0.000 *	50 (16.5%)	8 (36.4%)	0.000 *
D	138 (73.0%)	7 (18.4%)		221 (72.9%)	3 (13.6%)	
E	3 (1.6%)	0 (0%)		1 (0.3%)	0 (0.0%)	
NLI (neurologic level of injury)	9.60 ± 8.14	10.31 ± 7.14	0.612	10.52 ± 8.57	8.87 ± 6.23	0.241
Motor						
Motor level	10.54 ± 8.66	10.46 ± 7.07	0.95	11.90 ± 8.72	8.96 ± 6.17	0.040 *
UER	20.06 ± 6.68	18.15 ± 8.51	0.193	20.07 ± 5.21	14.91 ± 9.00	0.012 *
UEL	19.13 ± 6.97	18.59 ± 8.15	0.667	20.07 ± 5.21	15.30 ± 8.77	0.017 *
UEMS	39.07 ± 12.75	36.74 ± 16.54	0.41	40.15 ± 9.93	30.22 ± 17.65	0.014 *
LER	18.22 ± 8.71	6.21 ± 8.08	0.000 *	16.18 ± 7.42	5.96 ± 7.97	0.000 *
LEL	17.84 ± 8.63	6.32 ± 8.59	0.000 *	16.13 ± 7.49	5.39 ± 7.67	0.000 *
LEMS	35.72 ± 16.71	12.50 ± 16.48	0.000 *	32.31 ± 14.40	11.35 ± 15.54	0.000 *
Motor score, total	74.76 ± 22.42	48.89 ± 20.97	0.000 *	72.45 ± 18.69	41.57 ± 28.48	0.000 *
Sensory						
Sensory level	14.19 ± 10.44	12.69 ± 7.36	0.285	12.07 ± 9.30	11.83 ± 7.14	0.875
LTR	45.76 ± 10.40	39.62 ± 12.57	0.001 *	39.17 ± 11.06	34.04 ± 11.40	0.032 *
LTL	45.62 ± 10.61	39.15 ± 12.49	0.001 *	39.28 ± 11.11	33.70 ± 10.87	0.020 *
LT, total	91.38 ± 20.56	78.77 ± 25.00	0.001 *	78.44 ± 21.92	67.74 ± 22.15	0.024 *
PPR	45.72 ± 10.28	40.08 ± 12.29	0.003 *	38.38 ± 11.54	33.83 ± 12.64	0.069
PPL	45.90 ± 10.59	39.82 ± 12.17	0.002 *	38.80 ± 11.42	33.61 ± 11.94	0.036 *
PP, total	91.62 ± 20.35	79.90 ± 24.42	0.002 *	77.17 ± 22.51	67.43 ± 24.44	0.046 *
Sensory score, total	183.00 ± 40.56	158.67 ± 49.18	0.001 *	155.61 ± 43.84	135.17 ± 45.96	0.031 *
K-MBI						
Self-care	2.90 ± 1.90	2.33 ± 1.95	0.088 *	3.12 ± 1.72	2.33 ± 1.97	0.308
Bathing	1.79 ± 1.61	0.64 ± 0.84	0.000 *	2.15 ± 1.64	1.67 ± 1.51	0.502
Feeding	5.87 ± 3.91	5.10 ± 4.27	0.268	6.12 ± 3.60	6.00 ± 4.73	0.941
Toileting	4.05 ± 3.63	1.31 ± 1.45	0.000 *	4.44 ± 3.41	1.83 ± 1.84	0.016 *
Stair climbing	1.62 ± 3.04	0.05 ± 0.32	0.000 *	1.56 ± 2.87	0.00 ± 0.00	0.001 *
Dressing	4.23 ± 3.29	2.36 ± 2.08	0.000 *	5.12 ± 3.05	1.83 ± 1.84	0.014 *

Table 1. Cont.

Parameters	DKUH (n = 238)			CNUH (n = 385)		
	Non-PU (n = 199)	PU (n = 39)	p Value	Non-PU (n = 362)	PU (n = 23)	p Value
Bowel management	6.33 ± 4.13	2.51 ± 3.53	0.000 *	6.83 ± 4.07	2.33 ± 3.88	0.015 *
Bladder management	5.04 ± 4.70	1.08 ± 2.93	0.000 *	5.76 ± 4.12	1.17 ± 2.04	0.001 *
Ambulation	4.91 ± 5.40	0.69 ± 1.15	0.000 *	5.07 ± 4.60	1.50 ± 1.64	0.002 *
Transfer	6.79 ± 5.42	2.08 ± 2.26	0.000 *	7.27 ± 5.08	3.67 ± 3.62	0.102
Total	43.53 ± 30.17	18.15 ± 14.92	0.000 *	46.19 ± 27.48	22.33 ± 17.93	0.044 *
FIM						
Eating	4.13 ± 2.28	3.87 ± 2.54	0.556	4.50 ± 2.12	4.00 ± 4.24	0.773
Grooming	3.94 ± 2.21	3.33 ± 2.13	0.114	3.56 ± 1.92	2.50 ± 2.12	0.472
Bathing	2.63 ± 1.63	1.64 ± 0.78	0.000 *	2.94 ± 1.59	1.50 ± 0.71	0.228
Dressing upper body	3.49 ± 1.94	2.67 ± 1.71	0.015 *	3.72 ± 1.97	4.00 ± 4.24	0.865
Dressing lower body	3.07 ± 1.91	1.59 ± 0.94	0.000 *	3.39 ± 1.88	2.00 ± 1.41	0.330
Toileting	3.03 ± 2.00	1.64 ± 0.84	0.000 *	3.50 ± 1.95	1.50 ± 0.71	0.175
Self-care, total	20.29 ± 10.84	14.74 ± 7.72	0.000 *	21.61 ± 10.86	15.50 ± 13.44	0.466
Bladder control	3.88 ± 2.76	1.59 ± 1.70	0.000 *	4.56 ± 2.41	1.00 ± 0.00	0.000 *
Bowel control	4.46 ± 2.50	2.31 ± 1.94	0.000 *	4.78 ± 2.37	1.50 ± 0.71	0.009 *
Sphincter control, total	8.34 ± 4.88	3.90 ± 3.39	0.000 *	9.33 ± 4.72	2.50 ± 0.71	0.000 *
Transfer to bed/chair/wheelchair	3.33 ± 2.04	1.74 ± 0.85	0.000 *	3.06 ± 1.73	2.00 ± 1.41	0.420
Transfer to toilet	3.09 ± 2.04	1.51 ± 0.68	0.000 *	3.00 ± 1.78	1.50 ± 0.71	0.263
Transfer to tub/shower	2.93 ± 1.96	1.49 ± 0.64	0.000 *	2.83 ± 1.76	1.50 ± 0.71	0.311
Locomotion with walk/wheelchair	3.02 ± 1.93	1.44 ± 0.64	0.000 *	2.89 ± 1.64	2.00 ± 1.41	0.474
Locomotion to stairs	1.88 ± 1.67	1.05 ± 0.22	0.000 *	2.00 ± 1.75	1.00 ± 0.00	0.440
Transfer/Locomotion, total	14.25 ± 9.15	7.23 ± 2.72	0.000 *	13.78 ± 8.16	8.00 ± 4.24	0.345
Comprehension	6.86 ± 0.61	6.72 ± 0.916	0.344	6.17 ± 1.76	4.50 ± 3.54	0.255
Expression	6.84 ± 0.66	6.69 ± 0.83	0.304	6.22 ± 1.73	4.50 ± 3.54	0.235
Social interaction	6.81 ± 0.78	6.67 ± 1.01	0.324	6.28 ± 1.64	4.50 ± 3.54	0.201
Problem solving	6.78 ± 0.81	6.67 ± 1.11	0.46	6.17 ± 1.76	4.50 ± 3.54	0.255
Memory	6.79 ± 0.74	6.72 ± 0.97	0.58	6.22 ± 1.73	4.50 ± 3.54	0.235
Cognition, total	33.98 ± 3.97	32.74 ± 6.36	0.248	31.06 ± 8.59	22.50 ± 17.68	0.235
FIM, total	76.86 ± 23.31	58.62 ± 13.85	0.000 *	75.78 ± 26.96	48.50 ± 36.06	0.201
Laboratory parameters						
White blood cells ($\times 10^3/\mu L$)	8.87 ± 2.07	9.25 ± 2.13	0.301	6.95 ± 1.71	7.40 ± 2.53	0.234
Red blood cells ($\times 10^6/\mu L$)	4.08 ± 0.39	3.83 ± 0.46	0.000 *	4.10 ± 0.47	3.96 ± 0.51	0.150
Hemoglobin (g/dL)	12.62 ± 1.26	12.06 ± 1.49	0.014 *	12.57 ± 1.38	11.82 ± 1.33	0.012 *
Hematocrit (%)	37.42 ± 3.49	35.35 ± 4.20	0.001 *	37.40 ± 3.85	35.44 ± 3.90	0.018 *
Mean corpuscular volume (fl)	91.77 ± 4.42	92.32 ± 4.22	0.471	91.41 ± 3.88	89.89 ± 4.81	0.074
Mean corpuscular hemoglobin (pg)	30.95 ± 1.66	31.50 ± 1.70	0.060	30.68 ± 1.52	29.91 ± 1.61	0.019 *
Mean corpuscular hemoglobin concentration (g/dL)	33.72 ± 0.75	34.13 ± 0.88	0.003 *	33.57 ± 0.69	33.29 ± 0.76	0.060
Platelets ($\times 10^3/\mu L$)	240.29 ± 56.55	211.94 ± 67.70	0.006 *	256.03 ± 63.97	284.55 ± 82.67	0.043 *
Neutrophils, diff. count (%)	60.50 ± 8.85	64.46 ± 8.60	0.016 *	61.70 ± 7.13	64.88 ± 9.49	0.060
Lymphocytes, diff. count (%)	28.24 ± 7.71	24.38 ± 7.31	0.004 *	27.26 ± 6.53	23.59 ± 8.75	0.011
Monocytes, diff. count (%)	7.48 ± 1.88	7.51 ± 1.80	0.938	7.37 ± 1.52	7.65 ± 1.69	0.394
Eosinophils, diff. count (%)	3.33 ± 1.84	3.40 ± 2.29	0.842	3.07 ± 1.61	2.87 ± 1.51	0.578
Basophils, diff. count (%)	0.45 ± 0.26	0.45 ± 0.31	0.985	0.51 ± 0.19	0.53 ± 0.44	0.792
Neutrophils, diff. count ($\times 10^3/\mu L$)	4.46 ± 1.58	5.23 ± 2.14	0.010 *	4.47 ± 1.42	5.09 ± 2.41	0.238
Lymphocytes, diff. count ($\times 10^3/\mu L$)	1.84 ± 0.53	1.76 ± 0.61	0.420	1.74 ± 0.49	5.09 ± 2.41	0.028 *
Monocytes, diff. count ($\times 10^3/\mu L$)	0.52 ± 0.17	0.56 ± 0.16	0.149	0.50 ± 0.14	0.55 ± 0.19	0.222
Eosinophils, diff. count ($\times 10^3/\mu L$)	0.21 ± 0.11	0.24 ± 0.18	0.169	0.19 ± 0.11	0.19 ± 0.10	0.694
Basophils, diff. count ($\times 10^3/\mu L$)	0.03 ± 0.02	0.03 ± 0.02	0.470	0.03 ± 0.01	0.04 ± 0.03	0.602
Creatinine (mg/dL)	0.71 ± 0.20	0.71 ± 0.27	0.902	2.25 ± 5.50	0.85 ± 1.03	0.000 *
Blood urea nitrogen (mg/dL)	16.11 ± 3.87	17.44 ± 5.61	0.072	15.23 ± 10.68	13.57 ± 4.23	0.461

Note: Values are presented as the number of subjects (%) or means ± standard deviations. The p values of the non-PU and PU groups were determined by the chi-squared test and independent t test; * p < 0.05. Abbreviations: PU = pressure ulcer, ISNCSCI = International Standards for Neurological Classification of Spinal Cord Injury; K-MBI = Korean version of the Modified Barthel Index; FIM = Functional Independence Measure.

The distributions of patient data across the different datasets from the two hospitals are shown in Table 2. Notably, the "Lab" dataset was the most voluminous of all the datasets. Nevertheless, all the datasets were rigorously evaluated to optimize the machine learning models. The data revealed a marked difference in the composition of the datasets between the two hospitals. Primary analysis was performed using the comprehensive "Lab + ISNCSCI + K-MBI + FIM" dataset from DKUH. To increase the precision of external validation, distinct training and validation datasets were derived from the "Lab + ISNCSCI" collection of both DKUH and CNUH, thus facilitating cross-institutional validation. DKUH evaluated the performance of machine learning models using different dataset combinations, such as "Lab", "Lab + ISNCSCI", "Lab + ISNCSCI + K-MBI", and "Lab + ISNCSCI + K-MBI + FIM". In contrast, the CNUH evaluations focused primarily on the "Lab", "ISNCSCI", and "Lab + ISNCSCI" datasets due to significant data gaps in the K-MBI and FIM metrics.

Table 2. Number of patients in the dataset category.

Dataset	DKUH			CNUH		
	Non-PU	PU	Total	Non-PU	PU	Total
Lab	328	159 (253)	487	434	73 (92)	507
ISNCSCI	221	46 (55)	267	362	23 (24)	385
K-MBI	259	46 (59)	307	62	6 (6)	68
FIM	250	46 (59)	298	31	2 (2)	33
ISNCSCI + K-MBI	208	46 (48)	248	41	3 (3)	44
ISNCSCI + K-MBI + FIM	200	46 (46)	239	16	1 (1)	17
Lab + ISNCSCI	216	46 (55)	262	362	23 (24)	385
Lab + ISNCSCI + K-MBI	207	46 (48)	247	41	3 (3)	44
Lab + ISNCSCI + K-MBI + FIM	199	39 (46)	238	16	1 (1)	17

The numbers of patients satisfying each dataset in the two hospitals are presented. The numbers in parentheses represent the counts of PU events. Abbreviations: DKUH = Dankook University Hospital; CNUH = Chungnam National University Hospital; PU = pressure ulcer; Lab = laboratory data; ISNCSCI = International Standards for Neurological Classification of Spinal Cord Injury; K-MBI = Korean version of the Modified Barthel Index; FIM = Functional Independence Measure.

3.3. Predictive Performance of the Machine Learning Models

Table 3 delineates the predictive properties of various machine learning (ML) models across distinct dataset combinations at Dankook University Hospital (DKUH). A comparison across identical algorithms revealed that the "Lab + ISNCS + CI + K-MBI + FIM" amalgam dataset consistently surpassed the other datasets in terms of AUC values. Within the same dataset, algorithmic variations demonstrated different levels of performance; the GNN-GCN algorithm outperformed the "Lab" dataset, and the KNN algorithm outperformed the others in the "Lab + ISNCSCI" dataset, whereas the SVM algorithm consistently stood out in the "Lab + ISNCSCI + K-MBI" and "Lab + ISNCSCI + K-MBI + FIM" datasets. Remarkably, the SVM_linear algorithm in the "Lab + ISNCSCI + K-MBI + FIM" dataset achieved a pinnacle AUC of 0.904, an accuracy of 0.944, and an F1-score of 0.907.

Table 3. Performance comparison of machine learning algorithms in each dataset from DKUH.

Model	Measure	Dataset			
		Lab	Lab + ISNCSCI	Lab + ISNCSCI + K-MBI	Lab + ISNCSCI + K-MBI + FIM
GNN-GCN	Sensitivity	0.442 ± 0.143	0.367 ± 0.190	0.508 ± 0.107	0.494 ± 0.163
	Specificity	0.883 ± 0.034	0.886 ± 0.068	0.913 ± 0.043	0.960 ± 0.036
	Accuracy	0.808 ± 0.052	0.788 ± 0.041	0.837 ± 0.040	0.873 ± 0.040
	AUC	0.656 ± 0.077	0.626 ± 0.078	0.710 ± 0.058	0.727 ± 0.082
	F1-score	0.662 ± 0.084	0.622 ± 0.076	0.720 ± 0.064	0.754 ± 0.085
DNN	Sensitivity	0.420 ± 0.192	0.132 ± 0.101	0.472 ± 0.135	0.600 ± 0.129
	Specificity	0.903 ± 0.023	0.966 ± 0.031	0.920 ± 0.031	0.963 ± 0.035
	Accuracy	0.834 ± 0.040	0.810 ± 0.030	0.836 ± 0.034	0.895 ± 0.040
	AUC	0.647 ± 0.090	0.549 ± 0.053	0.696 ± 0.069	0.781 ± 0.069
	F1-score	0.662 ± 0.105	0.545 ± 0.076	0.707 ± 0.067	0.808 ± 0.071

Table 3. Cont.

Model	Measure	Dataset			
		Lab	Lab + ISNCSCI	Lab + ISNCSCI + K-MBI	Lab + ISNCSCI + K-MBI + FIM
SVM_linear	Sensitivity	0.106 ± 0.169	0.245 ± 0.160	0.560 ± 0.132	0.840 ± 0.110
	Specificity	0.898 ± 0.008	0.945 ± 0.035	0.893 ± 0.034	0.968 ± 0.026
	Accuracy	0.818 ± 0.015	0.813 ± 0.035	0.830 ± 0.039	0.944 ± 0.031
	AUC	0.532 ± 0.056	0.595 ± 0.077	0.727 ± 0.071	0.904 ± 0.058
	F1-score	0.502 ± 0.087	0.599 ± 0.104	0.723 ± 0.067	0.907 ± 0.052
SVM_RBF	Sensitivity	0.298 ± 0.144	0.278 ± 0.130	0.525 ± 0.139	0.492 ± 0.165
	Specificity	0.882 ± 0.024	0.935 ± 0.040	0.893 ± 0.040	0.930 ± 0.039
	Accuracy	0.798 ± 0.037	0.811 ± 0.037	0.824 ± 0.044	0.847 ± 0.043
	AUC	0.585 ± 0.062	0.606 ± 0.066	0.709 ± 0.075	0.711 ± 0.084
	F1-score	0.590 ± 0.077	0.619 ± 0.079	0.709 ± 0.072	0.723 ± 0.085
KNN	Sensitivity	0.208 ± 0.195	0.432 ± 0.148	0.282 ± 0.128	0.246 ± 0.127
	Specificity	0.894 ± 0.018	0.898 ± 0.059	0.893 ± 0.047	0.811 ± 0.043
	Accuracy	0.813 ± 0.031	0.810 ± 0.049	0.779 ± 0.044	0.811 ± 0.043
	AUC	0.559 ± 0.074	0.665 ± 0.074	0.588 ± 0.067	0.594 ± 0.067
	F1-score	0.551 ± 0.103	0.670 ± 0.074	0.593 ± 0.074	0.605 ± 0.086
Random Forest	Sensitivity	0.122 ± 0.131	0.262 ± 0.144	0.208 ± 0.133	0.073 ± 0.074
	Specificity	0.899 ± 0.008	0.933 ± 0.043	0.953 ± 0.042	0.990 ± 0.019
	Accuracy	0.820 ± 0.015	0.807 ± 0.030	0.813 ± 0.030	0.818 ± 0.021
	AUC	0.532 ± 0.040	0.597 ± 0.062	0.581 ± 0.058	0.532 ± 0.038
	F1-score	0.510 ± 0.068	0.602 ± 0.073	0.584 ± 0.074	0.511 ± 0.065
Logistic Regression	Sensitivity	0.380 ± 0.196	0.352 ± 0.153	0.438 ± 0.144	0.683 ± 0.163
	Specificity	0.907 ± 0.017	0.942 ± 0.040	0.918 ± 0.036	0.964 ± 0.029
	Accuracy	0.838 ± 0.031	0.831 ± 0.041	0.828 ± 0.036	0.911 ± 0.033
	AUC	0.630 ± 0.084	0.647 ± 0.077	0.678 ± 0.072	0.823 ± 0.078
	F1-score	0.643 ± 0.104	0.665 ± 0.083	0.689 ± 0.069	0.841 ± 0.065

Abbreviations: Lab = laboratory data; ISNCSCI = International Standards for Neurological Classification of Spinal Cord Injury; K-MBI = Korean version of the Modified Barthel Index; FIM = Functional Independence Measure.

Feature selection was used strategically to improve the predictive accuracy of our models. Figure 2 shows the t-SNE plots before and after this important feature selection process. As shown, the demarcation between the non-PU and PU groups became much more pronounced after feature selection, illustrating the critical role of feature selection in achieving clearer data differentiation.

Figure 3 shows the importance scores of the top 39 parameters identified by the SVM_linear model. These parameters are spread across several categories, including Lab, ISNCSCI, K-MBI, and FIM. The representation of each category in this ranking indicates its integral role in influencing the model's predictions. The most prominent parameter in this evaluation was "Ambulation" in the K-MBI, which received the highest importance score of 1.212, followed by lower body dressing, transfer to bed, chair, and wheelchair, eating, and bathing in the FIM. This score demonstrated the importance of the functional status of the upper and lower extremities in the modeling process. In addition, the balanced presence of clinical scales such as the K-MBI and FIM, combined with laboratory and neurological data from Lab and ISNCSCI, highlights the variety of factors considered important in this model. This combination of factors demonstrates the intricate blend of physical, cognitive, and biological considerations that the model accounts for when analyzing outcomes.

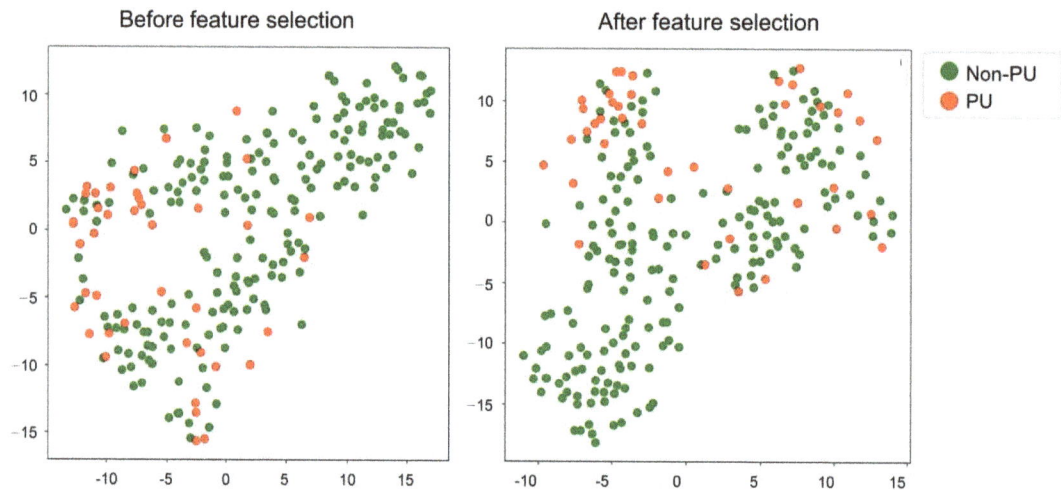

Figure 2. t-SNE plot before (**left**) and after (**right**) feature selection in the DKUH data.

In the CNUH dataset, Table 4 describes the predictive effectiveness of various machine learning models across different combinations of datasets and algorithms. Within each algorithm, the "ISNCSCI" dataset predominantly registered the highest AUC for the GNN-GCN, DNN, KNN, and random forest algorithms. Conversely, the "Lab + ISNCSCI" dataset included the SVM_linear, SVM_RBF, and logistic regression algorithms. When comparing different algorithms on the same dataset, the KNN algorithm consistently had the highest AUC in all three datasets. Overall, the KNN algorithm showed the best predictive performance on the "ISNCSCI" dataset, achieving an AUC of 0.737, an accuracy of 0.891 and an F1-score of 0.661.

Table 4. Performance comparison of machine learning algorithms in each dataset of CNUH data.

Model	Measure	Dataset		
		Lab	ISNCSCI	Lab + ISNCSCI
GNN-GCN	Sensitivity	0.180 ± 0.195	0.426 ± 0.218	0.362 ± 0.200
	Specificity	0.923 ± 0.036	0.947 ± 0.035	0.945 ± 0.037
	Accuracy	0.877 ± 0.034	0.914 ± 0.034	0.908 ± 0.033
	AUC	0.551 ± 0.096	0.686 ± 0.107	0.653 ± 0.097
	F1-score	0.538 ± 0.078	0.666 ± 0.092	0.635 ± 0.087
DNN	Sensitivity	0.108 ± 0.134	0.398 ± 0.214	0.388 ± 0.194
	Specificity	0.944 ± 0.031	0.947 ± 0.036	0.949 ± 0.033
	Accuracy	0.892 ± 0.031	0.913 ± 0.035	0.914 ± 0.028
	AUC	0.526 ± 0.068	0.672 ± 0.105	0.669 ± 0.092
	F1-score	0.523 ± 0.066	0.654 ± 0.099	0.654 ± 0.077
SVM_linear	Sensitivity	0.124 ± 0.132	0.416 ± 0.204	0.418 ± 0.181
	Specificity	0.961 ± 0.035	0.950 ± 0.027	0.925 ± 0.038
	Accuracy	0.909 ± 0.035	0.889 ± 0.032	0.894 ± 0.036
	AUC	0.543 ± 0.069	0.643 ± 0.072	0.672 ± 0.089
	F1-score	0.547 ± 0.084	0.614 ± 0.065	0.636 ± 0.081
SVM_RBF	Sensitivity	0.140 ± 0.173	0.362 ± 0.153	0.420 ± 0.214
	Specificity	0.944 ± 0.028	0.924 ± 0.035	0.957 ± 0.028
	Accuracy	0.894 ± 0.028	0.917 ± 0.025	0.924 ± 0.025
	AUC	0.542 ± 0.086	0.683 ± 0.098	0.689 ± 0.103
	F1-score	0.537 ± 0.083	0.661 ± 0.086	0.676 ± 0.085

Table 4. Cont.

Model	Measure	Dataset		
		Lab	ISNCSCI	Lab + ISNCSCI
KNN	Sensitivity	0.340 ± 0.175	0.562 ± 0.236	0.538 ± 0.223
	Specificity	0.875 ± 0.040	0.913 ± 0.030	0.910 ± 0.029
	Accuracy	0.842 ± 0.037	0.891 ± 0.027	0.887 ± 0.028
	AUC	0.607 ± 0.085	0.737 ± 0.114	0.724 ± 0.109
	F1-score	0.559 ± 0.053	0.661 ± 0.068	0.651 ± 0.069
Random Forest	Sensitivity	0.066 ± 0.114	0.386 ± 0.191	0.378 ± 0.194
	Specificity	0.996 ± 0.008	0.943 ± 0.031	0.945 ± 0.033
	Accuracy	0.938 ± 0.010	0.909 ± 0.028	0.910 ± 0.033
	AUC	0.531 ± 0.056	0.665 ± 0.093	0.662 ± 0.101
	F1-score	0.533 ± 0.083	0.646 ± 0.080	0.649 ± 0.093
Logistic Regression	Sensitivity	0.148 ± 0.160	0.408 ± 0.184	0.442 ± 0.191
	Specificity	0.941 ± 0.035	0.926 ± 0.033	0.928 ± 0.033
	Accuracy	0.892 ± 0.032	0.895 ± 0.032	0.898 ± 0.032
	AUC	0.545 ± 0.078	0.667 ± 0.093	0.685 ± 0.094
	F1-score	0.538 ± 0.070	0.636 ± 0.083	0.648 ± 0.082

The KNN model trained with the "ISNCSCI" dataset from CNUH demonstrated the highest performance, with an AUC of 0.737. Abbreviations: Lab = laboratory data; ISNCSCI = International Standards for Neurological Classification of Spinal Cord Injury.

The t-SNE plot before and after feature selection in the CNUH model is shown in Supplementary Figure S1. The non-PU and PU groups were more clearly classified after feature selection. The changes in the distribution patterns of the non-PU and PU groups after feature selection indicate notable changes. The eleven feature parameters were ranked by importance scores based on the outcome of the KNN model (Supplementary Figure S2), and the ASIA impairment scale (AIS) item of the ISNCSCI had the highest importance score of 0.19.

Figure 4 shows the receiver operating characteristic (ROC) curves for the optimal datasets from both DKUH and CNUH. With respect to the DKUH dataset, which comprises the Lab + ISNCSCI + K-MBI + FIM variables, the SVM_linear algorithm distinctly surpassed the other methods, with an AUC of 0.904, an accuracy of 94.4%, a sensitivity of 0.840, a specificity of 0.968, and an F1-score of 0.907. The CNUH dataset, which was based exclusively on ISNCSCI variables, exhibited more uniform results across different algorithms. Notably, the KNN algorithm had an AUC of 0.737, an accuracy of 89.1%, a sensitivity of 0.562, a specificity of 0.913, and an F1-score of 0.661. Overall, the performance at CNUH was more restrained than that at DKUH. The SVM_linear algorithm maintained its superior performance with only the ISNCSCI variables in the DKUH dataset, but its AUC and accuracy were considerably lower than those of the combination of the Lab + ISNCSCI + K-MBI + FIM variables and even the CNUH results (Supplementary Figure S3).

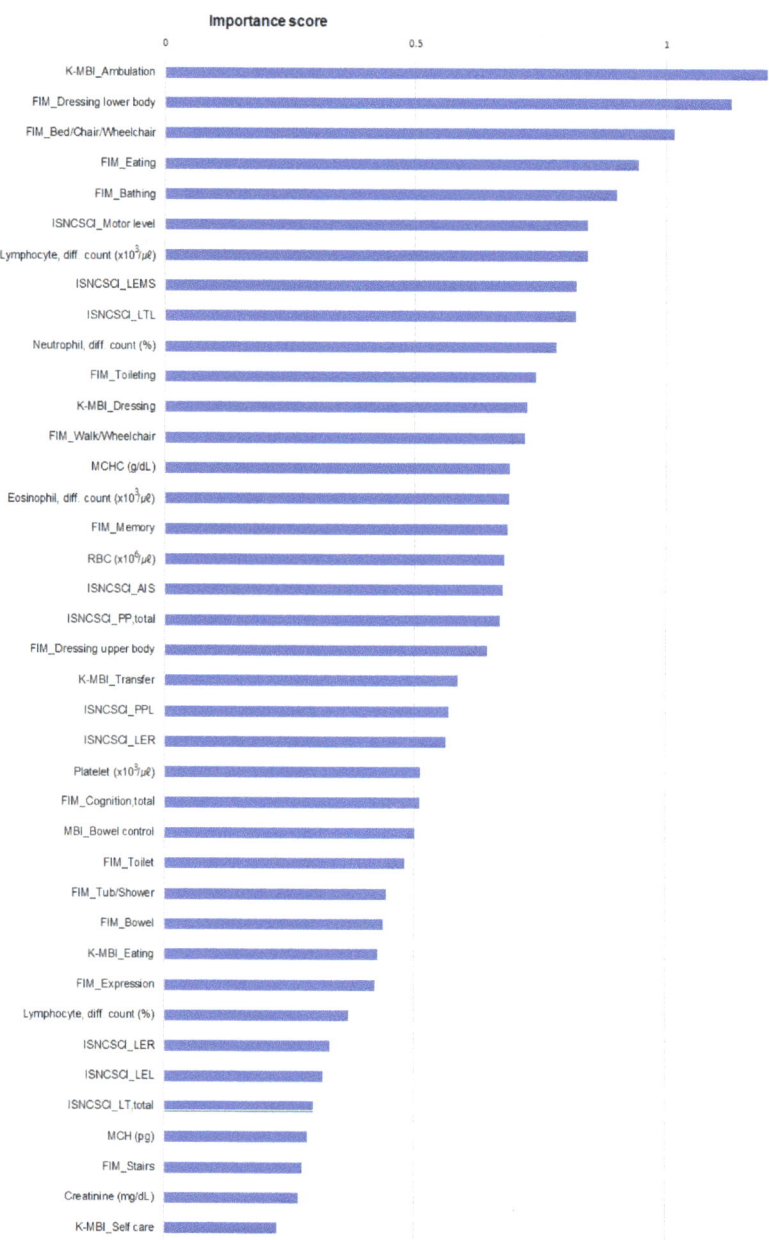

Figure 3. Importance scores of the top 39 featured parameters based on the outcome of the SVM_linear model. Abbreviations: K-MBI = Korean version of the Modified Barthel Index; FIM = Functional Independence Measure; ISNCSCI = International Standards for Neurological Classification of Spinal Cord Injury; LEMS = lower extremity, motor subscore; LTL = light touch, left; MCHC = mean corpuscular hemoglobin concentration; RBC = red blood cell; AIS = ASIA impairment scale; PPL = pinprick, left; LER = lower extremity, right; LEL = lower extremity, left; LT, total = light touch, total; MCH = mean corpuscular hemoglobin.

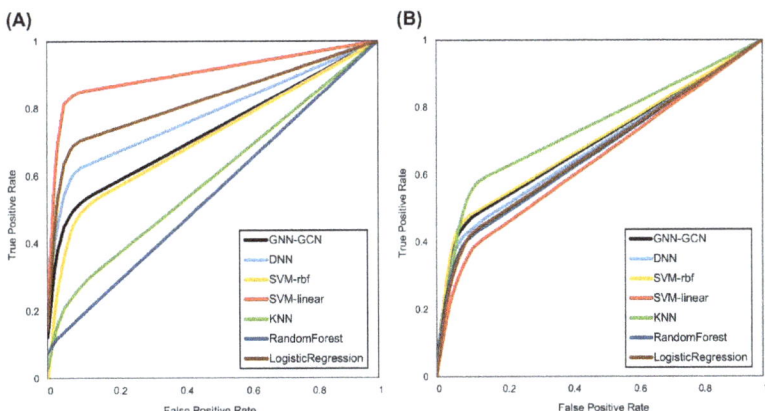

Figure 4. Receiver operating characteristic (ROC) curve of each machine learning algorithm in (**A**) DKUH using the Lab + ISNCSCI + K-MBI + FIM dataset and (**B**) CNUH using the ISNCSCI dataset.

Figure 5 shows the decision tree model employed to distinguish between the Non-PU and PU groups. The primary discriminator is "K-MBI: ambulation", with a threshold value of 2.338. Subjects who scored below this threshold were predominantly categorized using subsequent discriminators, notably "ISNCSCI: motor score of Rt. lower extremity" ($\leq$18.314) and "FIM: eating" ($\leq$5.033). In contrast, for those surpassing the "K-MBI: ambulation" threshold, "FIM: walk/wheelchair" ($\leq$3.445) and "ISNCSCI: motor score of Rt. lower extremity" ($\leq$7.388) emerged as salient discriminators. The tree further expands to encompass laboratory parameters such as platelet count, mean corpuscular hemoglobin, and eosinophil count, as well as multiple neurological and functional metrics. Each branch point denotes a unique criterion that aids in efficiently classifying subjects into the non-PU and PU groups.

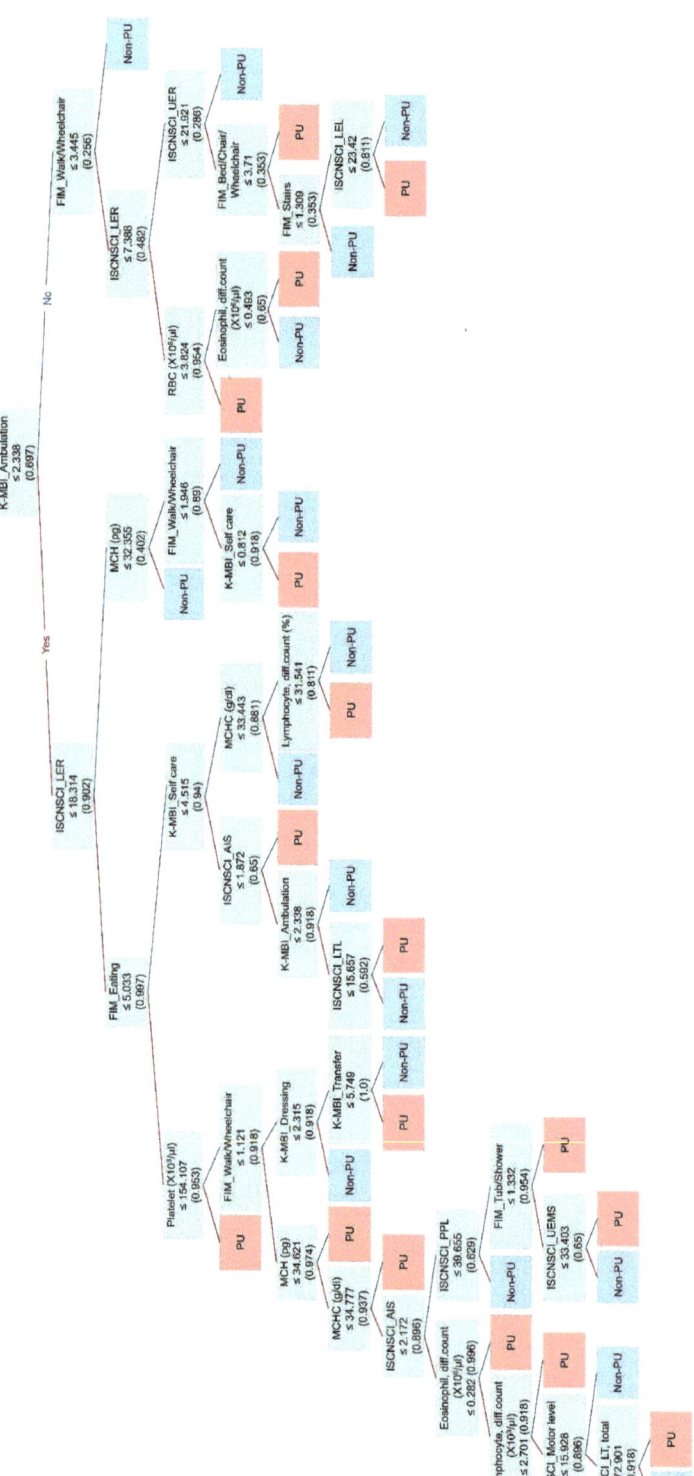

Figure 5. Decision tree of the SVM_linear model trained with the "'Lab + ISNCSCI + K-MBI + FIM" dataset of DKUH to classify the non-PU and PU groups. The "ambulation" subscale of the K-MBI was identified as the first single discriminator for determination of the two groups. The red line indicates "yes", and the blue line indicates "no". Abbreviations: K-MBI = Korean version of the Modified Barthel Index; ISNCSCI = International Standards for Neurological Classification of Spinal Cord Injury; FIM = Functional Independence Measure; LER = lower extremity, right; UER = upper extremity, right; AIS = ASIA Impairment Scale; LTL = light touch, left; LEL = lower extremity, left; PPL = pinprick, left; UEMS = Upper Extremity Motor Subscore; LT, total = light touch, total, MCH = mean corpuscular hemoglobin; MCHC = mean corpuscular hemoglobin concentration.

4. Discussion

In our quest to improve outcomes for patients with SCI, our study's application of ML techniques marks a shift from traditional areas of focus, including neurological and functional outcomes [30–35], to the proactive prevention of PUs. These prevalent yet preventable complications have a profound impact on the recovery and quality of life of patients with SCI [36]. Our innovative use of ML, ranging from SVM to DNN to GNN, has enabled us to delve into complex datasets and extract critical insights from nonlinear relationships for more accurate PU predictive modeling. This methodology underscores the potential of ML to go beyond the boundaries of conventional statistical analysis.

A key finding of our study was the differential performance of the linear SVM model across different datasets. The DKUH dataset, with its larger sample size and diverse baseline characteristics such as age range, injury severity, and neurological status, provided a different context for ML application than the CNUH dataset. This contrast in performance underscores the influence of specific dataset attributes on the success of ML models and highlights the need for data that encapsulate a broad range of patient scenarios to improve predictive accuracy in diverse clinical settings.

Furthermore, our analysis revealed the paramount importance of functional parameters, including walking (K-MBI), lower body dressing, transfers, eating and bathing (FIM), in predicting PUs (Figure 3). This finding highlights the dominance of functional data over neurological factors in risk assessment. The need for functional assessment is particularly pronounced in conditions such as spinal shock, where the neurological status may be uncertain. In addition to these functional indicators, our study also draws attention to the importance of pre-onset laboratory markers related to inflammation and anemia, such as lymphocyte, neutrophil and eosinophil counts, as well as MCHC and RBC counts, which is consistent with the findings of a previous study [37]. Although not primary predictors, their association with increased PU risk is consistent with previous research and underscores their importance in PU risk assessment.

As we move toward clinical application, we have developed a decision tree algorithm based on the results of our study. This algorithm incorporates key parameters identified as significant in predicting PUs, such as functional status indicators (e.g., mobility and self-care ability) and relevant laboratory markers (e.g., inflammatory, and hematological parameters). Designed as a user-friendly decision support tool, it systematically evaluates these factors to estimate PU risk, providing clinicians with a structured framework for early intervention. While the algorithm is promising, extensive validation in diverse clinical settings is essential to determine its utility and efficacy. Our preliminary external validation efforts have revealed variability in performance across datasets from different institutions, underscoring the challenges of creating a universally applicable ML-based prediction tool. These observations not only highlight the intricacies of ML model generalization, but also pave the way for further research to refine and adapt the algorithm for broader clinical use [38,39].

The limitations of our study are openly acknowledged, particularly with respect to the limited sample size and the brevity of the observation period. We recognize the potential of expansive data sources such as the National Spinal Cord Injury Statistical Center (NSCISC; https://www.nscisc.uab.edu/, accessed on 19 October 2021) and the National Institutes of Health (NIH) National Institute of Neurological Disorders and Stroke (NINDS; https://www.commondataelements.ninds.nih.gov/Spinal%20Cord%20Injury, accessed on 19 October 2021), although their use was limited by their mismatch with the acute and subacute phase specificity of our research, particularly the lack of time-sensitive laboratory data relevant to the onset of PUs. In addition, the design of our study needed a rigorous selection process to include only participants with unique records, limiting our dataset.

We envision that future studies include a wider network, integrate data from multiple centers, and account for the temporal progression of PUs. The exploration of hybrid machine learning frameworks that combine the strengths of different algorithms may hold the key to improving predictive accuracy. Our ultimate goal is to develop a reliable predictive framework that will not only facilitate the prevention and early treatment of PUs in clinical settings, but also have a tangible impact on the care and quality of life of patients with SCI. This framework will enable clinicians to intervene more effectively, potentially reducing the incidence of PUs and their associated complications. By improving early detection and intervention strategies, we aim to contribute to better health outcomes, increased independence, and overall well-being for patients with SCI.

5. Conclusions

In this study, we successfully developed a prediction model for PUs after SCI during the acute and subacute stages of the hospital stay using an ML algorithm, especially the SVM linear model. Our findings underscore the critical role of functional data, in addition to neurological and laboratory data, in the development of effective PU prediction models. Specifically, the five most important functional parameters identified were ambulation, lower body dressing, bed/chair/wheelchair transfers, eating, and bathing. These parameters, which are indicative of a patient's mobility and self-care capabilities, are critical in predicting PU risk. The integration of these functional aspects into our machine learning-driven models holds great promise for the early detection and prevention of PUs in clinical settings, potentially leading to improved patient care and outcomes for patients with SCI.

Supplementary Materials: The following supporting information can be downloaded at: https://www.mdpi.com/article/10.3390/jcm13040990/s1, Figure S1: tSNE plot before and after feature selection in CNUH data; Figure S2: Importance scores of the top 11 featured parameters based on the outcome of the KNN model in CNUH; Figure S3: Receiver operating characteristic (ROC) curve of each machine learning algorithm in DKUH using the ISNCSCI dataset.

Author Contributions: Conceptualization, H.-Y.J. and J.K.H.; methodology, J.K.H., M.L., and H.-Y.J.; software, M.L., and H.-Y.J.; validation, Y.K., M.L., S.-K.B., and H.-Y.J.; formal analysis, Y.K., M.L., Y.H., and H.-Y.J.; investigation, Y.K., M.L., and J.K.H.; resources, Y.K., S.-K.B., and J.K.H.; data curation, Y.K., S.Y.K., T.U.K., S.J.L., S.-K.B., and J.K.H.; writing—original draft preparation, Y.K., M.L., and J.K.H.; writing—review and editing, M.L. and J.K.H.; visualization, M.L., Y.H., and H.-Y.J.; supervision, S.P., H.-Y.J., and J.K.H.; project administration, S.P. and J.K.H.; funding acquisition, H.-Y.J. and J.K.H. All authors have read and agreed to the published version of the manuscript.

Funding: This study was supported by grants (2019R1A6A1A11034536 and RS-2023-00208315) through the National Research Foundation (NRF) and an Electronics and Telecommunications Research Institute (ETRI) grant [21YR2410, Development of image and medical intelligence core technology for rehabilitation diagnosis and treatment of brain and spinal cord diseases] funded by the Korean government.

Institutional Review Board Statement: The study was conducted according to the guidelines of the Declaration of Helsinki and approved by the Institutional Review Board of Dankook University Hospital (IRB No. 2021-05-021, approved on 20 May 2021).

Informed Consent Statement: Not applicable.

Data Availability Statement: The data presented in this study are available from the corresponding authors upon reasonable request.

Conflicts of Interest: The authors declare no conflicts of interest.

References

1. Ahuja, C.S.; Wilson, J.R.; Nori, S.; Kotter, M.R.N.; Druschel, C.; Curt, A.; Fehlings, M.G. Traumatic spinal cord injury. *Nat. Rev. Dis. Primers* **2017**, *3*, 17018. [CrossRef]
2. Chen, H.L.; Cai, J.Y.; Du, L.; Shen, H.W.; Yu, H.R.; Song, Y.P.; Zha, M.L. Incidence of Pressure Injury in Individuals With Spinal Cord Injury: A Systematic Review and Meta-analysis. *J. Wound Ostomy Cont. Nurs.* **2020**, *47*, 215–223. [CrossRef]
3. Zakrasek, E.C.; Creasey, G.; Crew, J.D. Pressure ulcers in people with spinal cord injury in developing nations. *Spinal Cord.* **2015**, *53*, 7–13. [CrossRef]
4. Gorecki, C.; Nixon, J.; Madill, A.; Firth, J.; Brown, J.M. What influences the impact of pressure ulcers on health-related quality of life? A qualitative patient-focused exploration of contributory factors. *J. Tissue Viability* **2012**, *21*, 3–12. [CrossRef] [PubMed]

5. Sen, C.K. Human Wound and Its Burden: Updated 2020 Compendium of Estimates. *Adv. Wound Care* **2021**, *10*, 281–292. [CrossRef] [PubMed]
6. Kruger, E.A.; Pires, M.; Ngann, Y.; Sterling, M.; Rubayi, S. Comprehensive management of pressure ulcers in spinal cord injury: Current concepts and future trends. *J. Spinal Cord. Med.* **2013**, *36*, 572–585. [CrossRef] [PubMed]
7. Consortium for Spinal Cord Medicine Clinical Practice. Pressure ulcer prevention and treatment following spinal cord injury: A clinical practice guideline for health-care professionals. *J. Spinal Cord. Med.* **2001**, *24* (Suppl. S1), S40–S101. [CrossRef] [PubMed]
8. Shiferaw, W.S.; Akalu, T.Y.; Mulugeta, H.; Aynalem, Y.A. The global burden of pressure ulcers among patients with spinal cord injury: A systematic review and meta-analysis. *BMC Musculoskelet. Disord.* **2020**, *21*, 334. [CrossRef] [PubMed]
9. Brienza, D.; Krishnan, S.; Karg, P.; Sowa, G.; Allegretti, A.L. Predictors of pressure ulcer incidence following traumatic spinal cord injury: A secondary analysis of a prospective longitudinal study. *Spinal Cord.* **2018**, *56*, 28–34. [CrossRef] [PubMed]
10. Verschueren, J.H.; Post, M.W.; de Groot, S.; van der Woude, L.H.; van Asbeck, F.W.; Rol, M. Occurrence and predictors of pressure ulcers during primary in-patient spinal cord injury rehabilitation. *Spinal Cord.* **2011**, *49*, 106–112. [CrossRef] [PubMed]
11. Gelis, A.; Dupeyron, A.; Legros, P.; Benaim, C.; Pelissier, J.; Fattal, C. Pressure ulcer risk factors in persons with SCI: Part I: Acute and rehabilitation stages. *Spinal Cord.* **2009**, *47*, 99–107. [CrossRef] [PubMed]
12. Mortenson, W.B.; Miller, W.C.; Team, S.R. A review of scales for assessing the risk of developing a pressure ulcer in individuals with SCI. *Spinal Cord.* **2008**, *46*, 168–175. [CrossRef] [PubMed]
13. Higgins, J.; Laramee, M.T.; Harrison, K.R.; Delparte, J.J.; Scovil, C.Y.; Flett, H.M.; Burns, A.S. The Spinal Cord Injury Pressure Ulcer Scale (SCIPUS): An assessment of validity using Rasch analysis. *Spinal Cord.* **2019**, *57*, 874–880. [CrossRef]
14. Ash, D. An exploration of the occurrence of pressure ulcers in a British spinal injuries unit. *J. Clin. Nurs.* **2002**, *11*, 470–478. [CrossRef] [PubMed]
15. Flett, H.M.; Delparte, J.J.; Scovil, C.Y.; Higgins, J.; Laramee, M.T.; Burns, A.S. Determining Pressure Injury Risk on Admission to Inpatient Spinal Cord Injury Rehabilitation: A Comparison of the FIM, Spinal Cord Injury Pressure Ulcer Scale, and Braden Scale. *Arch. Phys. Med. Rehabil.* **2019**, *100*, 1881–1887. [CrossRef] [PubMed]
16. Chan, M.S.; Avsar, P.; McEvoy, N.L.; Patton, D.; O'Connor, T.; Nugent, L.; Moore, Z. The role of proinflammatory cytokines in the detection of early pressure ulcer development: A systematic review. *J. Wound Care* **2023**, *32*, 83–91. [CrossRef] [PubMed]
17. Barrientos, S.; Brem, H.; Stojadinovic, O.; Tomic-Canic, M. Clinical application of growth factors and cytokines in wound healing. *Wound Repair. Regen.* **2014**, *22*, 569–578. [CrossRef] [PubMed]
18. Tran, J.P.; McLaughlin, J.M.; Li, R.T.; Phillips, L.G. Prevention of Pressure Ulcers in the Acute Care Setting: New Innovations and Technologies. *Plast. Reconstr. Surg.* **2016**, *138*, 232S–240S. [CrossRef]
19. Esteva, A.; Robicquet, A.; Ramsundar, B.; Kuleshov, V.; DePristo, M.; Chou, K.; Cui, C.; Corrado, G.; Thrun, S.; Dean, J. A guide to deep learning in healthcare. *Nat. Med.* **2019**, *25*, 24–29. [CrossRef]
20. Taye, M.M. Understanding of Machine Learning with Deep Learning: Architectures, Workflow, Applications and Future Directions. *Computers* **2023**, *12*, 91. [CrossRef]
21. Kato, C.; Uemura, O.; Sato, Y.; Tsuji, T. Decision Tree Analysis Accurately Predicts Discharge Destination After Spinal Cord Injury Rehabilitation. *Arch. Phys. Med. Rehabil.* **2024**, *105*, 88–94. [CrossRef]
22. Merali, Z.; Wang, J.Z.; Badhiwala, J.H.; Witiw, C.D.; Wilson, J.R.; Fehlings, M.G. A deep learning model for detection of cervical spinal cord compression in MRI scans. *Sci. Rep.* **2021**, *11*, 10473. [CrossRef] [PubMed]
23. McCoy, D.B.; Dupont, S.M.; Gros, C.; Cohen-Adad, J.; Huie, R.J.; Ferguson, A.; Duong-Fernandez, X.; Thomas, L.H.; Singh, V.; Narvid, J.; et al. Convolutional Neural Network-Based Automated Segmentation of the Spinal Cord and Contusion Injury: Deep Learning Biomarker Correlates of Motor Impairment in Acute Spinal Cord Injury. *AJNR Am. J. Neuroradiol.* **2019**, *40*, 737–744. [CrossRef] [PubMed]
24. Luther, S.L.; Thomason, S.S.; Sabharwal, S.; Finch, D.K.; McCart, J.; Toyinbo, P.; Bouayad, L.; Lapcevic, W.; Hahm, B.; Hauser, R.G.; et al. Machine learning to develop a predictive model of pressure injury in persons with spinal cord injury. *Spinal Cord.* **2023**, *61*, 513–520. [CrossRef] [PubMed]
25. Ghaffari-Rafi, A.; Peterson, C.; Leon-Rojas, J.E.; Tadokoro, N.; Lange, S.F.; Kaushal, M.; Tetreault, L.; Fehlings, M.G.; Martin, A.R. The Role of Magnetic Resonance Imaging to Inform Clinical Decision-Making in Acute Spinal Cord Injury: A Systematic Review and Meta-Analysis. *J. Clin. Med.* **2021**, *10*, 4948. [CrossRef] [PubMed]
26. Chandra, J.; Sheerin, F.; Lopez de Heredia, L.; Meagher, T.; King, D.; Belci, M.; Hughes, R.J. MRI in acute and subacute post-traumatic spinal cord injury: Pictorial review. *Spinal Cord.* **2012**, *50*, 2–7. [CrossRef] [PubMed]
27. Pedregosa, F.; Varoquaux, G.; Gramfort, A.; Michel, V.; Thirion, B.; Grisel, O.; Blondel, M.; Prettenhofer, P.; Weiss, R.; Dubourg, V.; et al. Scikit-learn: Machine Learning in Python. *J. Mach. Learn. Res.* **2011**, *12*, 2825–2830.
28. Choudhary, K.; DeCost, B.; Chen, C.; Jain, A.; Tavazza, F.; Cohn, R.; Park, C.W.; Choudhary, A.; Agrawal, A.; Billinge, S.J.L.; et al. Recent advances and applications of deep learning methods in materials science. *Npj Comput. Mater.* **2022**, *8*, 59. [CrossRef]
29. Paszke, A.; Gross, S.; Massa, F.; Lerer, A.; Bradbury, J.; Chanan, G.; Killeen, T.; Lin, Z.; Gimelshein, N.; Antiga, L. Pytorch: An imperative style, high-performance deep learning library. *Adv. Neural Inf. Process. Syst.* **2019**, *32*, 8026–8037.
30. Kapoor, D.; Xu, C. Spinal Cord Injury AIS Predictions Using Machine Learning. *eNeuro* **2023**, *10*. [CrossRef]
31. Kato, C.; Uemura, O.; Sato, Y.; Tsuji, T. Functional Outcome Prediction After Spinal Cord Injury Using Ensemble Machine Learning. *Arch. Phys. Med. Rehabil.* **2023**, *105*, 95–100. [CrossRef] [PubMed]

32. Okimatsu, S.; Maki, S.; Furuya, T.; Fujiyoshi, T.; Kitamura, M.; Inada, T.; Aramomi, M.; Yamauchi, T.; Miyamoto, T.; Inoue, T.; et al. Determining the short-term neurological prognosis for acute cervical spinal cord injury using machine learning. *J. Clin. Neurosci. Off. J. Neurosurg. Soc. Australas.* **2022**, *96*, 74–79. [CrossRef]
33. Fallah, N.; Noonan, V.K.; Waheed, Z.; Rivers, C.S.; Plashkes, T.; Bedi, M.; Etminan, M.; Thorogood, N.P.; Ailon, T.; Chan, E. Development of a machine learning algorithm for predicting in-hospital and 1-year mortality after traumatic spinal cord injury. *Spine J.* **2022**, *22*, 329–336. [CrossRef] [PubMed]
34. DeVries, Z.; Hoda, M.; Rivers, C.S.; Maher, A.; Wai, E.; Moravek, D.; Stratton, A.; Kingwell, S.; Fallah, N.; Paquet, J. Development of an unsupervised machine learning algorithm for the prognostication of walking ability in spinal cord injury patients. *Spine J.* **2020**, *20*, 213–224. [CrossRef]
35. Inoue, T.; Ichikawa, D.; Ueno, T.; Cheong, M.; Inoue, T.; Whetstone, W.D.; Endo, T.; Nizuma, K.; Tominaga, T. XGBoost, a machine learning method, predicts neurological recovery in patients with cervical spinal cord injury. *Neurotrauma Rep.* **2020**, *1*, 8–16. [CrossRef] [PubMed]
36. Haisma, J.A.; van der Woude, L.H.; Stam, H.J.; Bergen, M.P.; Sluis, T.A.; Post, M.W.; Bussmann, J.B. Complications following spinal cord injury: Occurrence and risk factors in a longitudinal study during and after inpatient rehabilitation. *J. Rehabil. Med.* **2007**, *39*, 393–398. [CrossRef] [PubMed]
37. Scivoletto, G.; Fuoco, U.; Morganti, B.; Cosentino, E.; Molinari, M. Pressure sores and blood and serum dysmetabolism in spinal cord injury patients. *Spinal Cord* **2004**, *42*, 473–476. [CrossRef] [PubMed]
38. Abdulazeem, H.; Whitelaw, S.; Schauberger, G.; Klug, S.J. A systematic review of clinical health conditions predicted by machine learning diagnostic and prognostic models trained or validated using real-world primary health care data. *PLoS ONE* **2023**, *18*, e0274276. [CrossRef]
39. Ho, S.Y.; Phua, K.; Wong, L.; Bin Goh, W.W. Extensions of the External Validation for Checking Learned Model Interpretability and Generalizability. *Patterns* **2020**, *1*, 100129. [CrossRef]

Disclaimer/Publisher's Note: The statements, opinions and data contained in all publications are solely those of the individual author(s) and contributor(s) and not of MDPI and/or the editor(s). MDPI and/or the editor(s) disclaim responsibility for any injury to people or property resulting from any ideas, methods, instructions or products referred to in the content.

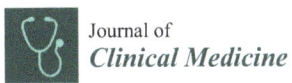
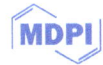

Article

Secondary Sarcopenia and Spinal Cord Injury: Clinical Associations and Health Outcomes

Anamaria Gherle [1,2,†], Carmen Delia Nistor-Cseppento [1,2,*], Diana-Carina Iovanovici [1,*], Iulia Ruxandra Cevei [3], Mariana Lidia Cevei [2,†], Danche Vasileva [4], Stefania Deac [1] and Dorina Stoicanescu [5]

[1] Doctoral School of Biomedical Sciences, Faculty of Medicine and Pharmacy, University of Oradea, 410087 Oradea, Romania; bl_anamaria@yahoo.com (A.G.); stefaniacristea95@yahoo.ro (S.D.)
[2] Department of Psycho-Neurosciences and Recovery, Faculty of Medicine and Pharmacy, University of Oradea, 410073 Oradea, Romania; cevei_mariana@yahoo.com
[3] Institute of Cardiovascular Diseases Timisoara, 13A Gheorghe Adam Street, 300310 Timisoara, Romania; iuliacevei@yahoo.com
[4] Faculty of Medical Sciences, Goce Delcev University, P5MX+HP6, 2000 Stip, North Macedonia; dance.vasileva@ugd.edu.mk
[5] Microscopic Morphology Department, "Victor Babes" University of Medicine and Pharmacy Timisoara, 300041 Timisoara, Romania; dstoicanescu@gmail.com
* Correspondence: delia_cseppento@yahoo.com (C.D.N.-C.); diana_iovanovici@yahoo.com (D.-C.I.); Tel.: +40-729901400 (C.D.N.-C.)
† These authors contributed equally to this work.

Abstract: Background: Sarcopenia and spinal cord injury (SCI) often coexist, but little is known about the associations. This study aimed to assess the impact of SCI on muscle and bone mass and the correlations between the clinical characteristics of SCI patients and sarcopenia. **Methods:** A total of 136 patients with SCI admitted to rehabilitation hospital were included in this study. The type and severity of injury (AIS), level of spasticity (MAS), bone mineral density and Appendicular Lean Muscle Mass (ALM) were assessed. Sarcopenia was diagnosed according to EWGSOP2 cut-off points for ALM. **Results:** Subjects were divided into two groups: Group S-SCI (N = 66, sarcopenia group) and Group NS-SCI (N = 70, without sarcopenia). Mean ALM values in the two groups were 0.49 and 0.65, respectively. A total of 75% of women and 42.9% of men developed sarcopenia. The mean age was 35.8 years in the sarcopenic patients and 41.5 in the non-sarcopenia group. Over 55% of AIS Grades A and B cases, 69.7% of MAS level 0 cases and 51.6% of the patients with osteoporosis had sarcopenia. The mean number of comorbidities was 2.7 in the sarcopenia group. **Conclusions:** Gender, type of injury, presence of multiple comorbidities and age were directly associated with sarcopenia; meanwhile, surprisingly, spasticity level and the presence of immobilization osteoporosis were not.

Keywords: spinal cord injury; sarcopenia; immobilization osteoporosis; spasticity

Citation: Gherle, A.; Nistor-Cseppento, C.D.; Iovanovici, D.-C.; Cevei, I.R.; Cevei, M.L.; Vasileva, D.; Deac, S.; Stoicanescu, D. Secondary Sarcopenia and Spinal Cord Injury: Clinical Associations and Health Outcomes. *J. Clin. Med.* **2024**, *13*, 885. https://doi.org/10.3390/jcm13030885

Academic Editor: Hideaki Nakajima

Received: 6 December 2023
Revised: 21 January 2024
Accepted: 31 January 2024
Published: 2 February 2024

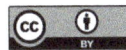

Copyright: © 2024 by the authors. Licensee MDPI, Basel, Switzerland. This article is an open access article distributed under the terms and conditions of the Creative Commons Attribution (CC BY) license (https://creativecommons.org/licenses/by/4.0/).

1. Introduction

The progressive loss of muscle mass and strength, with the impaired physical performance of individuals and associated with advancing age, has been defined as sarcopenia [1,2]. The term was first introduced by Rosenberg (1989) [3].

The etiology is multifactorial. Age-related decline, chronic diseases, presbyphagia, qualitative and quantitative muscle tissue impairment, hormonal changes and cellular metabolism (the imbalance between protein synthesis and degradation) are some of the factors involved in the occurrence of sarcopenia [4,5]. The loss of muscle mass and strength associated with the ageing process defines primary sarcopenia, which may contribute to a decrease in mobility, balance, coordination and the ability to perform activities of daily living [6]. Secondary sarcopenia is defined by the association of ageing with other evident factors or comorbidities [7].

In 2010, the European Working Group on Sarcopenia in Older People (EWGSOP) met to develop diagnostic criteria. They developed clear diagnostic criteria and a globally accepted definition for age-related sarcopenia. The working definition until 2018 was that sarcopenia is a syndrome characterized by the concurrent presence of both low muscle mass and low muscle function or low physical performance [6]; however, in early 2018, the EWGSOP2 re-convened to update the original definition and establish new cut-off points for sarcopenia, with the aim of highlighting the latest emerging scientific and clinical evidence that has accumulated over the past decade [8]. The conclusion reached by Cruz-Jentoft et al. in 2019 was that it is common among older adults but can also occur earlier in life [8].

Osteosarcopenia is defined by the concomitant presence of osteopenia/osteoporosis and sarcopenia. The etiology of osteosarcopenia is multifactorial, involving several factors, both genetic and environmental. In addition, a poor nutritional status and lack of physical activity, such as prolonged immobilization, are key risk factors for osteosarcopenia [9].

Spinal cord injuries (SCI) are typically characterized by a loss of function (motor and/or sensory) distal to the lesion and include multiple impairments: paralysis of voluntary muscles, altered sensory function, mobility disorders and joint contractures, abnormal muscle tone, pain and cardio-pulmonary deconditioning [10]. Road accidents are the most frequent causes of SCI, followed by falls resulting in bone fractures, gunshot wounds and sports. Several secondary long-term complications can occur after SCI, such as respiratory and cardiovascular complications, urinary and bowel complications, spasticity, bone disease and last but not least, loss of the skeletal muscles [11–13].

The loss of motor and/or sensory function leads to a reduction in physical activity which favors deconditioning [7]. Muscle unloading, lack of voluntary contraction, spasticity and injuries to small vessels cause changes in muscle fibers and histochemical changes in the muscle cells.

Patients with complete SCI can lose 20–55% of their muscle mass, while those with incomplete damage lose between 20 and 30% of their muscle mass [14].

The working definition of sarcopenia in patients with SCI is, to our knowledge, still not clear, and the current application of the definitions of sarcopenia in subjects with SCI requires further research [7].

The aim of this study was to evaluate the impact of SCI on muscle and bone mass, depending on a series of clinical characteristics of SCI patients.

2. Materials and Methods

2.1. Study Design

A cohort study was conducted from 2019 to 2022. Patients from the "Băile Felix Medical Rehabilitation Clinical Hospital" diagnosed with SCI were enrolled in this study. The study was approved by the local Ethics Committee (4016/30.04.2018) and was conducted in accordance with the principles of the Declaration of Helsinki. All participants provided their written consent before participating in this study.

2.2. Inclusion/Exclusion Criteria

Inclusion criteria were: patients with an established diagnosis of SCI from traumatic causes, aged 18 to 75 years, and at least 6 months since the traumatic event. Exclusion criteria for this study were: age under 18 years, SCI due to non-traumatic causes such as degenerative cervical myelopathy, tumors, birth defects, disruption of the blood supply to the spinal cord, multiple sclerosis, amyotrophic lateral sclerosis, infections and patients who could not undergo whole body dual X-ray absorptiometry (DXA) scanning.

2.3. Study Tools

This study used the revised ASIA scale (proposed by the American Spinal Injury Association) to assess the severity of SCI. This scale evaluates the motor score (by assessing key muscles) and the sensory score, by testing tactile and pain sensitivity such as a light touch and a pin prick (on dermatomes) (Figure 1) [15].

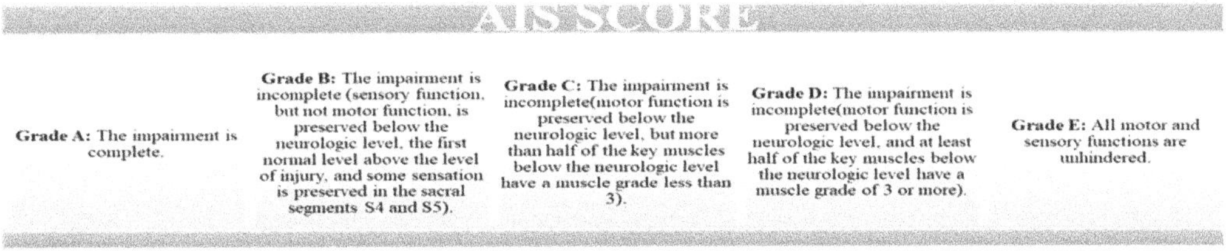

AIS SCORE

Grade A: The impairment is complete.

Grade B: The impairment is incomplete (sensory function, but not motor function, is preserved below the neurologic level, the first normal level above the level of injury, and some sensation is preserved in the sacral segments S4 and S5).

Grade C: The impairment is incomplete (motor function is preserved below the neurologic level, but more than half of the key muscles below the neurologic level have a muscle grade less than 3).

Grade D: The impairment is incomplete (motor function is preserved below the neurologic level, and at least half of the key muscles below the neurologic level have a muscle grade of 3 or more).

Grade E: All motor and sensory functions are unhindered.

Figure 1. American Spinal Injury Association Impairment scale (AIS).

The level of spasticity was assessed using the MAS [16]. The original Ashworth Scale is a numerical scale from 0 to 4. Lower scores indicate normal muscle tone, and higher scores represent spasticity [17]. The MAS adds 1+ to the scale to increase sensitivity (Figure 2) [18].

- 0: No increase in muscle tone
- 1: Slight increase in muscle tone, with a catch and release or minimal resistance at the end of the range of motion when an affected part(s) is moved in flexion or extension
- 1+: Slight increase in muscle tone, manifested as a catch, followed by minimal resistance through the remainder (less than half) of the range of motion
- 2: A marked increase in muscle tone throughout most of the range of motion, but affected part(s) are still easily moved
- 3: Considerable increase in muscle tone, passive movement difficult
- 4: Affected part(s) rigid in flexion or extension

Figure 2. The modified Ashworth Scale (MAS).

Bone mineral density was determined using DXA scans for all patients (Medix 90, Medilink Sarl, France). Skeletal muscle mass index (SMI) (appendicular skeletal muscle (ASM) to height^2: SMI = ASM/h^2; kg/m^2) [19] or ALM was determined via full-body DXA using whole body assessment. We established the diagnosis of sarcopenia according to the cut-off value recommended by EWGSOP2 for ALM. This cut-off value was 0.54. DXA indicates the total amount of lean tissue but does not measure muscle mass. ALM, derived from DXA scans, is the sum of lean tissue in the arms and legs. ALM alone or scaled to squared height (ALM/height^2) or body mass index (ALM/body mass index), was the most common parameter used as a proxy for muscle mass in our sarcopenia study [19]. Immobilization osteoporosis diagnosis was established using the Z-score for the lumbar spine and right and left hip via DXA, and according to the EWGSOP, the Z-score cut-off value is -1.5 [20].

A total of 206 SCI patients were recruited, as can be seen in the CONSORT flow chart shown in Figure 3, but only 136 met the inclusion criteria. After determining the ALM value, subjects were divided into two groups, according to the ALM values:

- Group S-SCI, which included 66 patients with SCI and ALM above the cut-off values (sarcopenia group).
- Group NS-SCI, which included 70 patients with SCI and ALM below the cut-off values (without sarcopenia).

The period of time since the SCI and the evaluation moment was calculated in months.

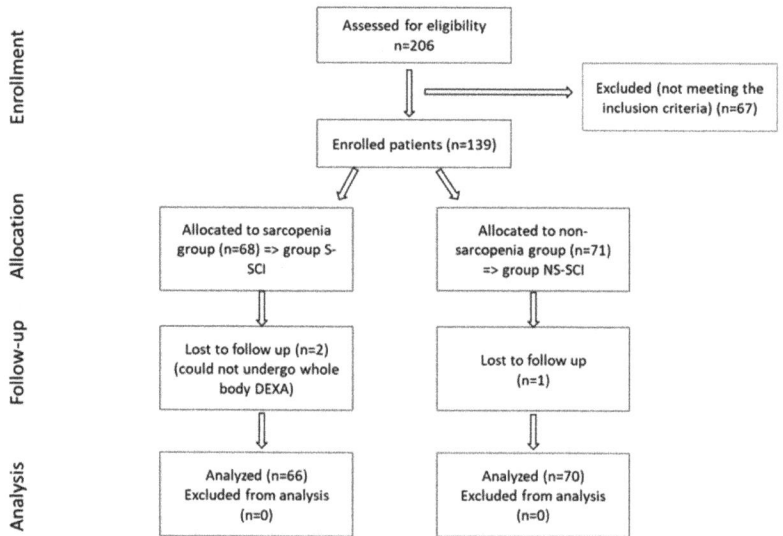

Figure 3. CONSORT flow diagram of the present study.

2.4. Sample Size

To calculate the sample size, we used the total number of patients admitted with a diagnosis of SCI (according to the inclusion criteria) during the period established in this study. The calculation formula that was used in this study to calculate the minimum sample was $n = t^2 pq/(x^2 + t^2 pq/N)$, where p is the probability of occurrence of the phenomenon, q is the counter-probability, $q = 1 - p$, t is the probability factor, x is the error limit, N is the community volume. The value of n is maximum if the product of pq is maximum ($p = q = 0.5$). The 95% probability corresponds to a value of $t = 1.96$. A limiting error of 0.1 was set. If N is large, above 10,000 (in our case N = 269), the ratio $t^2 pq/N$ is neglected. Applying the above formula yielded N = 96; the formula applies to studies where the target characteristic is an alternative.

2.5. Statistical Analysis

All statistical analysis was generated using the JASP software, version 0.18.0. The calculation of the p-values was performed using Student's t-test and the Mann–Whitney U test for numerical variables. The Poisson regression was used for count data and the chi-square test for nominal and ordinal variables. For accurate results, we conducted multiple comparisons; to control the false-positive rate, we conducted the Bonferroni correction when assessing the statistical significance of the results: we compared the obtained p-values with $\alpha^* = 0.05/k$, where k is the number of tests conducted.

2.6. Study Hypotheses

Given the latest research on sarcopenia and the fact that sarcopenia and SCI often coexist, but little is known about the associations between these two pathologies, our study aimed to assess the impact of SCI on muscle and bone mass and the correlations between a series of clinical characteristics of SCI patients, such as the neurological level of injury (NLI), the type of lesion (complete versus incomplete), AIS grade, level of spasticity measured with the MAS, period of time since the traumatic event and presence of complications and the prevalence of sarcopenia in these patients.

We hypothesized that more men than women would have SCI, according to the epidemiological studies in the literature [10], and that more women than men would be susceptible to having sarcopenia [21]. We also presumed that patients with a complete lesion would be more susceptible of developing sarcopenia versus patients with an incomplete lesion. We assumed that the presence of immobilization osteoporosis is directly related to the risk of developing secondary sarcopenia in patients with SCI, based on our clinical observations and experience, but also based on the literature review [20–22]. Regarding the period of time elapsed since SCI, we hypothesized that the mean time since injury was longer for the sarcopenia patients compared to those without sarcopenia [23].

3. Results

Sample Characteristics

The anthropometric data, number of months since SCI, NLI, AIS grade, MAS score, comorbidities, Z-score for immobilization osteoporosis, mean ALM values for both study groups (Group S-SCI, Group NS-SCI) are presented in Table 1. Mean ALM values in the two study groups were: 0.49 in the S-SCI group, and 0.65 in the NS-SCI group. A total of 48.52% of SCI patients were diagnosed with sarcopenia, while 51.47% were not.

Table 1. Baseline characteristics of the groups.

Parameter	Group S-SCI	Group NS-SCI	*p*-Value	SS/NS
ALM-value, M, SD	0.49 ± 0.042	0.65 ± 0.099	-	-
Patients N (%)	66 (48.529)	70 (51.471)	-	-
Age, M, SD (years)	35.83 ± 11.75	41.50 ± 14.36	0.013 *	SS
Female, N (%)	18 (75.00)	6 (25.00)	0.014 **	SS
Male, N (%)	48 (42.86)	64 (57.14)	0.131 **	NS
Number of months since SCI (M, SD)	55.17 ± 57.77	47.40 ± 33.17	0.620 ***	NS
Neurological level of injury				
Level Cervical, N (%)	27 (52.94)	24 (47.06)	0.674 **	NS
Level Thoracal, N (%)	33 (47.14)	37 (52.85)	0.633 **	NS
Level Lumbar, N (%)	6 (40)	9 (60)	0.439 **	NS
AIS Scale				
Grade A, N (%)	29 (55.77)	23 (44.23)	0.405 **	NS
Grade B, N (%)	23 (58.97)	16 (41.02)	0.262 **	NS
Grade C, N (%)	8 (28.57)	20 (71.43)	0.023 **	NS
Grade D, N (%)	6 (35.29)	11 (64.70)	0.225 **	NS
Modified Ashworth Scale				
Score 0, N (%)	23 (69.69)	10 (30.30)	0.024 **	NS
Score 1, N (%)	9 (42.85)	12 (57.14)	0.513 **	NS
Score 2, N (%)	17 (41.46)	24 (58.53)	0.274 **	NS
Score 3, N (%)	11 (40.74)	16 (59.25)	0.336 **	NS
Score 4, N (%)	6 (42.85)	8 (57.14)	0.583 **	NS
Comorbidities (M, SD)	2.667 ± 1.522	2.086 ± 1.164	0.028 **	SS
Immobilization Osteoporosis, Z-score				
Lumbar M, SD	−1.318 ± 1.182	−1.280 ± 0.976	-	
Right hip M, SD	−1.948 ± 0.945	−1.444 ± 1.454	-	
Left hip M, SD	−1.802 ± 1.330	−1.467 ± 1.233	-	

M: mean value; SD: standard deviation value; N: number of the patients; Group NS-SCI: patients with SCI, without sarcopenia; Group S-SCI: patients with SCI, and sarcopenia; AIS scale—American Spinal Injury Association Impairment Scale *p* values statistical significance (*, Student's *t*-test; **, chi-square test; *** Mann–Whitney U test); NS—without statistical significance; SS—statistically significant.

A total of 75% of women were diagnosed with sarcopenia. On the other hand, 42.9% of men were diagnosed with sarcopenia. A chi-square test in each gender group was performed to test these differences. Multiple comparisons were performed; therefore, the Bonferroni correction was used to control the false-positive rates: we compared the obtained p-values with $\alpha^* = 0.05/k$, where k is the number of tests conducted (k = 2 in this case). As the chi-square tests show, women are more likely to be diagnosed with sarcopenia ($p < 0.025$), whereas among men, these proportions do not seem to differ significantly. The computed log odds ratio showed that women were approximately 1.4 times (40%) more likely to be diagnosed with sarcopenia than men.

The mean age of the sarcopenic patients was lower than the mean age of the patients without sarcopenia (35.8 years and 41.5 years, respectively).

Descriptive statistics in Table 1 revealed that among the patients with a cervical (C)-level injury slightly more were diagnosed with sarcopenia (52.9%). Among the cases with a lumbar (L)-level injury, 40% of the patients were diagnosed with sarcopenia. Finally, among the patients with a thoracic (T)-level injury, slightly fewer were diagnosed with sarcopenia (47.1%). To test whether the frequency distributions of the SCI groups were similar across the lesion levels groups, we conducted a chi-square test within each lesion level group. Bonferroni correction was also used as we conducted multiple comparisons, to control the false-positive rate: we compared the obtained p-values with $\alpha^* = 0.05/k$, where k is the number of tests conducted (k = 3 in this case). The results are presented in Table 1. The data showed that the prevalence of sarcopenia did not vary across the three lesion level groups, as $p > 0.017$.

Descriptive statistics in Table 1 also showed that among the patients with AIS Grade A, slightly more were diagnosed with sarcopenia (55.8%). Of the patients with AIS Grade B, 59% were diagnosed with sarcopenia. Among the patients with AIS Grade C, 28.6% were diagnosed with sarcopenia, while 35.3% of the patients with AIS Grade D were diagnosed with sarcopenia. We conducted a chi-square test within each AIS grade group to test whether the frequency distributions of the SCI groups are similar across the AIS grade groups. As we conducted multiple comparisons, and to control the false-positive rate, we conducted the Bonferroni correction: we compared the obtained p-values with $\alpha^* = 0.05/k$, where k is the number of tests conducted (k = 4 in this case). The results are presented in Table 1. We did not find any statistically significant differences in the proportions of S-SCI and NS-SCI patients across the AIS grade groups ($p > 0.0125$).

Regarding the level of spasticity, our data showed that 69.7% of the patients with MAS level 0 were diagnosed with sarcopenia. Among patients with MAS level 1, 42.9% were diagnosed with sarcopenia, while 57.1% were not. Among patients with MAS level 2, 41.5% were diagnosed with sarcopenia and among those with MAS level 3, 40.7% had sarcopenia. Finally, among the patients with a level 4 on the MAS, 42.9% were diagnosed with sarcopenia. To test whether the frequency distributions of the SCI groups were similar across the Ashworth level groups, we conducted a chi-square test within each Ashworth level group.

We conducted the Bonferroni correction: we compared the obtained p-values with $\alpha^* = 0.05/k$, where k is the number of tests conducted (k = 5 in this case), as we conducted multiple comparisons and also to control the false-positive rate. We did not find any statistically significant differences in the proportions of S-SCI and NS-SCI patients across the Ashworth level groups ($p > 0.01$).

The minimum age in the NS-SCI group was 20 years, while in the S-SCI group it was 18 years; the maximum age in the NS-SCI group was 73 years, while in the S-SCI group it was 67 years. Statistical significance of these differences was tested conducting the t-test for independent samples. The results showed that patients with sarcopenia were significantly younger than those without sarcopenia, $p < 0.05$, and the effect size was medium (d = 0.431) (Figure 4a).

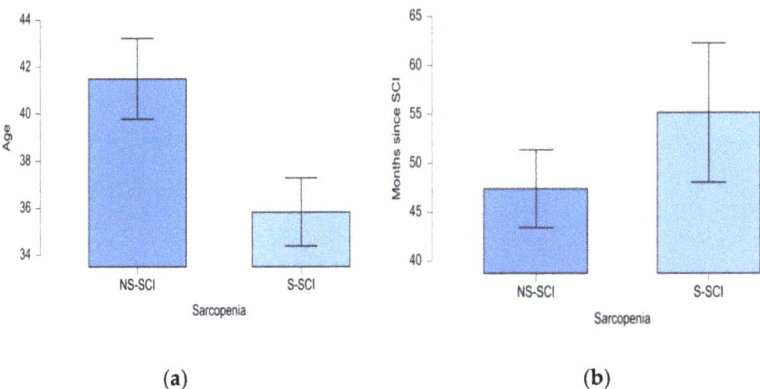

Figure 4. (**a**) Mean age (years) of patients in the two groups: NS-SCI and S-SCI. (**b**) Mean time (months) since SCI in the two groups: NS-SCI and S-SCI.

The mean time since the SCI was 55 months (ranging from 2 months to 312 months) in the sarcopenia group and about 47 months (ranging from 12 months to 132 months) in the non-sarcopenia group. The statistical significance of this difference was tested using the non-parametric Mann–Whitney U test, because the normality and equality of variances assumptions were not met by our data. According to the Mann–Whitney U test, our data do not support the hypothesis that the mean time since the SCI is longer for the sarcopenia patients compared to those without sarcopenia (W = 2379, $p > 0.05$, Figure 4b).

Data presented in Table 2 reveal that the mean Z-scores for the lumbar area (lumbar Z-score), the right hip (right hip Z-score) and the left hip (left hip Z-score) tend to be lower in the S-SCI group compared to the NS-SCI group.

Table 2. Descriptive statistics for Z-scores across the S-SCI and NS-SCI groups.

Region Z-Score	Group	M ± SD	MIN	MAX
Lumbar Z-score	Group NS-SCI	−1.280 ± 0.976	−3.500	1.400
	Group S-SCI	−1.318 ± 1.182	−4.600	1.900
Right hip Z-score	Group NS-SCI	−1.444 ± 1.454	−3.700	4.400
	Group S-SCI	−1.948 ± 0.945	−3.900	−0.100
Left hip Z-score	Group NS-SCI	−1.467 ± 1.233	−3.700	2.800
	Group S-SCI	−1.802 ± 1.330	−3.900	5.200

M: mean value; SD: standard deviation value; Group NS-SCI: patients with SCI, without sarcopenia; Group S-SCI: patients with SCI, and sarcopenia; MIN: minimum value of Z-score; MAX: maximum value of Z-score.

Moreover, 41% of the patients without osteoporosis were diagnosed with sarcopenia. Among the patients with osteoporosis, 51.6% were diagnosed with sarcopenia. We conducted a chi-square test within each group, to test whether the frequency distributions of the SCI groups were similar across patients with or without osteoporosis. The Bonferroni correction was used as we performed multiple comparisons, and also to control the false-positive rate: we compared the obtained p-values with $\alpha^* = 0.05/k$, where k is the number of tests conducted (k = 2 in this case). The results are presented in Table 3.

We did not find significant differences in the frequency distributions of immobilization osteoporosis across the groups of patients with and without sarcopenia ($p > 0.025$).

The mean number of comorbidities was 2 in the non-sarcopenia group (ranging between 0 and 6) and 2.7 in the sarcopenia group (ranging between 0 and 8) (Figure 5). The most common comorbidity in each group was hypertension. Among the patients without hypertension, the number of sarcopenic and non-sarcopenic patients was almost the same

(50.4% versus 49.6%). A total of 30.8% of the patients with hypertension were diagnosed with sarcopenia. To test whether the frequency distributions of the SCI groups were similar across patients with or without hypertension, we conducted a chi-square test within each group. We conducted the Bonferroni correction: we compared the obtained p-values with $\alpha^* = 0.05/k$, (k = number of conducted tests, two in this case). We did not find a statistically significant association between sarcopenia and the presence of hypertension ($p > 0.025$).

Table 3. Frequency of immobilization osteoporosis in the S-SCI and NS-SCI groups.

Immobilization Osteoporosis	Group NS-SCI	Group S-SCI	p-Value **
Yes, N (%)	47 (48.45)	50 (51.55)	0.761 ** NS
No, N (%)	23 (58.97)	16 (41.03)	0.262 ** NS

N: number of the patients; Group NS-SCI: patients with SCI, without sarcopenia; Group S-SCI: patients with SCI, and sarcopenia ; p-value statistical significance (**, chi-square); NS—without statistical significance.

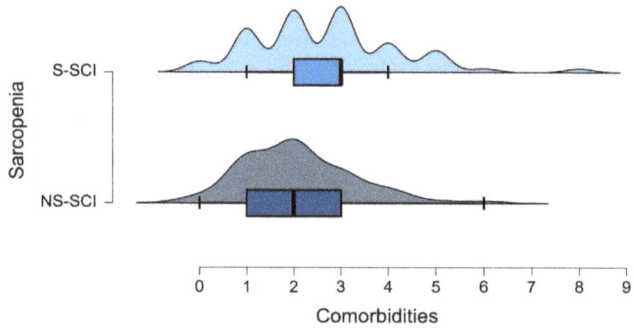

Figure 5. Density plot of the number of comorbidities across the groups of patients with and without sarcopenia.

Poisson regression (also known as a log-linear model) was used to test the association between sarcopenia and the number of comorbidities. The deviance goodness-of-fit test indicates that the model fits the data (D (134) = 107.858, $p = 0.953$). The tables below (Tables 4 and 5) show the model summary and the model coefficients.

Table 4. Model summary for the number of comorbidities.

Model	Deviance	AIC	BIC	df	χ^2	p-Value **
H_0	112.701	465.175	468.088	135		
H_1	107.858	462.332	468.157	134	4.843	0.028

H_0: the null hypothesis; H_1: the alternative hypothesis; χ^2: chi-square test; p-values statistical significance (**, chi-square); AIC: Akaike information criterion (AIC); BIC (Bayesian information criterion).

Table 5. Model coefficient for the number of comorbidities.

	Coefficients					95% Confidence Interval for B	
	B	Std. Error	Exp(B)	Z-Score	p-Value **	Lower Bound	Upper Bound
Intercept	0.735	0.083	2.086	8.882	<0.001	0.568	0.893
Sarcopenia (Yes)	0.246	0.112	1.279	2.195	0.028	0.027	0.466

p-values statistical significance (**, chi-square); Std. Error: standard error; B: regression coefficient.

The model summary table shows that there was a significant effect of sarcopenia on the number of comorbidities that patients were diagnosed with [χ^2 (1) = 4.843, $p < 0.05$].

Thus, the coefficients table reveals that the number of comorbidities is 1.279 times higher in patients with sarcopenia than in those without the disease. In other words, there is a 27.9% increase in the number of comorbidities among patients with sarcopenia compared to those without this condition.

4. Discussion

The goal of this study was to assess the impact of SCI on muscle and bone mass, and the correlations between different clinical characteristics of SCI patients and the presence of sarcopenia in these cases.

SCI is a severe and disabling disease, leading to loss of innervation of skeletal muscles, decreased motor function and significantly reducing the load on skeletal muscles, all these leading to atrophy. Skeletal muscle atrophy is accelerated by fractures, hormone level fluctuation, inflammation and oxidative stress damage. Muscle atrophy leads to impaired skeletal muscle function around and below the injury site [24]. In SCI, the inability or decreased ability to perform physical exercise are often associated with sarcopenia [25–27]. Leone et al. stated that neurogenic factors, musculoskeletal disuse and cellular/molecular events contribute to more rapid and debilitating levels of muscle and bone loss in individuals with SCI. The absolute causes of bone loss are not yet known; however, sarcopenia could be one of the causes [28]. Dionyssiotis et al. also considered that the pathophysiology of sarcopenia in SCI is complex. Although muscle mass does not predict muscle strength or physical performance, it is significantly correlated with these parameters and contributes to disability and frailty in old people. There are no guidelines or even recommendations regarding sarcopenia in SCI. Proper measurements of performance in SCI are not yet available [7]. Persistent neuromuscular paralysis leads to muscle atrophy related to both neurologic injury and functional immobility. Neuromuscular paralysis is one of the secondary causes of muscle atrophy and sarcopenia. Lean muscle mass has been correlated with strength and functional performance in healthy children, being considered a strong predictor of health and performance in all individuals. Muscle mass is frequently used as a surrogate for muscle strength, especially in young children [29,30].

The cross-sectional area of the skeletal muscle (which represents approximately 40% of the body weight) decreases fast in the following 1–17 months after a trauma. Muscular atrophy in patients with SCI is partially explained by the rapid changes in the quality of muscle proteins, activating proteolytic enzymes and proteases from mitochondria, the increase in the production of reactive oxygen species and the decrease in oxidative capacity [31,32]. Based on a previous study, Ishimoto et al. used only ASM as the criterion for identifying patients with sarcopenia. Their study revealed two clinical observations. Sarcopenia, obesity and sarcopenic obesity were prevalent among individuals with SCI and female gender, tetraplegia, motor-complete injury and inability to walk were identified as risk factors for muscle atrophy comparable to sarcopenia in persons with SCI [33]. Gater DR Jr et al. also stated that physiological changes occurring in the adipose tissue in SCI cases should be characterized as neurogenic obesity due to an obligatory sarcopenia, neurogenic osteoporosis, neurogenic anabolic deficiency, sympathetic dysfunction and blunted satiety associated with SCI [34]. According to these data, we expected to diagnose a high percentage of patients with sarcopenia, but, to our surprise, of all SCI cases, over 51% did not have sarcopenia. However, for the other 48.52% that were diagnosed with sarcopenia, the possible clinical implications that this condition raises are worth considering. The risk of frequent falling and the reduced ability or inability of a person with SCI to redress from a fall and lift from the floor, as well as other complications (e.g., cardiovascular disease occurrence, pulmonary disease) are crucial in patients with SCI. Sarcopenia synergistically worsens the adverse effects of the motor deficit in patients with SCI, leading to unfavorable health conditions, such as an increased risk of frailty and falls [35,36]. It can interfere with the capacity of a SCI patient to remain to some degree functional and can even influence the return of a SCI patient to a healthy, fulfilling independent lifestyle, which is the goal of every rehabilitation program. Therefore, the identification of modifiable risk factors associated with sarcopenia is of the utmost importance in order to prevent these adverse changes.

Comparing our results with the prevalence of sarcopenia in the general population, according to a meta-analysis of general population studies, published in 2017 by G Shafiee et al. the rate was 10% (95% CI: 8–12%) in men and 10% (95% CI: 8–13%) in women, respectively [37]; therefore, the prevalence of sarcopenia was high.

Comparing the two groups of patients with SCI (Group S-SCI and Group NS-SCI), there were statistically significant differences between the two study groups regarding gender, age and presence of comorbidities. Our results revealed that 75% of women suffering from SCI were diagnosed with sarcopenia. This finding was in line with the results of a study published by Hwang and Park (2022, N = 2697) that examined the prevalence of sarcopenia according to gender in young-old adults, reporting a higher prevalence of sarcopenia in females [38]. Ishimoto et al. [33], in a retrospective analysis (2023, N = 97), reported that female gender was a risk factor for sarcopenia. On the contrary, Zhang et al. in their published meta-analysis (2021) revealed no statistically significant difference in the pooled prevalence of sarcopenia in patients with heart failure between men and women [39]. Analyzing the effect of postoperative muscle loss and surgery-induced sarcopenia on the long-term outcomes of patients with gastric cancer, other authors found significant differences between genders, with more men having a rapid decrease in muscle mass, which impacted the overall survival [40].

However, our study revealed that women with SCI are more susceptible to developing sarcopenia. This could be due to the considerable sex-based differences in human skeletal muscle gene expression that regulates muscle mass, fiber composition and contractile function [41]. Considering the mentioned genetic traits, it is more likely that women would develop sarcopenia compared to men, androgens having a powerful anabolic effect that promotes muscle regeneration, while estrogen has muscle-protective effect through anti-inflammatory pathways that inhibit proteolysis [42]. On the other hand, the number of male patients was significantly higher compared to the number of female patients participating in this study, in agreement with previous studies [33]. Our results showed a significant association between gender and the likelihood of having sarcopenia. Despite the small sample size of female patients with SCI, they were more likely to develop sarcopenia. The computed log odds ratio showed that women with SCI are approximately 1.4 times (40%) more likely to be diagnosed with sarcopenia, which reinforces and strengthens the hypothesis issued at the beginning and is also in agreement with earlier observations [18]. A total of 42.9% of men were diagnosed with sarcopenia. Studies investigating muscle mass or sarcopenia and its correlation with the functional status of patients with SCI are few and at infrequent intervals. Previously, the somewhat few studies have shown that sarcopenia, obesity and sarcopenic obesity were prevalent among individuals with SCI; female gender, level of injury (tetraplegia) and a complete injury leading to inability to walk (AIS A, B) were identified as risk factors for sarcopenia in individuals with SCI [19,33].

The prevalence of sarcopenia may vary depending on the diagnostic criteria, definitions, study group, anthropometric values and measured parameters [8]. We need to be aware that we cannot perform a walking test with patients with disabilities, tetraplegia or paraplegia. We also lack the proper measurement of strength, assessed with hand dynamometers, because patients with tetraplegia cannot perform the handgrip test and for those with paraplegia it would be very difficult or even impossible, depending on the NLI. Therefore, it would be biased, not to mention the fact that patients with paraplegia who use a wheelchair may develop stronger upper limbs through the indirect training effect of their daily wheelchair activities.

Our results also revealed that patients with sarcopenia were significantly younger than those without sarcopenia. Primary sarcopenia is an age-related process associated with a loss of muscle mass [43,44]. This does not fit into the general frame of our study design, because patients with SCI participating in this study were, in general, young adults, with a mean age of 41 years in the NS-SCI group and 35 years in the S-SCI group; this reinforces the above mentioned hypothesis, and aligns with epidemiological studies regarding the average age at which SCIs occur, which was 37.6 years in a study from 2000 [45]. Another study published in 2023 by Tanaka et al. (N = 1039) found a statistically significantly higher mean age in the sarcopenic group compared with the non-sarcopenic one [46]. However, secondary sarcopenia occurs if other factors, besides aging, are evident in the study sample, as per our research [47].

Paradoxically, we did not find any significant correlations between the presence of immobilization osteoporosis and sarcopenia, which we would have expected, as the prevalence of secondary osteoporosis in SCI is high [48]. The presence of sarcopenia was found to be associated with reduced bone mineral density and osteoporosis [49]. Yoshimura et al., in a study published in 2017, examined the relationship between osteoporosis and sarcopenia (diagnosed according to AWGS criteria) based on the results of a survey of bone mineral density in 1099 participants and determined an osteoporosis prevalence of 24.9%. In addition, although 18.9% of these patients had sarcopenia, the prevalence of sarcopenia in the study group was 8.2% [50]. The prevalence of secondary conditions among patients with SCI depends on a variety of aspects; the severity and completeness of the injury are some of the most important ones. Gianna Rodriguez et al., in a study published in 2021 (N = 9081), investigated the risk of developing musculoskeletal comorbidities by comparing 9081 privately insured patients with 1,474,232 adults without SCI, and the results showed that adults with SCIs have a significantly higher incidence and risk for musculoskeletal comorbidities, as compared to adults without SCIs [43]. However, in our study, despite the lack of statistical significance, an important percentage of patients (46.84%) from the S-SCI group were diagnosed with secondary osteoporosis.

Considering the MAS scores, we expected that patients with a high degree of spasticity (who scored 3 or 4) would be less susceptible of developing sarcopenia. According to a study published in 2022 by Li et al. (N = 28) about sarcopenia following stroke, the authors demonstrated that spasticity in stroke survivors actually had a protective role against muscle loss in the lower limbs [51,52].

Many of the long-term outcomes of SCI are related to muscle and bone loss due to immobilization. The impact of SCI can vary depending on the NLI, but also on the type of lesion (complete/incomplete). There are short-term impacts and long-term impacts, as Leone et al. highlighted in a review article published in September 2023. Long-term impacts include sarcopenia and osteoporosis [28].

The last statistically significant difference between our study groups was the presence of comorbidities. On average, patients without sarcopenia had approximately 2 comorbidities associated with SCI, while patients with sarcopenia had approximately 2.7 comorbidities associated with SCI. Sarcopenia can be considered itself a comorbidity and is often studied in numerous clinical trials, and it seems that the presence of sarcopenia is associated with other secondary conditions such as respiratory disease, diabetes, dementia and cardiovascular disease [53].

Secondary health conditions affecting the sensory, respiratory, cardio-vascular, genitourinary and tegumentary system impact a SCI patient's life, being debilitating and potentially life-threatening [54]. Tallqvist et al. assessed the comorbidities and secondary health conditions (SHCs) among the Finnish population with SCI (2022, N = 884) and found that the prevalence of comorbidities and SHCs was common among elderly persons with SCI, with age being the strongest predictor for multimorbidity [55].

In our research, the most common comorbidity in both groups was hypertension; however, we did not find a statistically significant association between sarcopenia and the presence of hypertension. SCI instead can cause a variety of physiological changes. The sudden reduction in physical activity in individuals with SCI is translated into elevated risk of cardiovascular diseases; therefore, they are among the leading causes of death in the SCI population [56].

Kepler et al., in a retrospective case–control study published in 2015 (N = 92), investigated the effects of pre-existing hypertension in a number of patients with acute SCI and they found that chronic hypertension was an independent risk factor for poor outcomes in patients with acute SCI. This finding was independent of age and other comorbidities [57].

4.1. Strengths and Limitations of the Study

This is the first study in Romania, to our knowledge, that has evaluated sarcopenia in SCI patients and its correlation with gender, age, time elapsed since the onset of the disease, injury level and muscle tone. An important aspect to consider is the large number of patients recruited and evaluated.

Our study had certain limitations: (1) sarcopenia was diagnosed using only the ALM score, because some patients were tetraplegic and we could not use the Jamar dynamometer to determine muscle strength, and we also could not perform a walking test for these patients; the sarcopenia questionnaire, such as SARC-F [54], also could not be used; (2) the question remains as to whether the cut-off points for unaffected and able-bodied populations can be applied to SCI patients; (3) SCI with its pathophysiology may influence the validity of the results.

4.2. Future Directions

Future research is needed to establish clear definitions of sarcopenia in SCI patients with disabilities. Following SCI, many patients develop motor, but probably most importantly, functional impairments that can affect their daily living and reduce the quality of life [54]. In addition, in the chronic phase, multiple complications can occur. One of them can be secondary sarcopenia; the rehabilitation goals during this phase are to prevent further damage from the injury and to slow down or reverse the process of muscle loss. The general recommendation for the management of sarcopenia is to follow a resistance-based exercise program and to follow a high-protein diet [47].

There are several pharmacologic approaches to prevent or reduce muscle atrophy after SCI. Testosterone can increase muscle mass and strength in older individuals and a meta-analysis has confirmed its safety [55]. Acteoside-treated muscles had a significantly greater mass when compared to the vehicle treatment, which suggests that acteoside promotes skeletal muscle recovery and regeneration, potentially independently of exercise-induced myokine secretion [56]. Estrogen can also play a role in remodeling the extracellular matrix and muscle fiber expansion after unloading or not being used [57]. Imagery-based rehabilitation might be a promising therapeutic approach in patients with SCI [58].

The number of patients suffering from SCI increases year after year, and so do the secondary complications that can occur alongside it. The search for therapeutic modalities to improve the quality of patients' lives with SCI continues.

5. Conclusions

The study results showed that patients with sarcopenia were significantly younger than those without sarcopenia. The following clinical features of SCI patients: gender, the type of injury, the presence of multiple comorbidities and age were directly associated with sarcopenia, while, surprisingly enough, spasticity level and the presence of immobilization osteoporosis were not proved to be associated with sarcopenia. There was a statistically significant association between the ALM value and the gender, considerably more women with SCI developing sarcopenia. The number of male patients was significantly higher compared to the number of female cases participating in this study, but fewer men with SCI had sarcopenia. Optimizing muscle mass should be an important objective in the management of SCI patients.

Author Contributions: Conceptualization, A.G. and M.L.C.; methodology, C.D.N.-C., D.-C.I. and D.S.; software, A.G. and D.-C.I.; validation, M.L.C., I.R.C. and D.V.; formal analysis, A.G.; investigation, S.D.; resources, M.L.C. and I.R.C.; data curation, S.D. and I.R.C.; writing—original draft preparation, A.G. and C.D.N.-C.; writing—review and editing, C.D.N.-C.; visualization, M.L.C. and D.V.; supervision, D.S.; project administration, A.G.; funding acquisition, M.L.C. All authors have read and agreed to the published version of the manuscript.

Funding: This research received no external funding.

Institutional Review Board Statement: The study was approved by the local Ethics Committee (4016/30 April 2018) and was conducted in accordance with the principles of the Declaration of Helsinki.

Informed Consent Statement: Informed consent was obtained from all subjects involved in the study.

Data Availability Statement: Data of the patients are available in the medical archive of the hospital.

Acknowledgments: The authors would like to thank the University of Oradea, Oradea, Romania, for supporting the APC.

Conflicts of Interest: The authors declare no conflicts of interest.

References

1. Moga, T.D.; Nistor-Cseppento, C.D.; Bungau, S.G.; Tit, D.M.; Sabau, A.M.; Behl, T.; Nechifor, A.C.; Bungau, A.F.; Negrut, N. The Effects of the Catabolic Crisis on Patients Prolonged Immobility after COVID-19 Infection. *Medicina* **2022**, *58*, 828. [CrossRef]
2. Coletta, G.; Phillips, S.M. An elusive consensus definition of sarcopenia impedes research and clinical treatment: A narrative review. *Ageing Res. Rev.* **2023**, *86*, 101883. [CrossRef] [PubMed]
3. Rosenberg, I.H. Sarcopenia: Origins and clinical relevance. *Clin. Geriatr. Med.* **2011**, *27*, 337–339. [CrossRef] [PubMed]
4. Yuan, S.; Larsson, S.C. Epidemiology of sarcopenia: Prevalence, risk factors, and consequences. *Metabolism* **2023**, *144*, 155533. [CrossRef] [PubMed]
5. Cevei, M.; Onofrei, R.R.; Gherle, A.; Gug, C.; Stoicanescu, D. Rehabilitation of Post-COVID-19 Musculoskeletal Sequelae in Geriatric Patients: A Case Series Study. *Int. J. Environ. Res. Public Health* **2022**, *19*, 15350. [CrossRef] [PubMed]
6. Cruz-Jentoft, A.J.; Baeyens, J.P.; Bauer, J.M.; Boirie, Y.; Cederholm, T.; Landi, F.; Martin, F.C.; Michel, J.P.; Rolland, Y.; Schneider, S.M.; et al. Sarcopenia: European consensus on definition and diagnosis: Report of the European Working Group on Sarcopenia in Older People. *Age Ageing* **2010**, *39*, 412–423. [CrossRef] [PubMed]
7. Dionyssiotis, Y.; Skarantavos, G.; Petropoulou, K.; Galanos, A.; Rapidi, C.A.; Lyritis, G.P. Application of current sarcopenia definitions in spinal cord injury. *J. Musculoskelet. Neuronal Interact.* **2019**, *19*, 21–29. [PubMed]
8. Cruz-Jentoft, A.J.; Bahat, G.; Bauer, J.; Boirie, Y.; Bruyère, O.; Cederholm, T.; Cooper, C.; Landi, F.; Rolland, Y.; Sayer, A.A.; et al. Sarcopenia: Revised European consensus on definition and diagnosis. *Age Ageing* **2019**, *48*, 16–31. [CrossRef]
9. Polito, A.; Barnaba, L.; Ciarapica, D.; Azzini, E. Osteosarcopenia: A Narrative Review on Clinical Studies. *Int. J. Mol. Sci.* **2022**, *23*, 5591. [CrossRef]
10. Barbiellini Amidei, C.; Salmaso, L.; Bellio, S.; Saia, M. Epidemiology of traumatic spinal cord injury: A large population-based study. *Spinal Cord.* **2022**, *60*, 812–819. [CrossRef]
11. Shackleton, C.; Evans, R.; Shamley, D.; West, S.; Albertus, Y. Effectiveness of over-ground robotic locomotor training in improving walking performance, cardiovascular demands, secondary complications and user-satisfaction in individuals with spinal cord injuries: A systematic review. *J. Rehabil. Med.* **2019**, *51*, 723–733. [CrossRef]
12. Gorgey, A.S.; Dudley, G.A. Skeletal muscle atrophy and increased intramuscular fat after incomplete spinal cord injury. *Spinal Cord.* **2007**, *45*, 304–309. [CrossRef]
13. Nistor-Cseppento, C.D.; Gherle, A.; Negrut, N.; Bungau, S.G.; Sabau, A.M.; Radu, A.F.; Bungau, A.F.; Tit, D.M.; Uivaraseanu, B.; Ghitea, T.C.; et al. The Outcomes of Robotic Rehabilitation Assisted Devices Following Spinal Cord Injury and the Prevention of Secondary Associated Complications. *Medicina* **2022**, *58*, 1447. [CrossRef]
14. Kim, T.N.; Choi, K.M. Sarcopenia: Definition, epidemiology, and pathophysiology. *J. Bone Metab.* **2013**, *20*, 1–10. [CrossRef]
15. Roberts, T.T.; Leonard, G.R.; Cepela, D.J. Classifications In Brief: American Spinal Injury Association (ASIA) Impairment Scale. *Clin. Orthop. Relat. Res.* **2017**, *475*, 1499–1504. [CrossRef]
16. Meseguer-Henarejos, A.B.; Sánchez-Meca, J.; López-Pina, J.A.; Carles-Hernández, R. Inter- and intra-rater reliability of the Modified Ashworth Scale: A systematic review and meta-analysis. *Eur. J. Phys. Rehabil. Med.* **2018**, *54*, 576–590. [CrossRef]
17. Ashworth, B. Preliminary Trial of Carisoprodol in Multiple Sclerosis. *Practitioner* **1964**, *192*, 540–542. [PubMed]
18. Ansari, N.N.; Naghdi, S.; Arab, T.K.; Jalaie, S. The interrater and intrarater reliability of the Modified Ashworth Scale in the assessment of muscle spasticity: Limb and muscle group effect. *NeuroRehabilitation* **2008**, *23*, 231–237. [CrossRef] [PubMed]
19. Harvey, N.C.; Orwoll, E.; Kwok, T.; Karlsson, M.K.; Rosengren, B.E.; Ribom, E.; Cauley, J.A.; Cawthon, P.M.; Ensrud, K.; Liu, E.; et al. Sarcopenia Definitions as Predictors of Fracture Risk Independent of FRAX. *J. Bone Miner. Res.* **2021**, *36*, 1235–1244. [CrossRef]
20. Bagur, A.; Vega, E.; Mautalen, C. Discrimination of total body bone mineral density measured by dexa in vertebral osteoporosis. *Calcif. Tissue Int.* **1995**, *56*, 263–267. [CrossRef]
21. Melton, L.J.; Khosla, S.; Crowson, C.S.; O'Connor, M.K.; O'Fallon, W.M.; Riggs, B.L. Epidemiology of sarcopenia. *J. Am. Geriatr. Soc.* **2000**, *48*, 625–630. [CrossRef]

22. Clynes, M.A.; Gregson, C.L.; Bruyère, O.; Cooper, C.; Dennison, E.M. Osteosarcopenia: Where osteoporosis and sarcopenia collide. *Rheumatology* **2021**, *60*, 529–537. [CrossRef] [PubMed]
23. Moore, C.D.; Craven, B.C.; Thabane, L.; Laing, A.C.; Frank-Wilson, A.W.; Kontulainen, S.A.; Papaioannou, A.; Adachi, J.D.; Giangregorio, L.M. Lower-extremity muscle atrophy and fat infiltration after chronic spinal cord injury. *J. Musculoskelet. Neuronal Interact.* **2015**, *15*, 32–41. [PubMed]
24. Xu, X.; Talifu, Z.; Zhang, C.J.; Gao, F.; Ke, H.; Pan, Y.Z.; Gong, H.; Du, H.Y.; Yu, Y.; Jing, Y.L.; et al. Mechanism of skeletal muscle atrophy after spinal cord injury: A narrative review. *Front. Nutr.* **2023**, *10*, 1099743. [CrossRef] [PubMed]
25. Carda, S.; Cisari, C.; Invernizzi, M. Sarcopenia or muscle modifications in neurologic diseases: A lexical or patophysiological difference? *Eur. J. Phys. Rehabil. Med.* **2013**, *49*, 119–130.
26. Moga, T.D.; Moga, I.; Sabau, M.; Nistor-Cseppento, C.D.; Iovanovici, D.C.; Cavalu, S.; Dogaru, B.G. Sarcopenia, a major clinical problem in old age, potential causes, clinical consequences and therapeutic possibilities. *Balneo PRM Res. J.* **2022**, *13*, 492. [CrossRef]
27. Sirbu, E.; Onofrei, R.R.; Szasz, S.; Susan, M. Predictors of disability in patients with chronic low back pain. *Arch. Med. Sci.* **2023**, *19*, 94–100. [CrossRef] [PubMed]
28. Leone, G.E.; Shields, D.C.; Haque, A.; Banik, N.L. Rehabilitation: Neurogenic Bone Loss after Spinal Cord Injury. *Biomedicines* **2023**, *11*, 2581. [CrossRef] [PubMed]
29. Sadowsky, C.L. Targeting Sarcopenia as an Objective Clinical Outcome in the Care of Children with Spinal Cord-Related Paralysis: A Clinician's View. *Children* **2023**, *10*, 837. [CrossRef]
30. Cederholm, T.; Barazzoni, R.; Austin, P.; Ballmer, P.; Biolo, G.; Bischoff, S.C.; Compher, C.; Correia, I.; Higashiguchi, T.; Holst, M.; et al. ESPEN guidelines on definitions and terminology of clinical nutrition. *Clin. Nutr.* **2017**, *36*, 49–64. [CrossRef]
31. Alizadeh, A.; Dyck, S.M.; Karimi-Abdolrezaee, S. Traumatic Spinal Cord Injury: An Overview of Pathophysiology, Models and Acute Injury Mechanisms. *Front. Neurol.* **2019**, *10*, 282. [CrossRef]
32. Drasites, K.P.; Shams, R.; Zaman, V.; Matzelle, D.; Shields, D.C.; Garner, D.P.; Sole, C.J.; Haque, A.; Banik, N.L. Pathophysiology, Biomarkers, and Therapeutic Modalities Associated with Skeletal Muscle Loss Following Spinal Cord Injury. *Brain Sci.* **2020**, *10*, 933. [CrossRef]
33. Ishimoto, R.; Mutsuzaki, H.; Shimizu, Y.; Kishimoto, H.; Takeuchi, R.; Hada, Y. Prevalence of Sarcopenic Obesity and Factors Influencing Body Composition in Persons with Spinal Cord Injury in Japan. *Nutrients* **2023**, *15*, 437. [CrossRef]
34. Gater, D.R.; Farkas, G.J.; Tiozzo, E. Pathophysiology of Neurogenic Obesity After Spinal Cord Injury. *Top. Spinal Cord. Inj. Rehabil.* **2021**, *27*, 1–10. [CrossRef]
35. Yeung, S.S.Y.; Reijnierse, E.M.; Pham, V.K.; Trappenburg, M.C.; Lim, W.K.; Meskers, C.G.M.; Maier, A.B. Sarcopenia and its association with falls and fractures in older adults: A systematic review and meta-analysis. *J. Cachexia Sarcopenia Muscle* **2019**, *10*, 485–500. [CrossRef]
36. Inglis, T.; Banaszek, D.; Rivers, C.S.; Kurban, D.; Evaniew, N.; Fallah, N.; Waheed, Z.; Christie, S.; Fox, R.; Thiong, J.M.; et al. In-Hospital Mortality for the Elderly with Acute Traumatic Spinal Cord Injury. *J. Neurotrauma* **2020**, *37*, 2332–2342. [CrossRef]
37. Shafiee, G.; Keshtkar, A.; Soltani, A.; Ahadi, Z.; Larijani, B.; Heshmat, R. Prevalence of sarcopenia in the world: A systematic review and meta- analysis of general population studies. *J. Diabetes Metab. Disord.* **2017**, *16*, 21. [CrossRef] [PubMed]
38. Hwang, J.; Park, S. Gender-Specific Risk Factors and Prevalence for Sarcopenia among Community-Dwelling Young-Old Adults. *Int. J. Environ. Res. Public Health* **2022**, *19*, 7232. [CrossRef] [PubMed]
39. Zhang, Y.; Zhang, J.; Ni, W.; Yuan, X.; Zhang, H.; Li, P.; Xu, J.; Zhao, Z. Sarcopenia in heart failure: A systematic review and meta-analysis. *ESC Heart Fail.* **2021**, *8*, 1007–1017. [CrossRef] [PubMed]
40. Lee, J.K.; Park, Y.S.; Lee, K.; Youn, S.I.; Won, Y.; Min, S.H.; Ahn, S.H.; Park, D.J.; Kim, H.H. Prognostic significance of surgery-induced sarcopenia in the survival of gastric cancer patients: A sex-specific analysis. *J. Cachexia Sarcopenia Muscle* **2021**, *12*, 1897–1907. [CrossRef]
41. Haizlip, K.M.; Harrison, B.C.; Leinwand, L.A. Sex-based differences in skeletal muscle kinetics and fiber-type composition. *Physiology* **2015**, *30*, 30–39. [CrossRef] [PubMed]
42. Anderson, L.J.; Liu, H.; Garcia, J.M. Sex Differences in Muscle Wasting. *Adv. Exp. Med. Biol.* **2017**, *1043*, 153–197. [CrossRef]
43. Marzetti, E.; Calvani, R.; Tosato, M.; Cesari, M.; Di Bari, M.; Cherubini, A.; Collamati, A.; D'Angelo, E.; Pahor, M.; Bernabei, R.; et al. Sarcopenia: An overview. *Aging Clin. Exp. Res.* **2017**, *29*, 11–17. [CrossRef]
44. Nishikawa, H.; Fukunishi, S.; Asai, A.; Yokohama, K.; Nishiguchi, S.; Higuchi, K. Pathophysiology and mechanisms of primary sarcopenia (Review). *Int. J. Mol. Med.* **2021**, *48*. [CrossRef]
45. Wyndaele, M.; Wyndaele, J.J. Incidence, prevalence and epidemiology of spinal cord injury: What learns a worldwide literature survey? *Spinal Cord* **2006**, *44*, 523–529. [CrossRef]
46. Tanaka, Y.; Miyagi, M.; Inoue, G.; Hori, Y.; Inage, K.; Murata, K.; Fujimaki, H.; Kuroda, A.; Yokozeki, Y.; Inoue, S.; et al. Muscle strength rather than appendicular skeletal muscle mass might affect spinal sagittal alignment, low back pain, and health-related quality of life. *Sci. Rep.* **2023**, *13*, 9894. [CrossRef] [PubMed]
47. Supriya, R.; Singh, K.P.; Gao, Y.; Gu, Y.; Baker, J.S. Effect of Exercise on Secondary Sarcopenia: A Comprehensive Literature Review. *Biology* **2021**, *11*, 51. [CrossRef]
48. Varacallo, M.; Davis, D.D.; Pizzutillo, P. Osteoporosis in Spinal Cord. In juries. In *StatPearls [Internet]*; StatPearls Publishing: Treasure Island, FL, USA, 2023.

49. Verschueren, S.; Gielen, E.; O'Neill, T.W.; Pye, S.R.; Adams, J.E.; Ward, K.A.; Wu, F.C.; Szulc, P.; Laurent, M.; Claessens, F.; et al. Sarcopenia and its relationship with bone mineral density in middle-aged and elderly European men. *Osteoporos. Int.* **2013**, *24*, 87–98. [CrossRef]
50. Yoshimura, N.; Muraki, S.; Oka, H.; Iidaka, T.; Kodama, R.; Kawaguchi, H.; Nakamura, K.; Tanaka, S.; Akune, T. Is osteoporosis a predictor for future sarcopenia or vice versa? Four-year observations between the second and third ROAD study surveys. *Osteoporos. Int.* **2017**, *28*, 189–199. [CrossRef]
51. Mahitthiharn, K.; Kovindha, A.; Kaewchur, T.; Morse, L.R.; Pattanakuhar, S. Prevalence and influencing factors of spinal cord injury-related osteoporosis and fragility fractures in Thai people with chronic spinal cord injury: A cross-sectional, observational study. *J. Spinal Cord. Med.* **2023**, *46*, 458–465. [CrossRef]
52. Li, S.; Gonzalez-Buonomo, J.; Ghuman, J.; Huang, X.; Malik, A.; Yozbatiran, N.; Magat, E.; Francisco, G.E.; Wu, H.; Frontera, W.R. Aging after stroke: How to define post-stroke sarcopenia and what are its risk factors? *Eur. J. Phys. Rehabil. Med.* **2022**, *58*, 683–692. [CrossRef] [PubMed]
53. Pacifico, J.; Geerlings, M.A.J.; Reijnierse, E.M.; Phassouliotis, C.; Lim, W.K.; Maier, A.B. Prevalence of sarcopenia as a comorbid disease: A systematic review and meta-analysis. *Exp. Gerontol.* **2020**, *131*, 110801. [CrossRef] [PubMed]
54. Burns, A.S.; Marino, R.J.; Kalsi-Ryan, S.; Middleton, J.W.; Tetreault, L.A.; Dettori, J.R.; Mihalovich, K.E.; Fehlings, M.G. Type and Timing of Rehabilitation Following Acute and Subacute Spinal Cord Injury: A Systematic Review. *Glob. Spine J.* **2017**, *7*, 175S–194S. [CrossRef] [PubMed]
55. De Spiegeleer, A.; Beckwée, D.; Bautmans, I.; Petrovic, M.; Sarcopenia Guidelines Development Group of the Belgian Society of Geriatrics. Pharmacological Interventions to Improve Muscle Mass, Muscle Strength and Physical Performance in Older People: An Umbrella Review of Systematic Reviews and Meta-analyses. *Drugs Aging* **2018**, *35*, 719–734. [CrossRef] [PubMed]
56. Lee, J.H.; Jun, H.S. Role of Myokines in Regulating Skeletal Muscle Mass and Function. *Front. Physiol.* **2019**, *10*, 42. [CrossRef]
57. McClung, J.M.; Davis, J.M.; Wilson, M.A.; Goldsmith, E.C.; Carson, J.A. Estrogen status and skeletal muscle recovery from disuse atrophy. *J. Appl. Physiol.* **2006**, *100*, 2012–2023. [CrossRef]
58. Kaur, J.; Ghosh, S.; Singh, P.; Dwivedi, A.K.; Sahani, A.K.; Sinha, J.K. Cervical Spinal Lesion, Completeness of Injury, Stress, and Depression Reduce the Efficiency of Mental Imagery in People With Spinal Cord Injury. *Am. J. Phys. Med. Rehabil.* **2022**, *101*, 513–519. [CrossRef]

Disclaimer/Publisher's Note: The statements, opinions and data contained in all publications are solely those of the individual author(s) and contributor(s) and not of MDPI and/or the editor(s). MDPI and/or the editor(s) disclaim responsibility for any injury to people or property resulting from any ideas, methods, instructions or products referred to in the content.

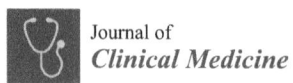 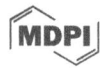

Article

Cognitive Reserve and Its Association with Cognitive and Mental Health Status following an Acute Spinal Cord Injury

Mohit Arora [1,2,*], Ilaria Pozzato [1,2], Candice McBain [1,2], Yvonne Tran [3], Danielle Sandalic [1,2], Daniel Myles [1,2], James Walter Middleton [1,2] and Ashley Craig [1,2]

1. The Kolling Institute, Faculty of Medicine and Health, The University of Sydney, Sydney, NSW 2000, Australia; danielle.sandalic@health.nsw.gov.au (D.S.); a.craig@sydney.edu.au (A.C.)
2. John Walsh Centre for Rehabilitation Research, Northern Sydney Local Health District, St Leonards, NSW 2065, Australia
3. Australian Institute of Health Innovation, Macquarie University, North Ryde, NSW 2113, Australia
* Correspondence: mohit.arora@sydney.edu.au

Abstract: Background: Mild cognitive impairment (MCI) is a common secondary condition associated with spinal cord injury (SCI). Cognitive reserve (CR) is believed to protect against cognitive decline and can be assessed by premorbid intelligence (pmIQ). Despite the potential utility of pmIQ as a complementary metric in the evaluation of MCI in SCI, this approach has been infrequently employed. The purpose of this study was to examine the association between MCI and pmIQ in adults with SCI with the aim of exploring the potential value of pmIQ as a marker of CR in this population. Methods: Cognitive function was assessed on three occasions in adults with SCI over a 12-month period post-injury, and pmIQ was assessed once at baseline. Demographic and mental health measures were also collected, and logistic regression was conducted to determine the strength of association between pmIQ and MCI while adjusting for factors such as mental health and age. Results: The regression analysis revealed that at the time of admission to SCI rehabilitation, the MCI assessed by a valid neurocognitive screen was strongly associated with pmIQ. That is, if a person has MCI, there was 5.4 greater odds ($p < 0.01$) that they will have poor pmIQ compared to a person without MCI after adjustment for age and mental health. Conclusions: The assessment of CR is an important area that should be considered to improve the process of diagnosing MCI in adults with an acute SCI and potentially facilitate earlier intervention to slow or prevent cognitive decline.

Keywords: spinal cord injury; cognitive impairment; cognitive reserve; depression; fatigue; rehabilitation

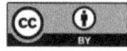

1. Introduction

Spinal cord injury (SCI) is a severe neurological injury resulting in substantial impairment, including loss of motor control and sensory and autonomic dysfunction [1]. Common physical secondary conditions include cardiovascular and respiratory dysfunction, pain, pressure injuries, urinary tract infections, and bowel complications, while psychological-based problems include fatigue, cognitive impairment, and mental health disorders [1–6]. The occurrence of mild cognitive impairment (MCI) after SCI is considered to be high, with best estimates suggesting rates of between 20 and 30% in the acute SCI adult population [4,7]. However, recent studies have highlighted a number of issues when assessing MCI after SCI [4,7,8]. These issues include: (i) broad estimates of the occurrence of MCI (ranging between 10–60%), derived from cross-sectional research conducted over the past 20 years; (ii) the lack of clarity about which cognitive domains are most affected by SCI [4]; (iii) the absence of a universally accepted definition for the identification of cognitive impairment following SCI [7]; (iv) the lack of a neurocognitive screen that has demonstrated structural validity for assessing MCI after SCI [7]; (v) the lack of cognitive performance norms for assessing MCI after SCI [7]; (vi) the lack of clarity around the contribution of environmental factors to cognitive performance during the acute and rehabilitation phases, and (vii) the problem of misdiagnosing cognitive impairment resulting from the application of norm-referenced assessments with little regard for measures of baseline or premorbid cognitive intelligence/cognitive reserve [8]. While these problems have been deliberated upon [4,7,8], they have not been resolved and therefore pose significant barriers to SCI adjustment and rehabilitation outcomes. This paper will specifically investigate the concerns posed by the seventh issue; that is, the importance of cognitive reserve (CR) following SCI and its relationship with post-cognitive performance, demographics such as age and education, and psychosocial factors, including depressive mood, anxiety, and fatigue.

The theory of CR refers to the brain's ability to maintain cognitive function despite age-related changes or brain damage and addresses the observation that people differ in how they fare after neurological injury [9,10]. For example, people with higher levels of CR may be less likely to experience cognitive decline or develop dementia as they age [10]. CR is based on the assumption that individual differences in post-neurological injury recovery are associated with cognitive abilities developed over the life span, which are believed to protect against and compensate for neurological damage caused by a traumatic injury (e.g., traumatic brain injury/TBI) or a disease process (e.g., Alzheimer's disease) [9,10]. Evidence suggests CR has strong convergent validity and reasonable discriminant validity and, therefore, can be considered a valid cognitive concept [9]. Evidence also suggests factors such as education and engagement in social and occupational activities increase CR, and these factors could therefore be used as measures of CR [9,10]. Premorbid intelligence is another important estimate of CR. An acceptable measure of premorbid intelligence (pmIQ) is the Test of Premorbid Functioning (TOPF), an objective lexical task. The premise is that vocabulary is highly correlated with cognitive function and, therefore, is considered a valid measure of global intelligence [8–12]. For example, research in individuals with a TBI found higher levels of premorbid intelligence (assessed by TOPF), and thus an assumed higher CR was related to more favourable neuropsychological outcomes [13]. We contend that diagnosing MCI based solely on population norms without recourse to the assessment of premorbid intelligence limits its application in SCI rehabilitation [8]. As an illustration of this assertion, in a study involving simulated data for 500,000 adults with SCI, norm-referenced and premorbid-intelligence methods of MCI screening were compared to examine the extent of MCI misclassification after SCI [8]. Results found that up to 20% of the simulated adults with SCI were potentially misclassified as having MCI. The study concluded that measures of premorbid intelligence (e.g., TOPF) should be included in the assessment of cognitive function after SCI in the absence of baseline and longitudinal cognitive screen measures [8].

Success of SCI rehabilitation is dependent to a certain extent upon the client having sufficient cognitive capacity to understand the complex instructions concerning medications, medical procedures, self-management, and ongoing self-care [1,7,8]. It is also crucial that these self-management skills learned in the rehabilitation phase can be translated into the community setting, such as managing caregivers when required. For this to occur, an evidence-based and effective system for classifying MCI is required. Therefore, the main aim of this study was to investigate the relationship between CR/pmIQ (assessed by TOPF) and post-SCI cognitive outcomes (assessed by the Neuropsychiatry Unit Cognitive Assessment Tool, NUCOG), as well as examine relationships between pmIQ and additional factors including age, education, level of injury, mental health, and fatigue. The main hypothesis is that TOPF scores will be strongly associated with neurocognitive scores post-SCI. Specifically, it was hypothesised that: (i) higher age, higher level of injury, lower years of education, lower pmIQ, higher depressive mood and anxiety, and higher fatigue will be related to lower neurocognitive scores; (ii) age, level of injury, and years of education will be related to CR (i.e., TOPF standard scores); (iii) adults with acute SCI who have lower neurocognitive scores after SCI and are therefore more likely to have MCI, will more likely have low scores on TOPF (i.e., low CR or pmIQ); (iv) psychosocial factors will influence the association between neurocognitive scores and TOPF scores assessed at admission to rehabilitation; so that those who have higher levels of depressive mood, anxiety, and fatigue will more likely have lower scores on TOPF (i.e., low CR or pmIQ).

2. Materials and Methods

2.1. Design

Full details of this study's protocol have been published [14]. The design involved an inception cohort longitudinal study that followed adults with an acute SCI from the first 24–48 h after their presentation to a hospital emergency department to discharge from rehabilitation (usually 4–6 months post-SCI) and up to 12 months post-SCI when living in the community.

2.2. Participants

Participants with SCI (n = 75) were recruited when engaged in SCI rehabilitation in one of the three specialised SCI units in Sydney, New South Wales, Australia. Inclusion criteria consisted of: (i) aged between 17 and 80 years; (ii) having an acute SCI of non-traumatic or traumatic origin; and (iii) having proficiency in English enabling them to complete all assessments. Exclusion criteria consisted of: (i) the existence of a severe mental disorder (e.g., bipolar disorder or psychosis); and (ii) the existence of a severe pre-morbid (i.e., presence of a serious medical condition that existed before the onset of an SCI) or concurrent severe TBI (i.e., loss of consciousness > 24 h, post-traumatic amnesia > 7 days, or a Glasgow Coma score of 3–8 usually assessed within 24 h of initial injury). Full compliance with the Code of Ethics of the World Medical Association occurred, and the local institutional human research ethics committee granted ethics approval. All participants provided informed consent prior to participating.

2.3. Study Measures

The protocol for this study provides full details of all the measures employed [14]. Participants were assessed three times (i.e., admission, discharge, and 12 months following SCI) during the study using multiple assessments, including cognitive and psychosocial measures. Baseline and discharge assessments were performed in one of three SCI units, and assessments at 12 months were performed in the community. However, only a limited number of measures believed to be relevant to the specific aims of this study are reported here. Socio-demographic measures included age, sex, and years of education. Injury characteristics included the level of injury and the American Spinal Injury Association Impairment Scale assessed by a medical specialist based on the International Standards for Neurological Classification of SCI (http://ais.emsci.org/, accessed 10 April 2023).

2.3.1. Neuropsychiatry Unit Cognitive Assessment Tool

Cognitive function was assessed by the NUCOG [7,15,16]. The NUCOG is a validated neurocognitive screen comprising 21 items in 5 cognitive domains: attention, visuoconstructional, memory, executive, and language. Scores for each of the domains range between 0 and 20, adding up to a total NUCOG score out of 100. Higher scores indicate higher levels of cognitive function.

Neuropsychologists and psychiatrists developed the NUCOG based on multiple neurocognitive tests, including the Stroop, Trail Making Test, and WAIS-4th Edition. The NUCOG has been shown to have criterion, convergent, and discriminant validity for a number of disorders, and to have acceptable reliability and specificity/sensitivity [16]. When applied to screening adults with SCI who have restricted hand function, it was necessary to adapt some items (e.g., drawing a reproduction) as per previous studies, where this has been shown to not alter the validity of NUCOG scores [7,15]. When face-to-face administration of the NUCOG was not possible (e.g., social distancing restrictions due to COVID-19), administration occurred via telehealth. Administration of the NUCOG via teleconferencing required additional adjustments to the NUCOG assessment procedures to satisfy the telehealth environment [7,15]. These procedural adjustments have been discussed elsewhere [7,15]. Although the NUCOG has been shown to have poor structural fit in the Memory and Language domains in an SCI sample, the overall NUCOG score has demonstrated adequate validity [7].

While the definition and criteria for determining the presence of MCI vary [7], in this study, to determine the possible presence of MCI, the total NUCOG mean (reported elsewhere; [15,16]) was used, with probable MCI defined as one standard deviation (SD) below a mean of 92.9 (SD = 4.9). Therefore, the MCI cut-off score of 88 (93 mean score minus 5 as one SD) was used, so that those scoring ≤ 88 were considered to have a probable MCI, while those scoring > 88 were considered not to be cognitively impaired.

2.3.2. Test of Premorbid Functioning

The TOPF was assessed only at admission and was employed to estimate pmIQ/CR [8,11,13]. Completing the TOPF involved reading a list of 70 phonemically irregular words and was scored according to its manual instructions. The TOPF score consisted of the number of words the participant read aloud with the correct pronunciation to derive the raw score, which was then transformed into age-corrected standard scores provided by the test [11]. The TOPF has demonstrated validity [9,10]. The TOPF has a range of scores from 40 to 160. A score of 101 is considered average, while scores above 101 indicate above-average cognitive functioning (superior CR), and scores below 101 indicate below-average cognitive functioning [17].

2.3.3. Patient Health Questionnaire—9 Items

Mood was assessed by the Patient Health Questionnaire-9 (PHQ-9) [18]. The PHQ-9 assesses each of the nine Diagnostic and Statistical Manual of Mental Disorders Fourth Edition (DSM-IV) criteria for major depressive disorder over the prior two-week period. Items range from 0 "not at all" to 3 "nearly every day" and are summed to establish depressive-symptom severity (0–4 no depressive symptoms; 5–9 mild depressive symptoms; 10–14 moderate depressive symptoms; 15–19 moderately severe depressive symptoms; and 20–27 severe depressive symptoms) [18]. The PHQ-9 has demonstrated validity [18,19].

2.3.4. Generalized Anxiety Disorder—7 Items

Anxiety was assessed using the Generalized Anxiety Disorder-7 (GAD-7) [20]. The GAD-7 is a seven-item psychometric instrument used to determine the severity of generalized anxiety disorder (GAD). Participants are asked to rate their anxiety symptoms as experienced over the prior two weeks. Responses include "not at all (0)", "several days (1)", "more than half the days (2)", and "nearly every day (3)". The scores of the seven items are summed to provide a total score. Total scores of 5, 10, and 15, respectively, represent cut-points for mild, moderate, and severe anxiety symptoms [20]. The GADS-7 has demonstrated validity [19,20].

2.3.5. Fatigue Severity Scale

Fatigue was assessed by the Fatigue Severity Scale (FSS) [21]. The FSS is a 9-item self-report scale that assesses the severity of fatigue and its effects on daily activities. Items are scored on a 7-point Likert scale (1 = strongly disagree to 7 = strongly agree). The higher the score, the more severe the fatigue. The FSS has demonstrated reliability and validity [21,22].

2.4. Analyses

Summary statistics were produced for the study variables. Pearson correlation analyses were conducted to determine relationships between age, sex, years of education, level of injury, and NUCOG scores with TOPF. Missing data for the TOPF and NUCOG variables were managed by listwise deletion of those participants who failed or could not be contacted to complete assessments in the second (discharge) and third (12 months) NUCOG assessments. Ten participants did not provide all NUCOG assessments or a TOPF assessment, leaving sixty-five participants for the logistic regression. For a small number of cases (less than 10%), item mean imputation was used for missing values in the psychosocial variables (GADS-7, PHQ-9, and FSS). The value of this technique is that it preserves statistical power but has less negative influence on variation than mean imputation (e.g., reducing standard error rates) than overall mean imputation [23]. Statistical power to find valid associations using multiple regression was calculated to be 98% given $n = 65$, $\alpha = 0.05$, number of predictors = 5, and an estimated effect size of 0.25 [24]. Crude odds ratio, sensitivity, and specificity values were calculated from the contingency table of MCI versus no MCI as a function of low TOPF ($\leq$101) versus high TOPF (>101).

Logistic regression with the dependent variable being the TOPF standardised score, dichotomised to include those scoring lower on the TOPF standardised score ($\leq$101) and those scoring higher (>101). A standardised TOPF score of 101 was selected to include those who scored just over 100 in the low TOPF sub-group, as arguably, a score of 100 or just over should not be considered superior CR [17].

Five independent factors were entered into the logistic regression. Given the sample size available for the regression analysis ($n = 65$), the number of independent variables able to be entered was limited to five [23]. Total NUCOG scores assessed at admission were entered in dichotomous form, that is, probable cognitive impairment ($\leq$88) versus probable no cognitive impairment (>88). Four continuous predictors were entered, consisting of age, PHQ-9, GADS-7, and FSS. The independent factors entered into the logistic regression were chosen because they have a theoretical basis for contributing to premorbid intelligence. For example, increased age (within the 17–80 age range) will be related to CR/ TOPF scores. Further, as higher pmIQ or CR is thought to be associated with better psychological outcomes, mental health measures were also included. Sex, years of education, and level of injury were not entered into the regression given restrictions on the number of independent variables. Restricting the number of independent factors entered into the regression complied with rules governing participants versus the number of independent variables entered [23]. Due to the limited sample size, logistic regression analysis was only conducted for admission to SCI rehabilitation. All analyses were performed using Statistica Version 13 (https://www.statistica.com, accessed 10 February 2023).

3. Results

Table 1 shows summary statistics and breakdown for the participants for socio-demographic, injury, TOPF, NUCOG, mental health, and fatigue factors. Table 1 shows participants classified with MCI had significantly fewer years of education ($p < 0.05$) and lower TOPF scores ($p < 0.01$). Participants classified as having MCI had significantly higher levels of depressive mood ($p < 0.05$) and anxiety ($p < 0.01$), though there were no differences in fatigue levels between these two sub-groups. For paraplegia, 17.6% (6 out of 34) had MCI, while 30.8% (12 out of 39) of those with tetraplegia had probable MCI (two missing values); however, this difference was not significant ($X^2 = 1.7$, df = 1, $p > 0.05$). No differences were found for age or sex between those with and without MCI.

Table 1. Parametric and breakdown statistics for socio-demographic ($n = 75$), injury characteristics, TOPF, NUCOG, PHQ-9, GADS-7, and FSS for 65 participants.

Variables	All Participants	Probable MCI (NUCOG $\leq$ 88)	No MCI (NUCOG > 88)
Sex (males, n (%))	58 (77.3)	16 (84.2)	42 (75)
Age in years, mean (SD)	51.0 (18.3)	50.3 (21.9)	51.4 (17.5)
Years of education, mean (SD)	14.5 (3.1)	12.5 (3.2)	15.1 (2.9) *
Paraplegia, n (%) [1]	34 (45.3)	--	--

Table 1. Cont.

Variables	All Participants	Probable MCI (NUCOG ≤ 88)	No MCI (NUCOG > 88)
AIS [1,2], n (%)			
Grade A	15 (20.5)	--	--
Grade B	7 (9.6)	--	--
Grade C	15 (20.5)	--	--
Grade D	35 (48.0)	--	--
Grade E	1 (1.4)	--	--
TOPF, mean (SD)	104.5 (14.3)	95.3 (13.4)	107.2 (13.7) **
NUCOG, mean (SD)			
At admission	91.2 (6.9)	81.5 (6.5)	94.5 (2.7)
At discharge [3]	92.5 (4.9)	85.2 (3.6)	94.6 (2.8)
At 12 months [4]	93.7 (5.3)	82.0 (5.3)	95.1 (3.3)
PHQ-9 at admission, mean (SD)	5.8 (5.0)	8.0 (7.0)	4.6 (3.7) *
GADS-7 at admission, mean (SD)	4.5 (4.2)	6.6 (5.8)	3.5 (2.9) **
FSS at admission, mean (SD)	32.4 (13.5)	32.0 (15.7)	32.7 (12.2)

Abbreviations: AIS: American Spinal Injury Association Impairment Scale; FSS: Fatigue Severity Scale; GADS-7: General Anxiety Disorder-7); NUCOG: The Neuropsychiatry Unit Cognitive Assessment Tool; PHQ-9: Patient Health Questionnaire-9; SD: Standard deviation; TOPF: Test of Premorbid Functioning. * $p < 0.01$ ** $p < 0.01$. [1] Two missing values for level of injury and AIS Grades: $n = 73$. [2] AIS grade definitions: Grade A: Complete: no motor or sensory function left below the lesion; Grade B: Incomplete. Sensory function, but not motor function, is preserved below the lesion, and some sensation is preserved in the sacral segments S4 and S5; Grade C: Incomplete. Motor function is preserved below the neurologic level, but more than half of the key muscles below the neurologic level have a muscle grade less than 3 (i.e., they are not strong enough to move against gravity); Grade D: The impairment is incomplete. Motor function is preserved below the neurologic level, and at least half of the key muscles below the neurologic level have a muscle grade of 3 or more (i.e., the joints can be moved against gravity); Grade E: The patient's functions are normal. All motor and sensory functions are unhindered. [3] $n = 41$; [4] $n = 29$.

3.1. Probable Rate of MCI

Based on $n = 75$ and the criteria employed for probable MCI in this study (NUCOG scores ≤ 88), the rate of MCI in this sample was 25.3% (19 out of 75) at admission to rehabilitation and 22% (9 out of 41) at discharge from rehabilitation (around 4–6 months post-SCI). Rates at 12 months are not reported given the low sample size at the 12-month assessment (ongoing data collection).

3.2. Probable Diagnostic Classification of MCI

Table 2 shows a contingency breakdown of the classification of probable MCI as well as misclassifications based on the MCI and TOPF criteria. Odds ratios that are greater than 1 indicate that the event is more likely to occur as the predictor increases. The crude odds ratio (i.e., not adjusted for potential factors that could influence the ratio) was calculated to be 4.85, suggesting that if a person with acute SCI has a NUCOG score > 88 (not cognitively impaired), then there is 4.85 greater odds that they will have a TOPF score of >101 (superior CR), compared to the odds of such a relationship in a person with a NUCOG score of ≤88 (cognitively impaired). The reverse relationship holds. This finding indicates there is a strong positive association between post-SCI cognitive outcomes and CR (or premorbid intelligence as assessed by TOPF). Sensitivity refers to the ability of the TOPF score, say ≤101, to also have a NUCOG score ≤ 88 or vice versa. The sensitivity, as shown in Table 2, is moderate at 71.4%, indicating a number of false negative results exist ($n = 17$ or 63% misclassification). Specificity refers to the ability of the TOPF score to be more likely associated with those who do not have MCI. The specificity, as shown in Table 2, is also not high at 66%; however, there are fewer false positives ($n = 4$ or 10.8%).

Table 2. Breakdown of classification and misclassification of MCI versus no cognitive impairment for admission to rehabilitation (one missing value).

TOPF	MCI (n), ≤88	No MCI (n), >88	Total
≤101	10	17	27
>101	4	33	37
Total	14	50	64

Abbreviations: MCI: mild cognitive impairment; TOPF: Test of Premorbid Functioning. $X^2 = 6.28$, df = 1, $p < 0.05$; odds ratio: 4.85; 95% confidence interval (CI): 1.32–17.79; $p < 0.01$. Sensitivity: 71.4%; 95% CI: 41.9–91.6%; specificity: 66.0%; 95% CI: 51.2–78.8%.

3.3. Association of Cognitive Reserve with Multiple Independent Factors in SCI

Table 3 shows Pearson correlations between the TOPF standard score (estimate of CR) and socio-demographic, injury, NUCOG, and predictor factors.

Table 3. Showing Pearson correlations between the study variables and TOPF.

Variable	TOPF Standardised Score
Age	0.52 **
Sex	0.14
Years of education	0.39 **
Level of injury	−0.15
NUCOG	
At admission	0.34 **
At discharge	0.43 *
At 12 months	0.54 **
PHQ-9, at admission	−0.16
GADS-7, at admission	−0.38 **
FSS, at admission	0.18

Abbreviations: FSS: Fatigue Severity Scale; GADS-7: General Anxiety Disorder-7); NUCOG: The Neuropsychiatry Unit Cognitive Assessment Tool; PHQ-9: Patient Health Questionnaire-9; TOPF: Test of Premorbid Functioning. * $p < 0.05$, ** $p < 0.01$.

Table 4 shows the results of the logistic regression between TOPF and NUCOG, age, PHQ-9, GADS-7, and FSS. The objective was to determine the adjusted association between CR (TOPF: ≤101 versus >101) and the probable presence of MCI (i.e., ≤88 versus no MCI > 88), age, mental health, and fatigue at admission. Table 4 shows, after including these variables, that a strong positive association exists between NUCOG and TOPF, with an odds ratio of 5.4 ($p = 0.05$). Odds ratios less than 1 indicate that it is more likely that as the independent factor increases, TOPF will be reduced (i.e., ≤101). Therefore, as age increases, the odds increase that CR decreases (odds ratio = 0.95, $p = 0.004$). That is, a 5% decrease in the odds of a TOPF > 101 with each additional year (0.95–1 × 100 = −0.05 × 100 = 5%). For depressive mood, the same association was found with an odds ratio of 0.76 (close to significance at $p = 0.06$), suggesting that as depressive mood increases, the odds are that TOPF scores will be lower. In contrast with the findings of correlation analyses, anxiety (GADS-7) was found to have a positive odds ratio of 1.69 with TOPF, suggesting that if a person with acute SCI has higher anxiety, there is 1.65 greater odds that they will have a TOPF > 101, compared to the odds of such a relationship in a person with a TOPF score ≤ 101. The relationship between TOPF and fatigue was also less than 1 (odds ratio = 0.98, $p = 0.57$) but was not significant.

Table 4. Logistic regression results for the association between the dependent binary TOPF variable (≤101 versus >101) with independent variables binary NUCOG (≤88 versus >88), age, mood (PHQ-9), anxiety (GADS-7), and fatigue (FSS).

Variable	Odds Ratio	95% CI	p	Log LRT	X^2	p
NUCOG MCI	5.4	1–29	0.05	−30.5	4.2	0.04
Age	0.95	0.92–0.99	0.02	−38.8	8.4	0.004
PHQ-9	0.76	0.56–1.0	0.06	−32.9	4.3	0.04
GADS-7	1.69	1.1–2.5	0.02	−35.1	7.5	0.01
FSS	0.98	0.93–1.0	0.57	−32.6	0.69	0.40

Abbreviations: CI: confidence interval; FSS: Fatigue Severity Scale; GADS-7: General Anxiety Disorder-7); LRT: Likelihood ratio test; MCI: mild cognitive impairment; NUCOG: The Neuropsychiatry Unit Cognitive Assessment Tool; *p*: probability; PHQ-9: Patient Health Questionnaire-9; TOPF: Test of Premorbid Functioning; X^2: chi-square.

4. Discussion

This study aimed to investigate the relationship between CR, as measured using the TOPF, and post-SCI cognitive outcomes using the NUCOG. The study also examined the potential value of CR as a marker of cognitive function in this population and explored relationships between CR and other factors such as age, education, level of injury, mental health, and fatigue. Our findings have important implications for improving the diagnosis and management of MCI in adults with SCI and suggest that assessing CR should become a standard component of evaluating neurocognitive status in this population.

Our hypothesis 1 was partially confirmed. Those with low neurocognitive scores (suggesting the presence of MCI) had an increased psychosocial burden [15]. Specifically, participants with MCI had significantly higher levels of depressive mood and anxiety but not fatigue. Participants with probable MCI also had fewer years of education and lower levels of CR compared to those without MCI. This finding confirms prior research that shows the presence of MCI is associated with an increased risk of secondary conditions such as depressive mood [15] and cardiovascular dysregulation [25]. Fatigue is a known problem in SCI [6], and our finding suggests it remains a challenge regardless of the presence of MCI. Past research has rarely found that demographic variables such as sex and injury variables are significantly related to neurocognitive scores [15]. Age has been found to be mildly related to MCI in a community sample of adults with SCI [15], but age was not significantly different between the MCI versus non-MCI sub-groups in this acute sample.

Prior research has shown that adults with SCI have problems in neural inhibitory function and perceptual encoding processes, as well as in executive functioning important for engaging in daily tasks [26]. As argued previously, adjusting to SCI, and understanding rehabilitation processes requires intensive learning and the use of adaptability skills to manage complications and improve adjustment to SCI. Deficits in cognitive performance [15,26] can impede outcomes, such as the use of computer assistive technology in the home environment [27], which can improve quality of life if used appropriately [28]. Therefore, it is important that neurocognitive screening be performed regularly after acute SCI, especially during intensive rehabilitation, to improve the detection rates of those with MCI. Strategies can then be developed to counter the negative influences associated with MCI [15].

Rates of MCI in adults with SCI have been shown to vary widely from 20–60% [4,7]. This variation is due to methodological issues, such as a lack of a universally accepted MCI definition, as well as assessments being conducted at different times post-SCI in past studies [4,8]. In the present study, a conservative definition of MCI was purposely employed; that is, MCI was defined as one SD below the mean for the population, and the rate was assessed at admission to rehabilitation just weeks after the injury. The MCI rate was found to be 25.3%. A slight decline in the MCI rate (22%) was found when MCI was assessed 4–6 months later when participants were discharged from rehabilitation into the community. There is not yet sufficient 12-month data to provide a reliable MCI rate. Nevertheless, this longitudinal data will be vital information for advancing how

MCI is understood and managed during SCI rehabilitation. For example, a one-off neurocognitive assessment does not provide information about whether the person assessed is declining or improving in their cognitive capacity [8]. To the best of our knowledge, there have been no longitudinal/prospective reports of neurocognitive function in adults with SCI. One suggestion to enhance the diagnostic accuracy of MCI is to incorporate multiple assessment methods. For example, combining cognitive tests with other techniques such as neuroimaging (e.g., MRI) or biomarkers (e.g., blood-based markers) can provide a more comprehensive evaluation of cognitive functioning post-SCI. This approach aims to improve the overall accuracy of MCI diagnosis by considering various aspects of cognitive impairment.

The crude odds ratio from Table 2 confirms our hypothesis that CR (i.e., TOPF scores) is strongly associated with post-SCI cognitive outcomes. As previously discussed, relying on normative values to classify MCI has its limitations, and thus the significance of this finding is contingent upon the establishment and evaluation of a universally accepted definition for MCI that can be used reliably. Nevertheless, the crude odds ratio of 4.85 reported in Section 3.2 suggests a strong relationship exists between neurocognitive scores and CR. One can conclude from this that if a participant has a low NUCOG score suggesting MCI, then the odds are high (4.85%) that they will also have low CR (i.e., a low TOPF score) compared to a participant who has a high NUCOG score. This is similar to CR research in areas such as TBI and dementia, which has found people with low CR have an increased occurrence of having poorer neurocognitive outcomes [9,10].

However, as highlighted in prior research [8], there remains a risk of misclassification of diagnoses [8,12]. In this study, 32.8% of cases were potentially misclassified, with 62.9% being false positives (17 out of 27) and 10.8% (4 out of 37) being false negatives. The sensitivity of a test refers to its capacity to identify an individual as positive when they are, with suggestions that an acceptable sensitivity should be at least 80% [29]. A very sensitive test suggests there should be few false negatives and, therefore, fewer true cases are missed [29]. In this study, the sensitivity was not high at 71.4%, with almost a third of cases being false positives. Various factors could have contributed to the high false positive rate, such as those who do not have English as their first language, and thus, the TOPF score could be biased toward a lower score. Further research is required to explore other possible contributors to false positives. The specificity of a test is concerned with how capable it is of correctly identifying people who are truly negative [29]. While the test had a low number of false negatives, it has also been suggested that an acceptable specificity is around 80% [29]. Contributors to false negatives likewise need further investigation. Strategies are needed to resolve the misclassification of MCI post-SCI, such as improving sensitivity and specificity. For example, employing prospective designs involving multiple assessments of neurocognitive data over time post-SCI and simultaneously assessing relationships to alternative measures such as pmIQ alongside norm-based neurocognitive assessment at different stages post-SCI [8].

The Pearson correlation analyses revealed that CR (TOPF standardised score) was positively and significantly associated with age. It should be remembered that the age range investigated in this study was between 17 and 80 years, with a mean age of around 51 years. Therefore, there will be less influence from decreased CR due to older age. Perhaps within this age range, older participants have accumulated greater CR, or the positive crude correlation between age and TOPF ($r = 0.52$) does not take into account the possible influence of other factors on this relationship between age and TOPF. Research is required to clarify the positive correlation between age and TOPF. TOPF was also positively associated with higher years of education, confirming prior research that found education to be a CR protective factor [10,12]. TOPF was also positively and significantly associated with NUCOG scores at admission, discharge, and after 12 months post-SCI; again, in line with prior research in which higher CR is positively related to better neurocognitive outcomes post-injury [10,13]. As hypothesised, TOPF was negatively correlated with depressive mood (PHQ-9) and anxiety (GADS-7), though the relationship with PHQ-9 was not significant.

These relationships have been shown elsewhere in TBI and dementia [10,12,13]. Fatigue was not related to CR.

The logistic regression tested the hypothesis that CR (high versus low TOPF scores) would be strongly associated with neurocognitive scores post-SCI, even after adjusting for age, mental health, and fatigue. The data suggest that CR and neurocognitive outcomes are strongly and positively associated with an odds ratio of 5.4, even after adjusting for other factors that may influence the relationship. Age and depressive mood were both found to have a negative relationship after adjusting for the other factors. That is, as TOPF scores decrease, the likelihood is that depressive mood and age will increase. The finding of depressive mood is important given that evidence strongly suggests that depression and other psychosocial barriers (e.g., poor self-efficacy) can be substantial challenges to adjustment after an SCI [30,31]. However, it was surprising that TOPF scores were positively associated with anxiety (GADS-7) with an odds ratio of 1.69, and this seems to contradict previous correlation analyses. It was hypothesised anxiety would have a negative relationship with CR. That is, a low TOPF score is more likely to be related to a higher anxiety score (as found in the crude correlational analysis). Further research will be needed to clarify this finding.

Study Limitation

The main limitation of this study is the lack of sufficient numbers in the longitudinal assessments at discharge and 12 months post-SCI (due to the COVID-19 pandemic). The study is still recruiting and continuing follow-up assessments to address this limitation.

In light of the COVID-19 restrictions, we accommodated the circumstances by conducting the NUCOG assessment via teleconferencing when necessary. However, it is essential to recognize that the adjustments made to test administration methods have the potential to influence the outcomes of the test. Specifically, participants' level of attention during teleconferencing-based testing may differ from that observed in in-person assessments. Consequently, it is crucial to consider the potential implications of these adjustments on the reliability and validity of the test results, particularly in relation to participants' attention levels. To address this limitation, we intend to conduct a comprehensive analysis in our future studies to assess any differences that may arise between in-person and remote administration methods.

Our study did not specifically focus on the direct effects of the pandemic. While we acknowledge that the pandemic may have influenced our results, it is challenging to disentangle its specific impact from the broader factors that might influence mental health post-SCI. Future research should explicitly focus on studying the direct effects of the pandemic on mental health and cognitive functioning to provide a more comprehensive understanding of these complex relationships.

5. Conclusions

These findings do provide helpful preliminary directions for improving the diagnosis of MCI after SCI. The relationship between CR and neurocognitive outcomes, after adjusting for potentially influential factors, has not been investigated previously after an SCI. The authors believe that the findings will lead to advances in SCI rehabilitation, such as the implementation of improved processes for assessing MCI after SCI, especially within the first 6 months post-injury. The findings also suggest that relying on a neurocognitive screen test conducted at one point in time is not sufficient, given the results of the logistic regression, where multiple factors were found to have a role in the relationship between CR and post-SCI cognitive outcomes. Lastly, the findings do indicate that CR/pmIQ should become a standard component of assessing neurocognitive status in adults with an SCI. These measures can help identify adults who may be at risk for cognitive decline and can be used clinically to evaluate the effectiveness of interventions aimed at enhancing CR.

Author Contributions: Conceptualisation: A.C., D.S., M.A., I.P. and J.W.M.; methodology: A.C., D.S., M.A., I.P., C.M. and Y.T.; validation: Y.T.; formal analysis: A.C. and M.A.; investigation: D.S., M.A., C.M., D.M. and I.P.; resources: A.C. and M.A.; data curation: M.A., C.M. and D.M.; writing—original draft preparation: A.C. and M.A.; writing—review and editing: J.W.M., I.P., D.S., D.M., C.M. and Y.T.; supervision: A.C., J.W.M. and M.A.; project administration: M.A., I.P. and C.M.; funding acquisition: A.C., M.A. and J.W.M. All authors have read and agreed to the published version of the manuscript.

Funding: This research was funded by icare New South Wales, Australia (2019), grant id G203704.

Institutional Review Board Statement: We certify that all applicable institutional and governmental regulations concerning the ethical use of human volunteers were followed during the course of this research. The study was approved by the Northern Sydney Local Health District Human Research Ethics Committee in 2019 (2019/ETH00592).

Informed Consent Statement: Informed consent was obtained from all participants involved in the study, and all participants gave their approval for their anonymised data to be published in group data format. No participants are able to be identified from the data published in this paper.

Data Availability Statement: The datasets generated are available from the corresponding author on reasonable request.

Acknowledgments: We acknowledge the valuable assistance of those who participated in the study and the rehabilitation teams in the three SCI Units involved.

Conflicts of Interest: The authors declare no conflict of interest. The funders had no role in the design of the study; in the collection, analyses, or interpretation of data; in the writing of the manuscript; or in the decision to publish the results.

References

1. Craig, A.; Tran, Y.; Arora, M.; Pozzato, I.; Middleton, J.W. Investigating Dynamics of the Spinal Cord Injury Adjustment Model: Mediation Model Analysis. *J. Clin. Med.* **2022**, *11*, 4557. [CrossRef]
2. Craig, A.; Tran, Y.; Guest, R.; Middleton, J. Trajectories of Self-Efficacy and Depressed Mood and Their Relationship in the First 12 Months Following Spinal Cord Injury. *Arch. Phys. Med. Rehabil.* **2019**, *100*, 441–447. [CrossRef] [PubMed]
3. Krassioukov, A.; Claydon, V.E. The clinical problems in cardiovascular control following spinal cord injury: An overview. *Prog. Brain Res.* **2006**, *152*, 223–229. [PubMed]
4. Sandalic, D.; Craig, A.; Tran, Y.; Arora, M.; Pozzato, I.; McBain, C.; Tonkin, H.; Simpson, G.; Gopinath, B.; Kaur, J.; et al. Cognitive Impairment in Individuals with Spinal Cord Injury: Findings of a Systematic Review with Robust Variance and Network Meta-analyses. *Neurology* **2022**, *99*, e1779–e1790. [CrossRef] [PubMed]
5. Siddall, P.J.; McClelland, J.M.; Rutkowski, S.B.; Cousins, M.J. A longitudinal study of the prevalence and characteristics of pain in the first 5 years following spinal cord injury. *Pain* **2003**, *103*, 249–257. [CrossRef]
6. Wijesuriya, N.; Tran, Y.; Middleton, J.; Craig, A. Impact of fatigue on the health-related quality of life in persons with spinal cord injury. *Arch. Phys. Med. Rehabil.* **2012**, *93*, 319–324. [CrossRef] [PubMed]
7. Sandalic, D.; Tran, Y.; Craig, A.; Arora, M.; Pozzato, I.; Simpson, G.; Gopinath, B.; Kaur, J.; Shetty, S.; Weber, G.; et al. The Need for a Specialized Neurocognitive Screen and Consistent Cognitive Impairment Criteria in Spinal Cord Injury: Analysis of the Suitability of the Neuropsychiatry Unit Cognitive Assessment Tool. *J. Clin. Med.* **2022**, *11*, 3344. [CrossRef]
8. Sandalic, D.; Tran, Y.; Arora, M.; Middleton, J.; McBain, C.; Myles, D.; Pozzato, I.; Craig, A. Improving Assessment of Cognitive Impairment after Spinal Cord Injury: Methods to Reduce the Risk of Reporting False Positives. *J. Clin. Med.* **2022**, *12*, 68. [CrossRef]
9. Harrison, S.L.; Sajjad, A.; Bramer, W.M.; Ikram, M.A.; Tiemeier, H.; Stephan, B.C. Exploring strategies to operationalize cognitive reserve: A systematic review of reviews. *J. Clin. Exp. Neuropsychol.* **2015**, *37*, 253–264. [CrossRef]
10. Stern, Y. Cognitive reserve. *Neuropsychologia* **2009**, *47*, 2015–2028. [CrossRef]
11. Clinical, P. *Advanced Clinical Solutions for WAIS-IV and WMS-IV: Administration and Scoring Manual*; The Psychological Corporation: San Antonio, TX, USA, 2009.
12. Gavett, B.E.; Ashendorf, L.; O'Bryant, S.E. When is it appropriate to infer cognitive impairment on the basis of premorbid IQ estimates? A simulation study. *Psychol. Assess.* **2022**, *34*, 390–396. [CrossRef] [PubMed]
13. Leary, J.B.; Kim, G.Y.; Bradley, C.L.; Hussain, U.Z.; Sacco, M.; Bernad, M.; Collins, J.; Dsurney, J.; Chan, L. The Association of Cognitive Reserve in Chronic-Phase Functional and Neuropsychological Outcomes Following Traumatic Brain Injury. *J. Head Trauma Rehabil.* **2018**, *33*, E28–E35. [CrossRef] [PubMed]
14. Sandalic, D.; Craig, A.; Arora, M.; Pozzato, I.; Simpson, G.; Gopinath, B.; Kaur, J.; Shetty, S.; Weber, G.; Cameron, I.; et al. A prospective cohort study investigating contributors to mild cognitive impairment in adults with spinal cord injury: Study protocol. *BMC Neurol.* **2020**, *20*, 341. [CrossRef] [PubMed]

15. Craig, A.; Guest, R.; Tran, Y.; Middleton, J. Cognitive Impairment and Mood States after Spinal Cord Injury. *J. Neurotrauma* **2017**, *34*, 1156–1163. [CrossRef] [PubMed]
16. Walterfang, M.; Siu, R.; Velakoulis, D. The NUCOG: Validity and reliability of a brief cognitive screening tool in neuropsychiatric patients. *Aust. N. Z. J. Psychiatry* **2006**, *40*, 995–1002. [CrossRef]
17. Delis, D.C.; Kaplan, E.; Kramer, J.H. *Delis-Kaplan Executive Function System (D-KEFS)*; The Psychological Corporation: San Antonio, TX, USA, 2001.
18. Kroenke, K.; Spitzer, R.L.; Williams, J.B. The PHQ-9: Validity of a brief depression severity measure. *J. Gen. Intern. Med.* **2001**, *16*, 606–613. [CrossRef]
19. Teymoori, A.; Gorbunova, A.; Haghish, F.E.; Real, R.; Zeldovich, M.; Wu, Y.J.; Polinder, S.; Asendorf, T.; Menon, D.; Center-Tbi, I.; et al. Factorial Structure and Validity of Depression (PHQ-9) and Anxiety (GAD-7) Scales after Traumatic Brain Injury. *J. Clin. Med.* **2020**, *9*, 873. [CrossRef]
20. Spitzer, R.L.; Kroenke, K.; Williams, J.B.; Löwe, B. A brief measure for assessing generalized anxiety disorder: The GAD-7. *Arch. Intern. Med.* **2006**, *166*, 1092–1097. [CrossRef]
21. Krupp, L.B.; LaRocca, N.G.; Muir-Nash, J.; Steinberg, A.D. The fatigue severity scale. Application to patients with multiple sclerosis and systemic lupus erythematosus. *Arch. Neurol.* **1989**, *46*, 1121–1123. [CrossRef]
22. Nadarajah, M.; Mazlan, M.; Abdul-Latif, L.; Goh, H.T. Test-retest reliability, internal consistency and concurrent validity of Fatigue Severity Scale in measuring post-stroke fatigue. *Eur. J. Phys. Rehabil. Med.* **2017**, *53*, 703–709. [CrossRef]
23. Tabachnick, B.G.; Fidell, L.S. *Using Multivariate Statistics*; Harper & Row, Publishers, Inc.: New York, NY, USA, 1989.
24. Faul, F.; Erdfelder, E.; Buchner, A.; Lang, A. *G* Power (Version 3.1. 9.6)*; University of Kiel: Kiel, Germany, 2020.
25. Nightingale, T.E.; Zheng, M.M.Z.; Sachdeva, R.; Phillips, A.A.; Krassioukov, A.V. Diverse cognitive impairment after spinal cord injury is associated with orthostatic hypotension symptom burden. *Physiol. Behav.* **2020**, *213*, 112742. [CrossRef]
26. Lazzaro, I.; Tran, Y.; Wijesuriya, N.; Craig, A. Central correlates of impaired information processing in people with spinal cord injury. *J. Clin. Neurophysiol.* **2013**, *30*, 59–65. [CrossRef]
27. Craig, A.; Moses, P.; Tran, Y.; McIsaac, P.; Kirkup, L. The effectiveness of a hands-free environmental control system for the profoundly disabled. *Arch. Phys. Med. Rehabil.* **2002**, *83*, 1455–1458. [CrossRef]
28. Baldassin, V.; Shimizu, H.E.; Fachin-Martins, E. Computer assistive technology and associations with quality of life for individuals with spinal cord injury: A systematic review. *Qual. Life Res. Int. J. Qual. Life Asp. Treat. Care Rehabil.* **2018**, *27*, 597–607. [CrossRef]
29. Loong, T.W. Understanding sensitivity and specificity with the right side of the brain. *BMJ* **2003**, *327*, 716–719. [CrossRef] [PubMed]
30. Craig, A.; Hancock, K.; Chang, E.; Dickson, H. The effectiveness of group psychological intervention in enhancing perceptions of control following spinal cord injury. *Aust. N. Z. J. Psychiatry* **1998**, *32*, 112–118. [CrossRef] [PubMed]
31. Craig, A.R.; Hancock, K.; Chang, E.; Dickson, H. Immunizing against depression and anxiety after spinal cord injury. *Arch. Phys. Med. Rehabil.* **1998**, *79*, 375–377. [CrossRef] [PubMed]

Disclaimer/Publisher's Note: The statements, opinions and data contained in all publications are solely those of the individual author(s) and contributor(s) and not of MDPI and/or the editor(s). MDPI and/or the editor(s) disclaim responsibility for any injury to people or property resulting from any ideas, methods, instructions or products referred to in the content.

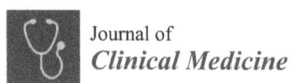

Article

Psychological Screening, Standards and Spinal Cord Injury: Introducing Change in NHS England Commissioned Services

Jane Duff [1,*], Rebecca Ellis [2], Sally Kaiser [3] and Lucy C Grant [1]

1. Department of Clinical Psychology, National Spinal Injuries Centre, Stoke Mandeville Hospital, Buckinghamshire Healthcare NHS Trust, Aylesbury HP21 8AL, UK; janeduff@nhs.net (J.D.)
2. Department of Clinical Health Psychology, Yorkshire Regional Spinal Injuries Centre, Mid Yorkshire NHS Trust, Wakefield WF1 4DG, UK; rebecca.ellis40@nhs.net
3. Department of Clinical Psychology, Midlands Centre for Spinal Injuries, The Robert Jones and Agnes Hunt Orthopaedic Hospital NHS Foundation Trust, Oswestry SY10 7AG, UK; sally.kaiser@nhs.net
* Correspondence: bht.nsicpsychology@nhs.net; Tel.: +44-(0)-1296-838355

Abstract: Psychologist resourcing across the United Kingdom (UK) spinal cord injury centres (SCICs) varies considerably, which has detrimentally impacted standardising service provision for people with spinal cord injuries/disorders (PwSCI/D) compared with other nations. This paper presents the outcome of a project involving the Spinal Cord Injury Psychology Advisory Group (SCIPAG) and NHS England Clinical Reference Group/SCI transformation groups to agree upon screening and standards and shares data from the National Spinal Injuries Centre (NSIC) and the Yorkshire and Midlands Regional SCICs. Inpatients completed the GAD-7, the PHQ-9, and the short form of the Appraisals of DisAbility: Primary and Secondary Scale (ADAPSSsf), assessing adjustment. A total of 646 participants were included, with 43% scoring above the clinical threshold on at least one of the measures on admission. A subset of 272 participants also completed discharge measures and 42% remained above the threshold on discharge, demonstrating sustained psychological need. This paper provides support for services to move to a screen-and-assessment model supplemented by referral options for those with changing needs or who present with difficulties outside the remit of screening. The findings also support the efficacy of universal screening across the system and consideration of screening and standards for psychological care by the wider psychology community.

Keywords: spinal cord injury; spinal cord disorders; mental health; clinical psychology; rehabilitation; screening; health psychology; quality improvement; psychiatry; ISCoS

Citation: Duff, J.; Ellis, R.; Kaiser, S.; Grant, L.C. Psychological Screening, Standards and Spinal Cord Injury: Introducing Change in NHS England Commissioned Services. *J. Clin. Med.* **2023**, *12*, 7667. https://doi.org/10.3390/jcm12247667

Academic Editor: Giacomo Mancini

Received: 30 October 2023
Revised: 6 December 2023
Accepted: 8 December 2023
Published: 13 December 2023

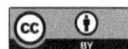

Copyright: © 2023 by the authors. Licensee MDPI, Basel, Switzerland. This article is an open access article distributed under the terms and conditions of the Creative Commons Attribution (CC BY) license (https://creativecommons.org/licenses/by/4.0/).

1. Introduction

There is a wealth of literature that identifies the role and impact that psychological factors can have on the outcome following a spinal cord injury/disorder (SCI/D). This includes, but is not exclusive to, rehabilitation gain and progress [1], surgical responsiveness [2], development of secondary health conditions [3,4], long-term quality of life and morbidity [5]. However, despite this awareness, as well as substantial research and some worldwide (though localised) initiatives, routine and systematic international recommendations for psychological health screening and standards for SCI/D care have been delayed compared with many other physical health conditions [6]. Comparison can be drawn most notably in the services for people who have experienced burns, stroke or cancer. For example, in the UK, The National Burn Care Review Committee recommended screening in 2001, which subsequently led to a pathway identifying "Levels of Psychological Care" for "watchful waiting" (Level 1) and psychological therapy/treatment (Level 2), with later developments including psychoeducation as part of the treatment pathway [7–9]. In oncology in the United States, work commenced in 1997, with a direct influence of this being the acknowledgement that many distressed patients are unrecognised and untreated. Pivotally, it was stated that the "management of a patient's psychological state is vital to the care of every patient at all stages of disease, irrespective of disease site or treatment...In fact, there is no other dimension of cancer that is quite so central to *every* patient" (*sic*) [10] (p. 109). Guidance was published by The National Comprehensive Cancer Network in 2003 [11]. In the UK, the National Institute for Health and Care Excellence (NICE) is the overarching body that approves centralised funding and, consequently, recommends a range of treatment protocols and medication. NICE guidance for improving palliative care cancer services was published in 2004 and included a recommendation to ensure "all patients undergo systematic psychological assessment at key points and have access to appropriate psychological support...[and] a four-level model of screening and professional psychological assessment and intervention" [12] (p. 9).

Similarly, with regard to stroke, the Physical Health and Disability Special Interest Group of the British Psychological Society commenced standard setting and screening in 1999, with publication in 2002 [13]. The guidance identified a service specification, mechanisms for monitoring quality and outcome, and recommended staffing levels. In 2016, the Intercollegiate Stroke Working Party produced the fifth NICE-accredited edition, which provided over 150 pages of comprehensive interdisciplinary guidance and measurement of outcomes, including goal setting, intensity of therapy and self-management. The recommended psychological service was a "matched care model" in which all patients are assessed and provided with needs-based treatment. The "matched care model" is stratified and includes an initial triage so that people commence at the level of treatment needed, which could be the highest and most intense. A further enhancement of this is "the matched collaborative care model", which includes collaborative goal setting and self-management training. It is different from the "stepped care model" commonly used in mental health services, where people usually commence at the lowest intervention, which tends to be more generic, and is often a group skills-based or online treatment with stepping up in treatment intensity and access to individual therapy if symptoms fail to improve.

The introduction of standards and screening in each of these conditions has led to several developments. In cancer and burns services, there was recognition that culture and the routine of healthcare delivery could enhance or reduce someone's psychological response, with the development of training and education for multi-disciplinary staff to detect and respond to psychological risk factors. In cancer services, the application of standardised psychometric scales enhanced the understanding of "caseness" and cultural sensitivity, as well as the recognition of psychologist staffing resource limitations [11]. Similarly, in stroke services, standards enabled significant service expansion due to the specificity of the recommendations and the ability of services to review, benchmark and evidence their needs.

Regarding SCI/D, the 1999 Paralyzed Veterans of America "Spinal Cord Medicine Consumer Guide on Depression" was possibly the first widely available consumer publication aimed at normalising emotional response to injury. Several attempts were made in the intervening years, as outlined in the foreword of the subsequent guidance, to gain funding for the necessary consensus and recommendations for screening, assessment, and treatment regarding anxiety, major depressive disorder, substance use, post-traumatic stress disorder (PTSD)/acute stress disorder and suicide [14]. Although unavoidably delayed, the rigor and detailed nature of the 2021 Clinical Practice Guideline (CPG) provides a comprehensive review of the literature; grades evidence for a recommended treatment; and unites information on psychological, pharmacological and MDT interventions. The CPG dovetails with two other bodies of work from the USA: a series of SCIRehab publications examining the details of psychological treatment and outcome [15] and professional practice standards [16].

Work on the US professional practice standards for psychologists and social workers commenced in 1990. There were various reviews and iterations over time prior to the most recent (2016) version anchoring psychosocial intervention as an inherent part of the biopsychosocial model in rehabilitation. The standards recommended staffing levels and that "psychologists and social workers should be core members of the interdisciplinary treatment team" [16] (p. 135), and the expectation that every inpatient across the lifespan receive psychological health screening and assessment commensurate with the timescale of other team members, including treatment as required. The guidance recommends cognitive behavioural therapy (CBT) and coping effectiveness therapy (CET), rating these as having Level 2 evidence, as well as identifying a range of other interventions. The guidance also recommends a written plan for psychosocial review after discharge and the need for follow-up outpatient screening across the lifespan.

In Australia, psychosocial care guidelines for New South Wales State SCI services were first published in 2008, with later editions in 2013 and 2023 [17,18]. As with the US guidance, a comprehensive psychological assessment for all inpatients was recommended, with a timescale of within 5 days of admission to rehabilitation. The guidance mandated that treatment be provided as required, with CBT being highlighted as an evidence-based intervention and that a psychological review occur prior to discharge, with mood screenings 6 and 12 months after returning to community living. The guidance was accompanied in 2016 by an "Emotional Wellbeing Toolkit: A clinicians guide to working with SCI" which provided measures of psychological screening for mood, PTSD, pain, psychosis, alcohol and substance use, with accompanying clinician tips for these and other concerns, such as suicidality and self-harm, challenging behaviour, traumatic brain injury and dementia [19]. A key element of the toolkit was the recognition that psychosocial care is "everyone's business" [19] (p. 1) and inherent within every healthcare clinician's role in SCI/D.

Psychosocial rehabilitation guidelines, which integrate peer counselling as an intervention alongside healthcare clinicians, were published by the Asian Spinal Cord Network in 2015 [20]. Crucially, the guidelines also identified the likelihood of variable provision because of resource limitations and recommended the provision of psychoeducational material about adjustment as an intervention in the absence of peer counsellors or healthcare clinicians with a psychosocial role. The guidance is partly based on a "stepped care model", with the peer counsellor identifying the need for formal individual psychological assessment and treatment. The family system of the PwSCI/D and their needs are recognised as part of the intervention in Levels 3 and 4, and the guidance names the importance of integrating sexual counselling as routine.

The Netherlands commenced psychological screening in 2018, with inpatients being administered a range of brief measures within two weeks of admission as an inpatient or on commencing an outpatient rehabilitation programme. The programme aimed to evaluate 80% of the people identified; however, an audit found that due to staffing constraints and logistics, only 64% of patients completed the measures [21]. Developed as part of the screening, the programme adopted a national approach of flagging those needing follow-up, with patient responses on each measure being RAG (red, amber, green) rated. Several benefits of screening were identified: timely recognition of psychological problems; screening measures, as administered by a psychologist, providing an introduction to broader psychosocial issues regarding self-efficacy and resilience rather than just a pathological focus; screening enabling more targeted treatment and use of personnel; and, of perhaps greatest significance, increased identification and recognition of psychological issues amongst other rehabilitation team members [21].

Despite the evidenced progress of these individual nations, international agreement on psychological screening and the psychological measures to use has been severely delayed compared with other areas of care for PwSCI/D. The delay has no doubt been impacted by the substantial rigor and time required for such an initiative and the absence of resourcing, as well as the lack of a Psychosocial Special Interest Group (SIG) within the International Spinal Cord Society (ISCoS) until 2018, to co-ordinate and champion the need. However, progress has been swift since the inception of the SIG, with the Basic Psychology Data Set screening recommendations being published in 2023 [22], and work having already commenced on the Advanced Data Set.

The absence of a systematised international consensus on screening and standards of psychological care has significantly impeded psychosocial care in some nations. One of these has been the UK, with a report on SCICs in England in 2023 showing huge differences in services and psychologist-to-inpatient ratios varying from 1:15 to 1:100 [23], with the lowest provision in Sheffield, Salisbury, Southport and the National Spinal Injuries Centre (NSIC) at Stoke Mandeville. The 2008 rehabilitation standards include one reference regarding the need to assess depressed mood [24] but, in contrast to many of the initiatives of other nations, did not include an expectation that assessment would be universal, that a psychologist should be included as a core member of the rehabilitation team, or that there be a timescale for screening and assessment. The current SCI/D service specification lists psychometric assessment at mobilisation and again at discharge as one of the key indicators and includes a reference to the employment of clinical psychologists with specialist expertise in SCI/D care and their involvement in MDT and treatment decision-making meetings [25,26]. However, this is the limit of the scope, and it does not specify the nature of the psychometric screen or assessment.

In 2014, the first author was part of a working group which agreed national psychology screening measures. These were not implemented due to the delayed revision of the NHS England Database; however, this enabled the UK and Ireland Spinal Cord Injury Psychology Advisory Group (SCIPAG) to revise, in 2019, the mood screen from the Hospital Anxiety and Depression Scale [27] to the Patient Health Questionnaire-9 for depression [28] and Generalised Anxiety Disorder-7 [29], with each NHS England commissioned SCIC agreeing to opt in where able and screen on admission and discharge from April 2021. Alongside this development, in March 2020, a small working group of SCIPAG, which comprised the first author and third author, clinical psychologists working in the Yorkshire and Welsh SCICs, and two people with lived experience from the Back Up Trust and Spinal Injuries Association, commenced work on psychological care standards.

There is a significant capacity gap for access to specialised SCI/D rehabilitation in the SCICs commissioned by NHS England. The 2021 annual Database report showed that only 36% of PwSCI/D were admitted to inpatient rehabilitation [30]. The trend of roughly one-third of newly injured PwSCI/D receiving rehabilitation through outpatient services of the SCIC and one-third through another NHS provider (most commonly a district general hospital or neurorehabilitation service) has been present for some time. However, these figures are likely to be an underestimate of need, given the Database captures referrals rather than nationally mandated reporting of PwSCI/D incidence. The UK Spinal Injuries Association estimates there to be seven new PwSCI/Ds each day and 2500 injuries per annum [31]. In 2020, in part to address the access gap, NHS England and SCI/D CRG broadened the scope of SCICs to include responsibility for all PwSCI/D within each service's catchment area and developed seven transformation workstreams to set standards and recommendations across the care pathway. The first author, as the chair of SCIPAG and a member of the SCI/D Clinical Reference Group (CRG, which oversees service provision for NHS England), led the workstream for psychological and mental health needs [23], which ratified the previously agreed screening measures and introduced several other recommendations; the first author also contributed to this work the psychology standards developed as part of SCIPAG (Appendix A) [32].

At the inception of the workstreams in October 2020, most of the psychology services within the eight NHS England commissioned SCICs did not have the staffing resources to assess every patient on admission and/or discharge, and the dominant model was based on referral rather than screening. To assess the referral versus screening gap and evidence the need for a changed model within its own service, the NSIC at Stoke Mandeville completed a retrospective audit of 166 inpatients between November 2020 and April 2022 and compared referral with screening data on the PHQ-9 [28]; the GAD-7 [29]; and the short form of the Appraisals of DisAbility Primary and Secondary Scale (ADAPSSsf), which measures adjustment [33]. Thirty percent of inpatients had a positive screen on at least one of these measures at admission; by discharge, 27% of the same inpatients had a positive screen and, crucially, had not been referred to the psychology service during their admission [34]. Each of the centres involved in this research had a slightly different service model. The NSIC at Stoke Mandeville had a 33:1 patient-to-clinical-psychologist ratio with a referral model and "watchful wait" monitoring through the MDT for those who screened in but had not been referred. The Yorkshire Regional Spinal Injuries Centre (YRSIC) had a 27:1 ratio and aimed to screen and assess every patient within 2 weeks of admission; however, after the implementation of screening, this centre experienced staffing difficulties and was operating on a referral model for the period of this study. The Midlands Centre for Spinal Injuries (MCSI) had a 29:1 ratio and either used MDT screening or the screen was combined with a psychological assessment with screening over the first 4 weeks of an inpatient's admission but did assess all first-time admissions for rehabilitation.

As referenced earlier, screening has been implemented by many psychology services as a means of discerning initial needs, augmented with a referral process in recognition that adjustment is not a linear process [4,14,35]. One of the influencers for the rise of screening across services rather than a clinician-led referral has been the recognition that "physicians continue to use personal experience as part of their decision-making process and are subject to a wide range of influences, despite the recent emphasis on the use of EBM [evidence-based medicine]" [36] (p. 184) and that "non-clinical influences on decision-making may be the most important, and up to now largely unrecognized obstacle to the practice of EBM", with a range of patient-related factors, as well as unconscious bias being present [36] (p. 179). Although the above references physician decision making, it is well known that all healthcare clinicians need to be sensitive to and aware of the risk of a uni-professional approach. A survey of MDT staff training needs was conducted by the NSIC at Stoke Mandeville: seven NHS hospitals that refer into the service, as well as private providers and third-sector organisations. Across 13/15 key areas of psychological care, respondents indicated low confidence and the need for training to develop their awareness of patient's psychological needs [37]. It was knowledge of these issues that influenced SCIPAG to implement the option to screen to augment the dominant MDT referral model within services in April 2021.

The psychology standards and psychological and mental health workstream were significantly influenced by the body of international work outlined earlier and aimed to incorporate the key learnings and initiatives within an evidence-based, system-wide model for NHS England SCI/D services. Appendix A, Supplementary Tables S1 and S2, and Supplementary Figure S1 reference the details of the recommendations for system-wide change: these include agreement regarding standards; adoption of a screening and matched collaborative care pathway (in which all PwSCI/D receive assessment and different levels of intervention based on their level of psychological complexity); an MDT curriculum (for enhancing knowledge and recognition of psychological care needs); and identified several developments, most crucially the need for workforce parity across SCICs to achieve implementation.

In light of the recent advances in standardising psychology provision for PwSCI/D, the current study sought to compare the introduction of screening across three NHS England commissioned SCICs: NSIC at Stoke Mandeville, MCSI and YRSIC. This study aimed to understand the incidence of psychological needs on admission and discharge from inpatient rehabilitation and to consider, in light of the standards, any recommendations for services that are working within a referral model. It was also hoped that the results could be used to inform the staffing resources needed to embed the standards and service changes within the participating centres and across all UK SCICs and to raise awareness of the psychological screening needs for the two-thirds of PwSCI/D not admitted to specialist SCIC rehabilitation. To aid the reader's understanding of the NHS in England, acronyms and a brief contextual explanation can be found in Abbreviation.

2. Materials and Methods

2.1. Study Design and Procedure

This study employed a multicentre retrospective cohort design. Two centres, namely, the NSIC and YRSIC, collected data via a "screen and refer" model, in which all inpatients received a psychometric screen at admission, but only those referred to the centres' respective psychology teams received a psychological intervention. The remaining centre, namely, the MCSI, operated an "assessment and screen" model, in which all inpatients were provided with a psychological assessment, which included psychometric screening as part of this.

Data collected at the NSIC were extracted from the psychological health domain of the Stoke Mandeville Spinal Needs Assessment Checklist (SMS-NAC), which is a self-report, MDT-administered, validated measure [38] used to assess inpatients' knowledge, skills, and physical or verbal independence across 10 domains of rehabilitation for SCI/D. The SMS-NAC should be administered within 2 weeks of admission to the rehabilitation centre to aid goal setting, and within four weeks of discharge to provide an outcome measure. Data from the NSIC were collected between January 2020 and September 2023 for all inpatients with SCI/D who had completed an adult version of the SMS-NAC at admission. Data from the YRSIC were collected between January 2019 and September 2023 as part of the Psychology Service screening proforma administered to all inpatients with SCI/D; the screening ranged from 2–67 days, with a mean time of 19 days for this study sample.

Data from the MCSI were collected between October 2021 and September 2023. Prior to mid-February 2023, demographic and psychometric information were extracted from the relevant sections of the adult version of the SMS-NAC, which was administered by a member of the inpatient's MDT. After this date, psychometric measures were instead administered by the centre's assistant psychologist to aid the completion rate. Measures were administered within three weeks of inpatients' admission to the SCIC.

2.2. Participants

PwSCI/D with an age at injury of at least 16 years who were admitted to an SCIC for first-time rehabilitation were eligible for inclusion in this study. Individuals with significant cognitive or language impairment who were unable to understand the screening measures were excluded. Overall, 759 participants across the 3 centres met inclusion criteria, while 113 did not complete screening measures and were excluded from this study. Of the total number of included participants with admission measures ($n = 646$), 272 had also completed discharge measures. Where necessary, incomplete demographic information was supplemented by checking participants' electronic patient notes.

2.3. Ethics

Retrospective data from the 3 SCICs were collected individually; however, participants' identifiable information was removed from their datasets by authors S.K. and R.E. prior to sending it to authors L.C.G. and J.D. for data collation and analyses. De-identified demographic information and psychometric data (comprising total scores on the PHQ-9 [28], the GAD-7 [29] and the short form ADAPSSsf [33]) were shared via secure email.

Participant consent was not required due to the data being collected as part of standard clinical care. All relevant approvals were completed prior to data transfer to ensure anonymous and ethical data sharing. The NHS England Health Research Authority provided approval for anonymised data sharing, and all research and governmental protocols were adhered to for the duration of this study.

2.4. Study Variables

Psychometric data for analyses comprised the PHQ-9, GAD-7 and ADAPSSsf. The PHQ-9 was used to screen for the presence of depressive symptoms at admission and prior to discharge. Participants indicate on a 4-point Likert scale, from 0 ("Not at all") to 3 ("Nearly everyday"), how often over the previous two weeks they had experienced each item. The total score, ranging from 0 to 27, is calculated by summing all items. Scores of 0–4 indicate subclinical depression, scores of 5–9 indicate mild depression, scores of 10–14 suggest moderate depression, scores 15–19 suggest moderately severe depression and scores of 20–27 indicate severe depression. The PHQ-9 has been validated for use in SCI/D inpatient rehabilitation and demonstrates good diagnostic accuracy and reliability [39,40].

The GAD-7 measure was used to assess the presence of anxiety symptoms. As with the PHQ-9, participants indicate how often over the last two weeks they had experienced each item using a 4-point Likert scale. The total score, ranging from 0 to 21, is calculated by summing all items. Total scores can be subdivided into categories depending on severity, with 0–4 indicating sub-clinical anxiety, scores of 5–9 suggesting mild anxiety, scores of 10–14 suggesting moderate anxiety and scores of 15–21 indicating severe anxiety. The GAD-7 has been validated for use in primary health populations [41], including good validity and reliability for use in the SCI/D population [42,43].

The ADAPSSsf was used to assess participants' appraisals of their injury and provide an indication of adjustment to SCI/D. The ADAPSSsf consists of 6 items, 3 of which relate to negative appraisals and are included in the "Loss/Catastrophic Negativity" subscale, and 3 which relate to positive appraisals and are included in the "Resilience" subscale. "Loss" items are measured on a 6-point Likert scale from 1 ("Strongly Disagree") to 6 ("Strongly Agree"), where higher scores indicate a greater sense of loss and more negative appraisal of injury. "Resilience" items are reverse scored, such that higher scores indicate less resilience and more negative appraisal of injury. A total score, ranging from 6 to 36, is calculated by summing each item. The ADAPSSsf shows good validity and reliability for use in SCI/D [33,40].

In line with recommendations from the literature, scores were considered above the threshold if they were ≥ 11 on the PHQ-9 [39], ≥ 8 on the GAD-7 [43] and ≥ 22 on the ADAPSSsf [33]. For each measure, scoring above the threshold indicates that a clinician-led mental health assessment is required to determine a diagnosis. Participants with missing responses on some of the psychometric measures were still included in the analyses as long as at least one of the measures had been fully completed.

2.5. Coding and Statistical Analyses

Minor differences existed between the samples in relation to the demographic information that was collected and recorded. De-identified data from the MCSI and YRSIC were therefore coded in line with the NSIC at Stoke Mandeville sample to ensure consistency and homogeneity. Demographic data not reported by all three samples were removed from the analysis.

For categorical data, chi-square tests of association were performed to compare the demographics between the 3 samples, as well as between participants scoring above compared with below the threshold on the PHQ-9, the GAD-7 and the ADAPSSsf. For continuous data, one-way ANOVAs were used to evaluate whether differences existed for age at injury and time since injury between the samples, as well as for participants who scored above compared with below the threshold on the PHQ-9, the GAD-7 and the ADAPSSsf. Calculations were conducted using all participants' admission data in addition to the participants with both admission and discharge data.

Additional analyses were conducted using a subgroup of participants that completed the admission and discharge measures to compare within-sample psychometrics at each time point. Paired-sample t-tests were used to determine whether mean differences existed between participants' admission and discharge scores for all screening measures. Finally, multiple linear regression analysis was used to examine whether the score at admission or demographic variables were predictive of the score at discharge for each of the measures.

Prior to commencing the analyses, statistical assumptions were first tested to ensure the reliability and validity of the results. For all statistical tests, IBM SPSS Statistics for Windows Version 17.0 was used, and the significance level was set at $p < 0.01$.

3. Results

3.1. Admission Data

Demographics and descriptive statistics for all participants are presented in Table 1. All participants completed at least one of the screening measures on admission. Forty-three percent ($n = 281$) of participants demonstrated psychological need by scoring above the threshold on at least one of the measures. Admission severity classifications for the PHQ-9, GAD-7 and ADAPSSsf are presented in Figure 1a–c. The psychometric properties for all three measures are shown in Table 2.

Table 1. Participant demographics and descriptive statistics across samples for all participants.

		N (% Total Number)			
		NSIC	MCSI	YRSIC	Combined
Total		438	87	121	646
Sex	Male	297 (68)	62 (71)	76 (63)	435 (67)
	Female	141 (32)	25 (29)	45 (37)	211 (33)
Ethnicity	White	266 (61)	54 (63)	106 (88) *	426 (66)
	Black	30 (7)	3 (3)	1 (1)	34 (5)
	Asian	24 (5)	1 (1)	6 (5)	31 (5)
	Mixed	4 (1)	1 (1)	1 (1)	6 (1)
	Other	3 (1)	0 (0)	3 (2)	6 (1)
	Not stated	111 (25)	28 (32)	4 (3)	143 (22)
Cause of injury	Traumatic	221 (51)	58 (67)	46 (38) *	325 (51)
	Non-traumatic	217 (49)	29 (33)	75 (62)	321 (49)
Level of injury	Tetraplegia (A/B/C)	89 (20)	28 (32)	37 (31)	154 (24)
	Paraplegia (A/B/C)	168 (39)	24 (28)	46 (38)	238 (37)
	All levels D	181 (41)	32 (37)	26 (21) *	239 (37)
	Not stated	0 (0)	3 (3)	12 (10)	15 (2)
Psychometrics	PHQ-9	432 (99)	85 (98)	115 (95)	632 (98)
	GAD-7	432 (99)	86 (99)	118 (98)	636 (98)
	ADAPSSsf	423 (97)	83 (95)	110 (91)	616 (95)
		Mean (St. Dev.)			
		NSIC	MCSI	YRSIC	Combined
Age at injury (years)		54.64 (17.56) *	58.36 (19.14)	60.23 (16.20)	56.19 (17.66)
Time since injury (years)		0.41 (0.42)	0.37 (0.17)	0.21 (0.30) *	0.37 (0.38)
PHQ-9 total score		6.38 (5.86)	4.95 (4.81)	7.03 (6.56)	6.31 (5.88)
GAD-7 total score		4.44 (5.16)	2.92 (3.70)	4.96 (5.67)	4.33 (5.12)
ADAPSSsf total score		19.18 (6.60)	18.78 (6.18)	19.05 (6.59)	19.11 (6.59)

Note: * indicates significance.

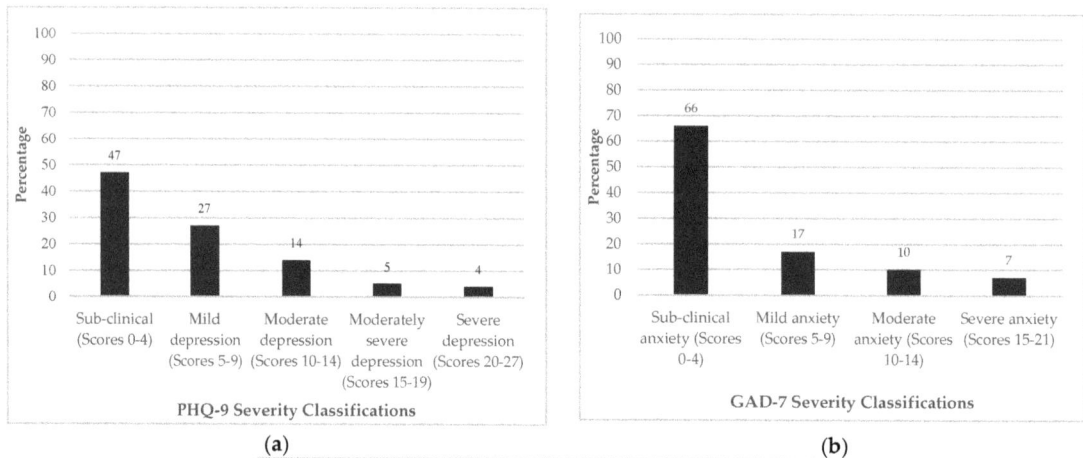

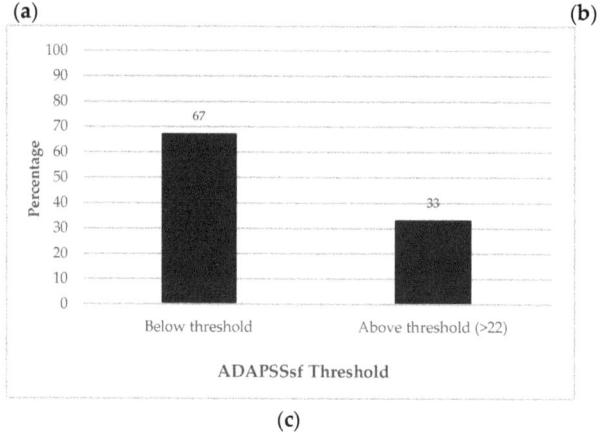

Figure 1. Combined sample percentage severity classifications at admission only for (**a**) PHQ-9, (**b**) GAD-7 and (**c**) ADAPSSsf.

Table 2. Psychometric properties for combined sample for those with admission measures.

		Combined Sample N (% Excluding Missing Values)
Psychometrics	PHQ-9	632
	GAD-7	636
	ADAPSSsf	616
Above threshold	PHQ-9 (≥ 11)	138 (22)
	GAD-7 (≥ 8)	142 (22)
	ADAPSSsf (≥ 22)	206 (33)
		Combined Sample Mean (St. Dev.)
PHQ-9	Above threshold	15.54 (3.90)
	Below threshold	3.72 (3.09)
GAD-7	Above threshold	12.60 (3.56)
	Below threshold	1.95 (2.18)
ADAPSSsf	Above threshold	26.50 (3.53)
	Below threshold	15.39 (4.20)

When comparing demographics across samples, there was a small overrepresentation of individuals identifying as "White" ethnicity in the YRSIC sample ($\chi^2(10) = 50.28$, $p < 0.01$, $V = 0.197$). Additionally, there was a small underrepresentation of traumatic injuries ($\chi^2(2) = 16.63$, $p < 0.01$, $V = 0.160$) and a small-to-moderate underrepresentation of incomplete ASIA D injuries ($\chi^2(6) = 60.26$, $p < 0.01$, $V = 0.216$) in the YRSIC sample. The YRSIC sample also had a significantly shorter time since injury ($F(1,2) = 13.67$, $p < 0.01$), while the NSIC sample was significantly younger at injury compared with the other samples ($F(1,2) = 5.66$, $p = 0.004$).

A small overrepresentation of females scoring above the threshold on both the PHQ-9 ($\chi^2(1) = 8.02$, $p = 0.005$, $V = 0.113$) and GAD-7 ($\chi^2(1) = 7.31$, $p = 0.007$, $V = 0.107$) was observed. Individuals scoring above the threshold on the PHQ-9 ($F(1630) = 6.73$, $p = 0.01$) were significantly younger at injury ($M_{above} = 52.85$, $M_{below} = 57.22$); however, no significant differences were found in either age at injury or time since injury for the GAD-7 or ADAPSSsf. No other significant differences were observed when comparing demographics for those above compared with below the threshold across the measures with respect to sex, ethnicity, cause of injury or level of injury.

3.2. Subgroup with Admission and Discharge Data

From the total sample, a subgroup of 272 participants had both admission and discharge data. When comparing the demographics of this subgroup to participants with only admission data, the only significant difference observed was for the level of injury, in which there was an overrepresentation in the subgroup individuals with paraplegic (A/B/C) injuries ($\chi^2(3) = 15.44$, $p = 0.001$, $V = 0.155$).

At admission, 46% ($n = 124$) of participants with admission and discharge data demonstrated psychological need by scoring above the threshold on at least one of the screening measures. By discharge, 42% ($n = 115$) still scored above the threshold on at least one of the measures. The total scores for those with both admission and discharge measures across samples are presented in Table 3. The admission and discharge severity classifications for the PHQ-9 and GAD-7 are presented in Table 4 and Figure 2a–c. Psychometric properties for all three measures are shown in Table 5.

Table 3. Participant PHQ-9, GAD-7 and ADAPSSsf score across samples for those with admission and discharge measures.

	Mean (St. Dev.)			
	NSIC	MCSI	YRSIC	Combined
PHQ-9 total—admission	6.26 (5.73)	5.41 (5.21)	8.23 (6.95)	6.33 (5.80)
PHQ-9 total—discharge	5.35 (5.98)	2.89 (3.41)	6.30 (5.46)	5.19 (5.77)
GAD-7 total—admission	4.23 (5.14)	3.75 (4.67)	5.22 (6.19)	4.27 (5.18)
GAD-7 total—discharge	3.84 (5.09)	2.59 (4.03)	4.04 (3.07)	3.74 (4.85)
ADAPSSsf total—admission	19.44 (6.77)	20.42 (6.31)	18.55 (7.13)	19.46 (6.75)
ADAPSSsf total—discharge	19.28 (6.47)	17.50 (5.83)	18.14 (6.80)	19.01 (6.44)

For the combined sample, there was a small underrepresentation of people with incomplete ASIA D injuries scoring above the GAD-7 threshold at discharge ($\chi^2(2) = 11.90$, $p = 0.003$, $V = 0.210$). However, there were no other significant differences for those scoring above compared with below the threshold for either the PHQ-9, GAD-7 or ADAPSSsf with respect to sex, ethnicity or cause of injury.

Table 4. PHQ-9 and GAD-7 severity classifications for combined sample for those with admission and discharge measures.

		Combined Sample N (%)	
		Admission	Discharge
PHQ-9 severity	Total N	266	270
	Sub-clinical	126 (47)	157 (58)
	Mild depression	71 (27)	63 (23)
	Moderate depression	41 (15)	29 (11)
	Moderately severe depression	18 (7)	11 (4)
	Severe depression	10 (4)	10 (4)
GAD-7 severity	Total N	267	269
	Sub-clinical anxiety	174 (65)	181 (67)
	Mild anxiety	44 (17)	50 (19)
	Moderate anxiety	32 (12)	26 (10)
	Severe anxiety	17 (6)	12 (4)

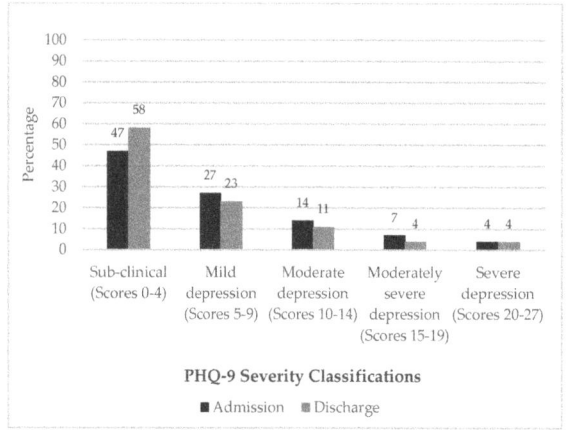

(a)

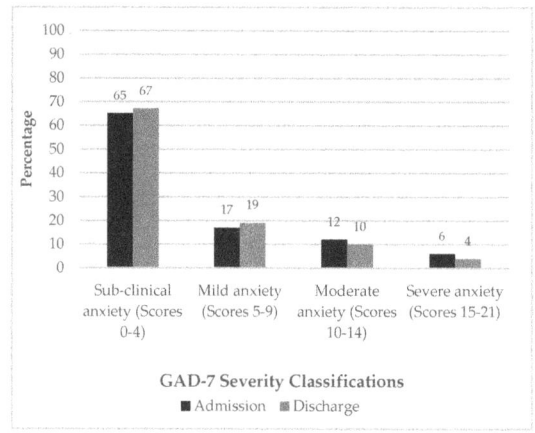

(b)

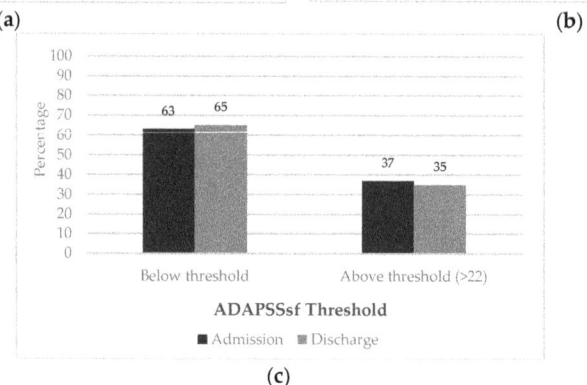

(c)

Figure 2. Combined sample percentage severity classifications at admission and discharge for (**a**) PHQ-9, (**b**) GAD-7 and (**c**) ADAPSSsf.

Table 5. Psychometric properties for combined sample for those with admission and discharge measures.

		Combined Sample N (% Excluding Missing Values)	
		Admission	Discharge
Psychometrics	PHQ-9	266	270
	GAD-7	267	269
	ADAPSSsf	267	267
Above threshold	PHQ-9	61 (23)	38 (14)
	GAD-7	60 (23)	44 (16)
	ADAPSSsf	98 (37)	94 (35)
		Combined Sample Mean (St. Dev.)	
		Admission	Discharge
PHQ-9	Above threshold	15.11 (3.83)	16.68 (4.65)
	Below threshold	3.72 (3.08)	3.31 (3.17)
GAD-7	Above threshold	12.63 (3.63)	12.89 (4.05)
	Below threshold	1.84 (2.15)	1.95 (2.31)
ADAPSSsf	Above threshold	26.49 (3.73)	25.72 (3.63)
	Below threshold	15.38 (4.30)	15.36 (4.37)

There were no significant differences in age at injury nor time since injury between the combined samples. However, participants scoring above the threshold at admission on the GAD-7 had a significantly longer time since injury (M_{above} = 0.48, M_{below} = 0.33), ($F(1265) = 8.54$, $p = 0.004$). Those scoring above threshold on the PHQ-9 at discharge were significantly younger at injury (M_{above} = 48.71, M_{below} = 57.45), ($F(1268) = 9.01$, $p = 0.003$). Similarly, those scoring above threshold on the GAD-7 at discharge had a significantly younger age at injury (M_{above} = 49.48, M_{below} = 57.33), ($F(1267) = 8.23$, $p = 0.004$).

The mean PHQ-9 score at admission ($M = 6.33$) was significantly greater than the mean score at discharge ($M = 5.19$), ($t = 3.36$, $p = 0.001$). However, there were no significant mean differences at admission compared with discharge for either the GAD-7 or the ADAPSSsf.

3.3. Regression Analyses

For the subgroup that contained admission and discharge measures, a multiple linear regression was calculated to determine whether the admission psychometric score or any demographic variables were predictive of the discharge score (Table 6). A priori power analysis indicated that a multiple regression with seven predictor variables would require a sample size of 142 to achieve a medium effect size of 0.15 with a significant criterion of $\alpha < 0.01$ and power = 0.80. Thus, the obtained sample size of subgroup participants ($n = 272$) exceeded this minimum requirement.

A higher admission score ($M = 6.32$, $SD = 5.81$) for the PHQ-9, higher level of injury (*Mode* = paraplegic A/B/C) and younger age at injury ($M = 56.28$, $SD = 16.90$) were significantly associated with a higher discharge score and explained approximately 38% of the variance ($F(7257) = 18.186$, $p < 0.001$, $R^2 = 0.331$). Similarly, the multiple regression for the GAD-7 was significant, with a higher admission score ($M = 3.80$, $SD = 4.88$), younger age at injury ($M = 56.14$, $SD = 16.80$) and higher level of injury (*Mode* = paraplegic A/B/C) predicting a higher discharge score and explained 38% of the variance ($F(7256) = 22.813$, $p < 0.001$, $R^2 = 0.384$). The strongest relationship was found for the ADAPSSsf, in which only the admission score ($M = 19.49$, $SD = 6.76$) explained 39% of the variance in the discharge score ($F(7256) = 23.760$, $p < 0.001$, $R^2 = 0.394$).

Table 6. Multiple regression on the predictive relationship between admission scores and demographic variables on discharge score for the PHQ-9, GAD-7 and ADAPPsf.

		Beta	SE	95% CI LB	95% CI UB	β	p
PHQ-9	Admission score	0.493	0.052	0.390	0.596	0.493	<0.001 *
	Level of injury	−1.243	0.410	−2.051	−0.435	−0.160	0.003 *
	Age at injury	−0.053	0.019	−0.090	−0.016	−0.154	0.005 *
	Ethnicity	−0.135	0.145	−0.422	0.151	−0.049	0.352
	Cause of injury	0.379	0.609	−0.820	1.577	0.033	0.534
	Time since injury	0.348	0.844	−1.315	2.011	0.022	0.681
	Sex	−0.090	0.662	−1.393	1.213	0.007	0.892
GAD-7	Admission score	0.473	0.048	0.379	0.567	0.504	<0.001 *
	Level of injury	−1.172	0.330	−1.822	−0.522	−0.181	<0.001 *
	Age at injury	−0.054	0.015	−0.084	−0.024	−0.186	<0.001 *
	Ethnicity	−0.072	0.118	−0.304	0.160	−0.031	0.541
	Cause of injury	0.533	0.491	−0.435	1.501	0.055	0.279
	Time since injury	0.724	0.688	−0.630	2.078	0.053	0.293
	Sex	0.245	0.532	−0.802	1.292	0.023	0.645
ADAPPsf	Admission score	0.574	0.047	0.481	0.667	0.604	<0.001 *
	Level of injury	−0.768	0.434	−0.89	−1.622	0.086	0.078
	Age at injury	0.004	0.020	−0.035	0.043	0.010	0.839
	Ethnicity	0.220	0.153	−0.81	0.521	0.072	0.152
	Cause of injury	0.028	0.641	−1.235	1.291	0.002	0.965
	Time since injury	0.991	0.896	−0.773	2.755	0.056	0.270
	Sex	0.012	0.687	−1.341	1.366	0.001	0.986

Note: * indicates significance.

4. Discussion

This study aimed to understand the incidence of psychological need following PwSCI/D's admission to specialist SCIC rehabilitation and at discharge. Additionally, this study sought to consider whether the current referral model used across most of the SCICs commissioned by NHS England should remain or whether all services should move to a mixed model of screening and referral, with screening being incorporated within routine psychological assessment on admission and intervention aligned with the matched collaborative care pathway.

A key finding was that between 43 and 46% (depending on whether the combined or subset data were used) of inpatients were above the threshold on at least one of the screening measures, indicating their psychological needs following admission to an SCIC. This was slightly higher than a prior study, which found that 32% of participants scored above the threshold on at least one measure [1]; however, the current study used the PHQ-9 and GAD-7 rather than the HADS and included data from three rather than one SCIC. Focussing specifically on the PHQ-9 and the GAD-7, 23% of individuals scored above the threshold on each measure, which very strongly supported the 22% occurrence of above-threshold symptoms of depression reported across a meta-analysis of 21 studies [44], and 21% occurrence for above threshold symptoms of anxiety in a cross-cultural combined inpatient and community study [43]. Additionally, and comparative to the current retrospective findings, a prospective study tracking inpatients from admission to discharge and through to community living found that the rate of any diagnosed mental disorder was 21.8% at admission and 17.3% at discharge from rehabilitation [45].

Compared with the measures that screen for mood, a higher occurrence of psychological need was evidenced for the ADAPSSsf, with 35% of individuals presenting with suspected adjustment difficulties. The inclusion of the ADAPSSsf in this study enhanced and underlined the fact that "the absence of mood disturbance is not necessarily an indicator of adjustment to SCI/D, as this is a complex process that develops as the person experiences new events and understanding of their condition and can take substantial time following transition into the community" [46] ("Interventions for Mental Health Disorders" section). This suggests that to best support the psychological health of PwSCI/D, screening must go beyond merely considering mood by recognising the significance of adjustment following injury and the complex and ever-developing interplay of each. Indeed, research by Guest et al. (2015) argued that even individuals who demonstrate resilience nevertheless continue to face significant challenges of daily living and adjustment to severe injury and its associated lifelong impairment [47]. Echoing the 35% estimated occurrence of adjustment problems in the current sample, Guest and colleagues (2015) similarly suggested that "a large minority of participants (just over 30%) remain highly vulnerable to problems such as maladaptive coping, hopelessness, and negativity in the longer term" [47] (p. 685).

A crucial outcome from this study was that admission scores on all three measures were predictive of the scores at discharge, suggesting that individuals' degree of psychological need upon entry to an SCIC will influence psychological health outcomes during their rehabilitation and through to discharge. This strongly supports the recommendations for SCICs and other providers to include early and routine psychometric screening as part of the psychological assessment and alongside referral to ensure individuals with psychological needs are recognised. The findings are augmented by previous research suggesting poorer physical rehabilitation outcomes if psychological needs are unrecognised [1], as well as early mortality and long-term adjustment difficulties from symptoms of depression and anxiety at 12 weeks following injury [5,48].

There was a significant reduction in PHQ-9 scores by discharge, which is similar to the findings by Craig et al. (2015) [45]. However, Kennedy et al.'s (2016) longitudinal study found that symptoms of depression and anxiety increased as discharge approached [5], and indeed the current study also revealed that individuals scoring above the PHQ-9 threshold at admission had higher mean scores at discharge. It is important to note the different contextual framework from Kennedy et al. (2016), whose discharge data from an SCIC were collected prior to 1995. Since this date, SCICs have seen the introduction of surgical intervention rather than conservative management, as well as recent demographic changes in the representation of "non-traumatic injuries", which may reflect some differences in results. A limiting factor in the current study was that psychological intervention was unable to be controlled for during the analyses, which may have accounted for the decrease in depression symptoms by discharge. However, if this were solely responsible for the change in scores, a significant reduction in the scores for the GAD-7 and ADAPSSsf might also have been expected. It is important to acknowledge that discharge from rehabilitation occurs at a time when a physical outcome is achieved rather than guided by psychological variables and that psychological adjustment often takes much longer and can be significantly delayed and influenced by someone's understanding of their condition and needs following the resumption of community living [46]. This underlines the importance of screening at regular follow-up reviews, as recommended in the USA [14], Australian [19] and current study's standards (Appendix A) and again reiterates the complexity of psychological need following a spinal cord injury, i.e., it encompasses more than simply the presence versus absence of mood disorder and very rarely follows a linear process. Indeed, the research on trajectories following spinal cord injury provides insight into the varying presentations, with Craig et al. (2019), Bombardier et al. (2021), Bonnano et al. (2012) and van Leeuwen et al. (2012) identifying different pathways for symptoms of depression and anxiety, including a "delayed" pathway in which individuals initially present below the threshold for depression or anxiety but deteriorate to clinical levels over time [4,15,36,49]. A previous study conducted at the NSIC at Stoke Mandeville found that although the patients' moods and ADAPSSsf scores improved by discharge, there was a deterioration in both at the 18-month follow-up [50].

Also identified was that those scoring above the threshold on the PHQ-9 and the GAD-7 at discharge were significantly younger at injury and that younger age at injury was predictive of psychometric measures at discharge. While this only accounted for an approximately 10-year mean age difference (48 years compared with 57 years), this finding may be useful to identify individuals at greater risk of mood disturbance. Indeed, prior research identified an inverse "U-shaped curve" regarding age and depression symptoms in individuals both with and without disability such that middle-aged individuals report more severe depression symptoms than either younger or older individuals [51]. As such, sustaining an injury when approaching middle age compared with later may facilitate or exacerbate depression symptoms in an already at-risk population. Another theory is that individuals with a younger age at injury could be behind their older counterparts in relation to employment, finances, and retirement planning, and therefore may be less prepared for such an adjustment and more susceptible to low mood disturbance. Hirsh et al. (2009) found that PwSCI/D aged between 45 and 54 were more likely to be employed following injury compared with the group aged between 55 and 64, which perhaps lends support to the theory that early middle-aged individuals still rely on the financial security of employment prior to retirement [52].

A finding specific to anxiety in the current study was that the participants who scored above the threshold at admission on the GAD-7 had a significantly longer time since injury. The major trauma pathway model states that inpatients should be admitted to SCIC rehabilitation about 1–2 weeks after injury, whereas the current sample had a delay of between 2 and 4 months, which can be understood in the context of the NHS England annual report regarding capacity issues discussed in the introduction. From this study, it is unclear when symptoms of anxiety developed and whether the symptoms were associated with a delay in admission. Systematic screening prior to SCIC admission by major trauma centres, which is one of the recommendations of the standards (Appendix A), would help to illuminate this. Anecdotal accounts from inpatients after SCIC admission and major trauma centre colleagues indicate concerns from inpatients about whether specialist SCIC services would be able to be accessed at all and a sense from the MDT in major trauma centres that inpatients are unable to fully engage in therapies as they wait for the highly prized specialised rehabilitation, as well as an assumption that patients express improved functional outcome from admission to such services, all of which could account for the results found in this study.

As identified in the introduction, screening in other conditions has led to pathway and service developments, including the identification of the need for an increased workforce [53]. In the short-term, screening in resource-constrained services may help to support more effective deployment of psychological resources. However, as commented, this would need to include screening for other variables, such as appraisals, as identified in the current study, as well as a range of other factors, rather than an over-reliance on mood measures to identify adjustment difficulties. Alongside this should be recognition that a range of psychological interventions are needed to face the challenge of such a life-changing event as an SCI/D [54]. Nevertheless, screening and retrospective analysis of referral data [34] have enabled the NSIC at Stoke Mandeville to engage in a "watchful wait" for those who were above the clinical threshold on either the PHQ-9, GAD-7 or ADAPSSsf, allowing for the mitigation of service constraints by providing group-based psychoeducation and through discussion of management and support strategies with MDT colleagues. More recently, the service has taken this a step further and aims to commence a "triage" for all admissions to augment screening and help identify those most in need of psychological assessment [55]. However, there is an accompanying acknowledgement that because of resource constraints, the likely corollary would be the reduction in the frequency of treatment sessions for those identified.

This study also highlights the variation in service provision across the three SCICs involved despite the introduction of screening, which emphasises the need for standards relating to psychological assessment and treatment, and the embedding of these within clinical practice to accompany the introduction of screening. The introduction to this paper identified the need for international rehabilitation standards and the consequent impact on psychological care. The World Health Organisation 2030 Package of Rehabilitation Interventions, which outlines a range of rehabilitation standards, including psychological guidance, for services and health ministries across the world, will significantly contribute to future service development and parity [56]. The systematic introduction of screening will aid many resource-constrained services to evidence the psychological needs and impact on service provision for PwSCI/D. This may include, as two of the SCICs in the current study demonstrated, MDT colleagues administering psychological health screening. As identified in the Netherlands, screening enhanced non-psychologist rehabilitation members' appreciation of psychological issues [21]. Bombardier et al.'s (2021) comprehensive overview of screening and intervention includes guidance regarding how MDT colleagues can structure rehabilitation for those identified with mood difficulties and are highly applicable when qualified psychological resources are lacking [14].

Limitations and Suggestions for Future Research

The current study sought to increase the generalisability of findings by examining data from three SCICs in England. Although there were some demographic differences between the samples, overall, these were small and limited in influence due to the large sample size. However, there was a significant amount of missing data for ethnicity in the NSIC and MCSI samples, which may have contributed to the findings of over-representation of "White" participants in the YRSIC sample. The high proportion of missing data may have also contributed to the lack of significant variation accounted for in discharge psychometric scores. This absence is concerning in several regards in relation to the efficacy of screening. In a study assessing rehabilitation outcome using the SMS-NAC, skills in the domains of physical healthcare and psychological healthcare were self-rated as lower for "Black" than "White" individuals on admission, indicating lesser self-perceived levels of knowledge and independence in these areas [57]. This finding was maintained at discharge, with the addition of lowered self-rated outcomes in community preparation for "Black" individuals. Outcomes on discharge for "White" individuals were also self-rated as significantly higher in the physical healthcare domain than those who identified as "Asian". Potential differences between ethnic groups are, therefore, of significant importance for both clinicians and researchers to consider in relation to rehabilitation provision and further emphasises the need for psychological screening and routine assessment to identify where issues may reduce someone's ability to engage and participate and impact their outcome.

The combined datasets across SCICs resulted in a large sample size. However, the subgroup with admission and discharge data was restricted in number due to a large proportion of missing discharge measures which led to difference within the aetiology of injury in the MCSI and YRSIC samples compared to national data. However, the proportions of traumatic and non-traumatic injuries in the combined sample were consistent with the annual report data, and the comparable occurrence of psychological need between the combined and sub-dataset of admission and discharge, as well as with prior research, should restore confidence in the results. Nonetheless, the reduction in completed measures at discharge emphasises the limited workforce capacity across SCIC psychology services; this causes a gap in resourcing, which is subsequently disrupting the regular recording of psychological and rehabilitation outcomes and requires consideration for the embedding of the screening and standards across the NHS England SCICs. In addition to limiting services' ability to accurately evaluate outcomes, PwSCI/D are at risk of unidentified psychological and/or rehabilitation needs negatively affecting adjustment and transition to community living.

Allied with this, participants who were not administered psychometric measures at admission were only recorded by the YRSIC sample, and even then, a large number did not provide a reason for the lack of data ($n = 42$). It was not possible, therefore, to determine whether certain groups were at greater risk of being missed, for example, short-stay admissions.

The current findings demonstrated the predictive influence of admission score on discharge score across all three measures. However, the level of injury also had a negative predictive effect on the discharge score for the measures that screened for mood such that people with higher levels of injury had higher depression and anxiety scores at discharge. This is in contrast to previous research that indicated the negligible influence of the level of injury on either depression or anxiety severity [58,59]. As such, the conflicting evidence requires further review.

A key limitation in the current study was that psychological treatment was not able to be controlled for during the analysis due to the retrospective design, which future research should consider. The influence of psychological intervention in relation to improvements in mood and appraisals from admission to discharge would have been useful to examine. Additionally, systematic screening compared with referral data could have further elucidated the need for model change. In addition, though out of scope for the current study, is the consideration of length of stay for individuals who screen positive/receive a psychological intervention, with recent research suggesting comparatively longer hospital admissions for people who screened positive on measures of mood and appraisals compared with those who did not [1]. Additionally, a limitation of the current study, and an area of much-needed research, is to focus not only on screening for those admitted for first-time rehabilitation but also on the needs of those who age with injury [60] and who undergo earlier physical decline associated with their injury than non-injured counterparts [61]. The recommendations of the standards and screening are for across the lifespan, and thus, it is hoped that this will be addressed in time. Indeed, another key area for the future is to survey across the system knowledge and implementation of the standards [62].

While the current findings were important for identifying mood and appraisals for PwSCI/D, future guidance and screening should also examine a range of other psychological concerns, and readers are directed to the work currently being undertaken as part of the ISCoS Advanced Psychological Dataset. The introduction of screening in the NHS England SCICs also included assessing pain, and future research should consider this area alongside mood and appraisals. Had pain data been included in the current sample, it could have illuminated the effect of pain on psychological needs, which would have added to the robustness of the findings. Additionally, this would have enabled clinicians and MDT to be more aware of the complex dynamic between pain and psychological need to better support PwSCI/D during rehabilitation [48].

5. Conclusions

This study has provided support for NHS England SCIC psychological services to systematically move to a screen and routine assessment model, with the inclusion of referral options for those whose needs change over time and/or present with difficulties outside the remit of screening. There is a range of evidence from other conditions supporting the advantages of such developments, though the scale of the task and embedding of the standards is significant given the current staffing variation across SCICs. This study also supports the adoption of screening across the system in recognition of the capacity demands in NHS England and the consideration of screening and standards for psychological care by the wider SCIPAG and the worldwide psychology community.

6. Patents

The Stoke Mandeville Spinal Needs Assessment Checklist (SMS-NAC) is the intellectual property of and invention of the Department of Clinical Psychology of the National Spinal Injuries Centre, Stoke Mandeville Hospital, Buckinghamshire Healthcare NHS Trust, Aylesbury, UK (UK Copyright Services Registration Number 284732791). The NSIC Psychological Care Pathway is the intellectual property of the Department of Clinical Psychology of the National Spinal Injuries Centre, Stoke Mandeville Hospital, Buckinghamshire Healthcare NHS Trust, Aylesbury, UK (UK Copyright Services Registration Number 284734611), and provided the basis for the Psychological Health and Wellbeing Matched Collaborative Care Intervention Pathway (Supplementary Table S1). Please contact bht.nsicpsychology@nhs.net to seek permission for use.

Supplementary Materials: The following supporting information can be downloaded from https://www.mdpi.com/article/10.3390/jcm12247667/s1, Figure S1: Preadmission Outreach Pathway; Table S1: Psychological Health and Wellbeing Matched Collaborative Care Intervention Pathway; Table S2: SCI MDT Education Curriculum.

Author Contributions: Conceptualisation, J.D., R.E. and S.K.; methodology, J.D., R.E., S.K. and L.C.G.; formal analysis, L.C.G.; writing—original draft preparation, J.D. and L.C.G.; writing—review and editing, J.D., R.E., S.K. and L.C.G. All authors read and agreed to the published version of the manuscript.

Funding: This research received no external funding.

Institutional Review Board Statement: This study was conducted in accordance with the Declaration of Helsinki and approved by the NHS England Health Research Authority (protocol code 331385, approved 18 August 2023).

Informed Consent Statement: The data in the paper were collected as part of routine service evaluation and were used to improve patient care and for future research. Therefore, individual written inpatient consent was not required.

Data Availability Statement: The data used in the current study were part of a standard clinical database that contains identifiable patient information and are, therefore, not publicly available. Anonymised data can be made available upon reasonable request to Buckinghamshire Healthcare NHS Trust.

Acknowledgments: We thank all participants whose screening data were used in this research and the respective research teams for their support with ethical data transfer. We thank and acknowledge the contribution of a range of people in this work: Andy Masters, the Back Up Trust; Dave Bracher, the Spinal Injuries Association; Nigel Wainwright, YRSIC; Jenny Moses, Welsh Spinal Injuries Centre; current and past members of SCIPAG. Thanks also to the Psychological and Mental Health Workstream members and David Cummings for his conceptualisation and leadership of the seven transformation workstreams. We acknowledge the contribution of past and present colleagues in the NSIC Department of Clinical Psychology, in particular Amy Black's support with revisions for this study, and the wider NSIC team at Stoke Mandeville Hospital.

Conflicts of Interest: The authors declare no conflict of interest.

Abbreviation

Acronym description and short explanation.

Acronym	Meaning
ADAPPSsf	Appraisals of DisAbility Primary and Secondary Scale short form. This is a six-item scale that assesses a participant's appraisal of their injury and provides an indication of adjustment to SCI/D and screens for a full-scale version
CPG	Clinical Practice Guideline
CRG	Clinical Reference Group, which oversees the service provision for a range of health conditions for NHS England and sets the service specification and standards for care
EBM	Evidence-based medicine
GAD-7	General Anxiety Disorder-7 is a seven-item measure used to assess the presence of anxiety symptoms
ISCoS	The International Spinal Cord Society
MCSI	Midlands Centre for Spinal Injuries
MDT	Multidisciplinary Team
NHS	National Health Service, which is the universal health care provider in the UK; the NHS provision is devolved into separate bodies for England, Wales, Scotland and Northern Ireland
NICE	National Institute for Health and Care Excellence is an overarching body that creates recommendations for treatment protocols and medication
NSIC	National Spinal Injuries Centre at Stoke Mandeville
PHQ-9	Patient Health Questionnaire is a nine-item measure used to assess the presence of depression symptoms
PwSCI/D	People with spinal cord injuries/disorders
SCI/D	Spinal cord injuries/disorders
SCICs	Spinal cord injury centres provide inpatient rehabilitation in the UK
SCIPAG	UK and Ireland Spinal Cord Injury Psychology Advisory Group review and promote psychological service provision and care standards across the SCICs
SIG	Special interest group
SMS-NAC	Stoke Mandeville Spinal Needs Assessment Checklist, which is used to assess inpatient's knowledge, skills, and physical or verbal independence across 10 domains of rehabilitation for SCI/D
YRSIC	Yorkshire Regional Spinal Injuries Centre

Appendix A. Standards Recommendations for System-Wide Change with Table

The below information outlines the mental health standards for implementation in UK Spinal Cord Injury Services. Table A1 also highlights the timeline for implementation of the standards and relevant citations.

Standards:

1. Adoption across all providers of a matched collaborative care pathway (see also Supplementary Table S1). The NSIC Stoke Mandeville Psychological Care Pathway (UK Copyright Service 284734611) proposed foundation needs for all PwSCI/D and identified the need for a clinician and peer-facilitated coping effectiveness group intervention to aid self-management, alongside psychoeducation and consideration of psychosexual and family counselling, with four specific interventions depending on needs [63]. The workstream enhanced this by adding screening thresholds for the interventions and renamed it the "psychological health and wellbeing matched collaborative care intervention pathway" to aid system-wide adoption and comparison between SCICs and others in the pathway regarding complexity and workforce need.
2. Adoption across all providers of an MDT curriculum, with basic (Level 1) skills needed by all healthcare professionals who have contact with PwSCI/D, with someone trained to advanced (Level 2) skills within each team/clinical area (Supplementary Table S2).
3. A preadmission outreach pathway to ensure the parity of admission for people with complex mental health needs (Supplementary Figure S1).

4. Implementation of psychological health screening on admission, discharge, readmission and outpatient review across the sector.
5. The workstream acknowledged the variety of resourcing across the SCICs and other providers as a limiting factor for the implementation of the standards. Therefore, it was recommended that all services be resourced similarly and to at least the staffing of the current best ratio (London SCIC 1:15) and/or aligned with other SCI providers in the network, such as neurorehabilitation services given the complexity of need [64]. The workstream anticipated that some services would be nonadherent because of staffing variation and recommended yearly audits by SCIPAG/peer review, and where service gaps are identified, an action plan should be implemented.
6. The workstream recommended support to consult, finalise and publish the broader evidence-based standards that had been commenced by SCIPAG.
7. Three key areas for development were identified across the sector:
    i. SCIC Outpatient Services—The workstream referenced the need for psychological support for adjustment to injury to be about 40% (not including those referred to community mental health services) and noted the high prevalence of persistent pain and the current gap in services for PwSCI/D [50,65]. The workstream recommended the development of an MDT clinic and estimated that 60–70% of people presenting with persistent pain would need an associated psychological review.
    ii. Traumatic Brain Injury (TBI) provision within SCICs. The workstream acknowledged that whilst SCICs manage the needs of those with co-morbid mild TBIs, those with more severe injuries often fall between neurorehabilitation and SCI/D rehabilitation services. Recommended future development should focus on (a) scoping local services and developing links, providing an integrated pathway for those with moderate TBI and SCI/D by embedding neuro-rehabilitation expertise within SCICs and vice versa, including joint training events and rotational arrangements for therapists and nurses in the first instance, and (b) progress to the employment of staff skilled in managing moderate TBI in SCICs.
    iii. Psychiatry provision. The workstream recommended the following: (a) services should foster links with local specialist mental health services, particularly liaison psychiatry services; (b) have service level arrangements with or embed liaison psychiatry services within SCI/D services; (c) improve the training of staff to better manage mental health complexity on SCI/D units through the adoption of the MDT curriculum identified (Supplementary Table S2); (d) arrange collaborative and parallel working practices for people with co-occurring complex mental health and spinal cord injury rehabilitation needs, such as repatriation arrangements; (e) agree on responsible clinician arrangements with local specialist services for people detained under the Mental Health Act [66]; and (f) the development of wheelchair-accessible services across mental health units for PwSCI/D.

Table A1. Quality standards summary and timings for implementation.

Timing	Quality Standard Summary	References
Onset of injury/acute care	Psychological health screen (PHQ-5) within 4 weeks of injury.	[14,18,64,67,68]
	Assessment prior to SCIC/rehabilitation transfer to include screening measures and structured clinical interview with information about known mental health and forensic history, any barriers or additional needs for engagement in rehabilitation, and past and present mental health professional involvement. To be completed where relevant: MOCA, AMTS, 6CIT or another recognised cognitive test if the person has a pre-existing or current cognitive impairment. An assessment of alcohol, tobacco, and recreational drug history and current use. A mental capacity assessment.	[14,18,67,69,70]

Table A1. Cont.

Timing	Quality Standard Summary	References
	Amendment of the NHS England Database to recategorise the current category "mental health" and instead categorise using self-harm/suicide attempt/neglect, severe and enduring mental health/psychosis/schizophrenia, depression/anxiety, substance use, neurodevelopmental diagnosis or dementia.	-
	Implement pre-admission outreach flowchart across SCICs and yearly audit of its use by SCIPAG/peer review.	-
Admission to SCIC/rehabilitation	All inpatients to have access to specialist evidence-based psychological treatment intervention and include trauma-based intervention.	[14–18,20,25,26,63,64,67,68,70–74]
	Implementation of the psychometric screening measures across all parts of the pathway and for all levels and completeness of SCI/D.	[14,17,18,67]
	Implementation of the Psychological Health and Wellbeing Matched Collaborative Care Intervention Pathway (Supplementary Table S1) across SCICs and service provision alignment. Yearly audit of implementation and complexity of inpatient needs.	[63,69,71]
	Documented pathway for access to liaison psychiatry and other specialist services.	[14,18,20,25,26,63,64,67,69,73,75–77]
	Outcome comparison by SCIC and other services to track group trajectory profiles by complexity with revision of pathway as required.	-
	Initial contact from a psychosocial team member within 5 days of inpatient admission.	[14,18,67,71]
	Inpatient access to specialist psychological assessment and therapy within 10 working days of admission and include psychological health screen with psychometrically validated tools.	[14–16,18,20,63,67,69,70,73,75–78]
	Where suicidality is present, risk assessment, personal safety plan and treatment plan are to be established.	[14,18,48,67,73,77]
	Where motivation/engagement/progress in rehabilitation is limiting progress/change, psychological assessment and intervention should be provided.	[14,15,18,71,75]
	Peer support and peer mentoring should be available for all inpatients and the psychosocial care team leading on recruitment and organisation of this model within the SCIC.	[18,20,25,26,63,64,67,70,73]
	Provision of support services for the psychological/emotional needs of families/carers, including referrals.	[18,25,26,63,64,69,71,73]
	Adoption of the SCI MDT Education Curriculum (Supplementary Table S2) to align healthcare clinicians working in SCICs to be able to identify and support patients' psychosocial needs, e.g., mood, adjustment issues, risk, substance use, cognition, and behaviours that challenge and know how to escalate for specialist psychological intervention as needed. All staff to have basic (Tier 1) skills and some staff to have advanced (Tier 2) skills.	[14,18,63,67,69,71,73,78]
	Inpatients, families and carers are to be offered support on self-management skills and empowered to advocate for their needs and seek support.	[15,18,64,67,71,73,76,78]
Discharge from rehabilitation	Psychological health psychometric screening and psychological assessment are to be repeated prior to discharge.	[14,18,25,26,67,69,73,78]
	Comprehensive psychological discharge planning, including referrals to relevant services.	[14,18,25,26,67,69,73]
	Onward referral made as required to the BackUp Trust peer mentoring or Spinal Injuries Association counselling service.	[18,64]
Follow-up	Psychological health screen (PHQ-4) and substance/alcohol use screen to take place across four time points/ranges: 6–12 weeks post-discharge, 6 months, annually for 5 years, and then every 2 years or as required.	[14,16,18,25,26,64,67,69,70,78]
SCIC/ hospital readmission	All secondary rehabilitation admissions of PwSCI/D are to be administered a short form psychological health screen (PHQ-4). A referral is to be made to the SCIC psychological services for full assessment if there is a positive screen.	[14,18,67,71,73,77]

References

1. Wallace, M.; Duff, J.; Grant, L.C. The influence of psychological need on rehabilitation outcomes for people with spinal cord injury. *Spinal Cord* **2023**, *61*, 83–92. [CrossRef] [PubMed]
2. Strøm, J.; Bjerrum, M.B.; Nielsen, C.V.; Thisted, C.N.; Nielsen, T.L.; Laursen, M.; Jørgensen, L.B. Anxiety and depression in spine surgery-a systematic integrative review. *Spine J.* **2018**, *18*, 1272–1285. [CrossRef]
3. van Diemen, T.; Crul, T.; van Nes, I.; SELF-SCI Group; Geertzen, J.H.; Post, M.W. Associations between self-efficacy and secondary health conditions in people living with spinal cord injury: A systematic review and meta-analysis. *Arch. Phys. Med. Rehabil.* **2017**, *98*, 2566–2577. [CrossRef] [PubMed]
4. Craig, A.; Tran, Y.; Guest, R.; Middleton, J. Trajectories of self-efficacy and depressed mood and their relationship in the first 12 months following spinal cord injury. *Arch. Phys. Med. Rehabil.* **2019**, *100*, 441–447. [CrossRef] [PubMed]
5. Kennedy, P.; Kilvert, A.; Hasson, L. A 21-year longitudinal analysis of impact, coping, and appraisals following spinal cord injury. *Rehabil. Psychol.* **2016**, *61*, 92–101. [CrossRef]
6. Psychological Professions Network. Maximising the Impact of Psychological Practice in Physical Healthcare: Discussion Paper. 2020. Available online: https://www.ppn.nhs.uk/resources/ppn-publications/34-maximising-the-impact-of-psychological-practice-in-physical-healthcare-discussion-paper/file (accessed on 4 September 2023).
7. Nichols, K. *Psychological Care for Ill and Injured People—A Clinical Guide*; Open University Press: Maidenhead, UK, 2003.
8. Nichols, K. Why is psychology still failing the average patient? *Psychologist* **2005**, *18*, 26–27.
9. Wisely, J.A.; Hoyle, E.; Tarrier, N.; Edwards, J. Where to start? Attempting to meet the psychological needs of burned patients. *Burns* **2007**, *33*, 736–746. [CrossRef] [PubMed]
10. Holland, J.C. Preliminary guidelines for the treatment of distress. *Oncology* **1997**, *11*, 109–114.
11. Grassi, L.; Caruso, R.; Sabato, S.; Massarenti, S.; Nanni, M.G.; The UniFe Psychiatry Working Group Coauthors. Psychosocial screening and assessment in oncology and palliative care settings. *Front. Psychol.* **2015**, *5*, 1485. [CrossRef]
12. National Institute for Clinical Excellence. *Improving Supportive and Palliative Care for Adults with Cancer: The Manual*; Guidance on Cancer Services; National Institute for Clinical Excellence: London, UK, 2004; ISBN 1-84257-579-1. Available online: https://www.nice.org.uk/guidance/csg4/resources/improving-supportive-and-palliative-care-for-adults-with-cancer-pdf-773375005 (accessed on 10 August 2023).
13. Psychological Services for Stroke Survivors and Their Families. In *The British Psychological Society, Division of Clinical Psychology and Division of Neuropsychology*; Briefing Paper No. 19; British Psychological Society: Leicester, UK, 2002.
14. Bombardier, C.H.; Azuero, C.B.; Fann, J.R.; Kautz, D.D.; Richards, J.S.; Sabharwal, S. Management of mental health disorders, substance use disorders, and suicide in adults with spinal cord injury: Clinical practice guideline for healthcare providers. *Top. Spinal Cord Inj. Rehabil.* **2021**, *27*, 152–224. [CrossRef]
15. Huston, T.; Gassaway, J.; Wilson, C.; Gordon, S.; Koval, J.; Schwebel, A. Psychology treatment time during inpatient spinal cord injury rehabilitation. *J. Spinal Cord Med.* **2011**, *34*, 196–204. [CrossRef]
16. Russell, H.F.; Richardson, E.J.; Bombardier, C.H.; Dixon, T.M.; Huston, T.A.; Rose, J.; Sheaffer, D.; Smith, S.A.; Ullrich, P.M. Professional standards of practice for psychologists, social workers, and counselors in SCI rehabilitation. *J. Spinal Cord Med.* **2016**, *39*, 127–145. [CrossRef] [PubMed]
17. Middleton, J.; Perry, K.N.; Craig, A. A clinical perspective on the need for psychosocial care guidelines in spinal cord injury rehabilitation. *Int. J. Phys. Med. Rehabil.* **2013**, *2*, 226. [CrossRef]
18. Psychosocial Care of Adults with Spinal Cord Injuries Guide. Available online: https://aci.health.nsw.gov.au/__data/assets/pdf_file/0006/891978/ACI-psychosocial-spinal-cord-injury-Recommendations.pdf (accessed on 7 September 2023).
19. NSW State Spinal Cord Injury Service. Strategy for the Psychosocial Care of People with Spinal Cord Injury. In *The Emotional Wellbeing Toolkit: A Clinician's Guide to Working with Spinal Cord Injury*; NSW State Spinal Cord Injury Service: Agency for Clinical Innovation: New South Wales, Australia, 2016. Available online: https://www.aci.health.nsw.gov.au/resources/spinal-cord-injury/psychosocial_strategy/emotional-wellbeing-toolkit (accessed on 10 August 2023).
20. The Asian Spinal Cord Network (ASCoN). Psychosocial Task Force. In *Psychosocial Guidelines in Spinal Cord Rehabilitation*; Jagadamba Press: Lalitpur, Nepal, 2015.
21. Kuiper, H.; van Leeuwen, C.M.C.; Stolwijk-Swüste, J.M.; Mulder, L.; Post, M.W.W. Implementatie van een psychologische screening bij revalidanten met een dwarslaesie. [Implementation of a psychological screening in rehabilitation inpatients with spinal cord injury]. *Ned. Tijdschr. Revalidatiegeneeskunde* **2020**, *42*, 21–25. Available online: https://www.kcrutrecht.nl/wp-content/uploads/2018/10/NTR-2020-5-Publicatie-H.-Kuiper-Implementatie-psych-screening-bij-dwarslaesie.pdf (accessed on 14 August 2023).
22. International Spinal Cord Injury Psychological Functioning Basic Data Set. Available online: https://www.iscos.org.uk/resource/resmgr/psychological_dataset_/psychological_functioning.pdf (accessed on 14 August 2023).
23. Duff, J. *Psychological and Mental Health Needs Standards for Adults with Spinal Cord Injury*; MASCIP, BSPRM, BASCIS: UK, 2023. Available online: https://spinal.co.uk/wp-content/uploads/2023/01/Psychological-and-Mental-Health-Standards-for-Adults-with-SCI-Final-Jan-2023.pdf (accessed on 7 September 2023).
24. Gall, A.; Horne, D.; Kennedy, P.; Turner-Stokes, L.; Tussler, D. *No. 9: Chronic Spinal Cord Injury: Management of Patients in Acute Hospital Settings: National Guidelines*; Concise Guidance to Good Practice; RCP, BSRM, MASCIP and BASCIS, 2008.

25. NHS England Spinal Cord Injury Services (Adults and Children); Specification Number 170119S; NHS: London, UK, 2020. Available online: https://www.england.nhs.uk/wp-content/uploads/2019/04/service-spec-spinal-cord-injury-services-all-ages.pdf (accessed on 7 September 2023).
26. NHS Standard Contract for Spinal Cord Injuries (All Ages), Specification Number D13/S/a, NHS England. Available online: https://www.england.nhs.uk/commissioning/wp-content/uploads/sites/12/2014/04/d13-spinal-cord-0414.pdf (accessed on 7 September 2023).
27. Zigmond, A.S.; Snaith, R.P. The Hospital Anxiety and Depression Scale. *Acta Psychiatr. Scand.* **1983**, *67*, 361–370. [CrossRef] [PubMed]
28. Spitzer, R.L.; Kroenke, K.; Williams, J.B.; Patient Health Questionnaire Primary Care Study Group. Validation and utility of a self-report version of PRIME-MD: The PHQ primary care study. *JAMA* **1999**, *282*, 1737–1744. [CrossRef]
29. Spitzer, R.L.; Kroenke, K.; Williams, J.B.; Löwe, B. A brief measure for assessing generalized anxiety disorder: The GAD-7. *Arch. Intern. Med.* **2006**, *166*, 1092–1097. [CrossRef] [PubMed]
30. NHS England. *National Spinal Cord Injury Database Annual Report*; NHS: London, UK, 2021.
31. Spinal Injuries Association (SIA). Available online: www.spinal.co.uk (accessed on 7 September 2023).
32. *Standards for Specialist Rehabilitation of Spinal Cord Injury*; MASCIP, BSPRM, BASCIS: UK, 2022. Available online: https://www.mascip.co.uk/wp-content/uploads/2022/12/SCIST-FINAL-2022.pdf (accessed on 7 September 2023).
33. Dean, R.E.; Kennedy, P. Measuring appraisals following acquired spinal cord injury: A preliminary psychometric analysis of the appraisals of disability. *Rehabil. Psychol.* **2009**, *54*, 222–231. [CrossRef]
34. Duff, J.; Grant, L.C. How to identify who needs psychological treatment and when: Addressing the gap through screening (*oral*). In Proceedings of the 24th Multidisciplinary Association of Spinal Cord Injury Professionals (MASCIP) Conference, Loughborough, UK, 17 November 2022.
35. Bonanno, G.A.; Kennedy, P.; Galatzer-Levy, I.R.; Lude, P.; Elfström, M.L. Trajectories of resilience, depression, and anxiety following spinal cord injury. *Rehabil. Psychol.* **2012**, *57*, 236–247. [CrossRef]
36. Hajjaj, F.M.; Salek, M.S.; Basra, M.K.; Finlay, A.Y. Non-clinical influences on clinical decision-making: A major challenge to evidence-based practice. *J. R. Soc. Med.* **2010**, *103*, 178–187. [CrossRef]
37. Gilchrist, H.; Grant, L.C.; Saleh, S.; Sarhan, F.; Duff, J. Identifying and meeting the psychological care training needs of healthcare clinicians and third sector partners (*poster*). In Proceedings of the 24th Multidisciplinary Association of Spinal Cord Injury Professionals (MASCIP) Conference, Loughborough, UK, 17 November 2022.
38. Berry, C.; Kennedy, P. A psychometric analysis of the Needs Assessment Checklist. *Spinal Cord* **2002**, *41*, 490–501. [CrossRef] [PubMed]
39. Bombardier, C.; Kalpakjian, C.; Graves, D.; Dyer, J.; Tate, D.; Fann, J. Validity of the Patient Health Questionnaire-9 in assessing major depressive disorder during inpatient spinal cord injury rehabilitation. *Arch. Phys. Med. Rehabil.* **2012**, *93*, 1838–1845. [CrossRef] [PubMed]
40. Russell, M.; Ames, H.; Dunn, C.; Beckwith, S.; Holmes, S.A. Appraisals of disability and psychological adjustment in veterans with spinal cord injuries. *J. Spinal Cord Med.* **2021**, *44*, 956–958. [CrossRef] [PubMed]
41. Roy-Byrne, P.; Veitengrubet, J.P.; Bystrisky, A.; Edlund, M.J.; Sullivan, G.; Craske, M.G.; Shaw Welch, S.; Rose, R.; Stein, M.B. Brief intervention for anxiety in primary care patients. *J. Am. Board Fam. Med.* **2009**, *22*, 175–186. [CrossRef]
42. Coker, J.; Cuthbert, J.; Ketchum, J.M.; Holicky, R.; Huston, R.; Charlifue, S. Re-inventing yourself after spinal cord injury: A site-specific randomized clinical trial. *Spinal Cord* **2019**, *57*, 282–292. [CrossRef] [PubMed]
43. Duff, J.; Grant, L.C.; Coker, J.; Monden, K.R. Anxiety in response to sustaining spinal cord injuries and disorders: When should clinicians be concerned? *Arch. Phys. Med. Rehabil.* **2023**, *104*, 1409–1417. [CrossRef]
44. Williams, R.; Murray, A. Prevalence of depression after spinal cord injury: A meta-analysis. *Arch. Phys. Med. Rehabil.* **2015**, *96*, 133–140. [CrossRef]
45. Craig, A.; Nicholson Perry, K.; Guest, R.; Tran, Y.; Dezarnaulds, A.; Hales, A.; Ephraums, C.; Middleton, J. Prospective study of the occurrence of psychological disorders and comorbidities after spinal cord injury. *Arch. Phys. Med. Rehabil.* **2015**, *96*, 1426–1434. [CrossRef]
46. Duff, J.; Jackson, K.; Bombardier, C.B.; Zebracki, K. Spinal Cord Injuries and Disorders, Chapter 32. In *Oxford Handbook of Rehabilitation Psychology*, 2nd ed.; Meade, M., Wegner, S., Bechtold, K., Eds.; Oxford University Press: Oxford, UK, *in press*.
47. Guest, R.; Craig, A.; Tran, Y.; Middleton, J. Factors predicting resilience in people with spinal cord injury during transition from inpatient rehabilitation to the community. *Spinal Cord* **2015**, *53*, 682–686. [CrossRef]
48. Kennedy, P.; Hasson, L. The relationship between pain and mood following spinal cord injury. *J. Spinal Cord Med.* **2017**, *40*, 275–279. [CrossRef]
49. van Leeuwen, C.M.; Hoekstra, T.; van Koppenhagen, C.F.; de Groot, S.; Post, M.W. Trajectories and predictors of the course of mental health after spinal cord injury. *Arch. Phys. Med. Rehabil.* **2012**, *93*, 2170–2176. [CrossRef] [PubMed]
50. Saleh, S.; Duff, J.; Wallace, M.; Proudlove, G.; Jones, K. Bridging the gap: Psychological outcomes after discharge (*poster*). In Proceedings of the 59th International Spinal Cord Injury (ISCoS) Virtual Conference, Tokyo, Japan, 1–5 September 2020.
51. Alschuler, K.N.; Jensen, M.P.; Sullivan-Singh, S.J.; Borson, S.; Smith, A.E.; Molton, I.R. The association of age, pain, and fatigue with physical functioning and depressive symptoms in persons with spinal cord injury. *J. Spinal Cord Med.* **2013**, *36*, 483–491. [CrossRef] [PubMed]

52. Hirsh, A.T.; Molton, I.R.; Johnson, K.L.; Bombardier, C.H.; Jensen, M.P. The relationship of chronological age, age at injury, and duration of injury to employment status in individuals with spinal cord injury. *Psychol. Inj. Law* **2009**, *2*, 263–275. [CrossRef]
53. Carlson, L.E.; Waller, A.; Mitchell, A.J. Screening for distress and unmet needs in patients with cancer: Review and recommendations. *J. Clin. Oncol.* **2012**, *30*, 1160–1177. [CrossRef] [PubMed]
54. Heinemann, A.W.; Wilson, C.S.; Huston, T.; Koval, J.; Gordon, S.; Gassaway, J.; Kreider, S.E.; Whiteneck, G. Relationship of psychology inpatient rehabilitation services and patient characteristics to outcomes following spinal cord injury: The SCIRehab project. *J. Spinal Cord Med.* **2012**, *35*, 578–592. [CrossRef] [PubMed]
55. Carlson, L.E. Screening alone is not enough: The importance of appropriate triage, referral, and evidence-based treatment of distress and common problems. *J. Clin. Oncol.* **2013**, *31*, 3616–3617. [CrossRef]
56. Rauch, A.; Negrini, S.; Cieza, A. Toward strengthening rehabilitation in health systems: Methods used to develop a WHO Package of Rehabilitation Interventions. *Arch. Phys. Med. Rehabil.* **2019**, *100*, 2205–2211. [CrossRef]
57. Kennedy, P.; Kilvert, A.; Hasson, L. Ethnicity and rehabilitation outcomes: The Needs Assessment Checklist. *Spinal Cord* **2015**, *53*, 334–339. [CrossRef]
58. Migilorini, C.E.; New, P.W.; Tonge, B.J. Comparison of depression, anxiety and stress in persons with traumatic and non-traumatic post-acute spinal cord injury. *Spinal Cord* **2009**, *47*, 783–788. [CrossRef]
59. Khandelwal, A.; Shafer, L.A.; Ethans, K. Does severity of spinal cord injury predict likelihood of suffering chronically from severe depression and anxiety? *Spinal Cord Ser. Cases* **2022**, *8*, 58. [CrossRef]
60. Cijsouw, A.; Adriaansen, J.J.; Tepper, M.; Dijksta, C.A.; van Linden, S.; ALLRISC; de Groot, S.; Post, M.W. Associations between disability-management self-efficacy, participation and life satisfaction in people with long-standing spinal cord injury. *Spinal Cord* **2017**, *55*, 47–51. [CrossRef] [PubMed]
61. Savic, G.; DeVivo, M.; Frankel, H.; Jamous, M.A.; Soni, B.M.; Charlifue, S. Long-term survival after traumatic spinal cord injury: A 70-year British study. *Spinal Cord* **2017**, *55*, 651–658. [CrossRef] [PubMed]
62. Gray, A.A.; Madrigal-Bauguss, J.A.; Russell, H.F.; Rose, J. Dissemination and use of the professional standards of practice for psychologists, social workers, and counselors in spinal cord injury rehabilitation. *J. Spinal Cord Med.* **2020**, *43*, 871–877. [CrossRef] [PubMed]
63. Craig, A.; Duff, J.; Middleton, J. Spinal cord injuries. In *Comprehensive Clinical Psychology*, 2nd ed.; Asmundson, G.J.G., Ed.; Elsevier: New York, NY, USA, 2022; Volume 8, pp. 301–328.
64. British Society of Rehabilitation Medicine. *BSRM Standards for Rehabilitation Services, Mapped on to the National Service Framework for Long-Term Conditions*; BSRM: London, UK, 2009. Available online: https://www.headway.org.uk/media/3321/bsrm-standards-for-rehabilitation-services.pdf (accessed on 10 August 2023).
65. Siddall, P.J.; McClelland, J.M.; Rutkowski, S.B.; Cousins, M.J. A longitudinal study of the prevalence and characteristics of pain in the first 5 years following spinal cord injury. *Pain* **2003**, *103*, 249–257. [CrossRef]
66. Mental Health Act 1983. Available online: https://www.legislation.gov.uk/ukpga/1983/20/contents (accessed on 10 August 2023).
67. Craig, A.; Perry, K.N. *Guide for Health Care Professionals on the Psychosocial Care for Spinal Cord Injury*, 2nd ed.; Spinal Cord Injury Service: Sydney, Australia, 2013. Available online: https://www.aci.health.nsw.gov.au/__data/assets/pdf_file/0019/155233/Guide-Psychosocial-Care.pdf (accessed on 10 August 2023).
68. Department of Health. The National Service Framework for Long-Term Conditions. 2005. Available online: https://assets.publishing.service.gov.uk/media/5a756bede5274a1baf95e73b/National_Service_Framework_for_Long_Term_Conditions.pdf (accessed on 10 August 2023).
69. NHS Improvement & NICE—Stroke Psychological Care after Stroke. Available online: https://www.nice.org.uk/media/default/sharedlearning/531_strokepsychologicalsupportfinal.pdf (accessed on 10 August 2023).
70. Dorstyn, D.S.; Mathias, J.L.; Denson, L.A. Psychological intervention during spinal rehabilitation: A preliminary study. *Spinal Cord* **2010**, *48*, 756–761. [CrossRef]
71. Royal College of Physicians National Clinical Guidelines for Stroke. Available online: https://www.rcplondon.ac.uk/guidelines-policy/stroke-guidelines-2016 (accessed on 10 August 2023).
72. National Institute for Clinical Excellence. *Post-Traumatic Stress Disorder*; NG116; National Institute for Clinical Excellence: London, UK, 2018. Available online: https://www.nice.org.uk/guidance/NG116 (accessed on 10 August 2023).
73. Royal College of Nursing Response to Psychological Best Practice in Inpatient Services of Older People. Available online: https://www.rcn.org.uk/about-us/our-influencing-work/policy-briefings/CONR-0317 (accessed on 10 August 2023).
74. Agency for Clinical Innovation Trauma-Informed Care and Practice in Mental Health Services. Available online: https://aci.health.nsw.gov.au/networks/mental-health/trauma-informed-care (accessed on 10 August 2023).
75. Distel, D.F.; Amodeo, M.; Joshi, S.; Abramoff, B.A. Cognitive dysfunction in persons with chronic spinal cord injuries. *Phys. Med. Rehabil. Clin.* **2020**, *31*, 345–368. [CrossRef]
76. Stroke Foundation Australian Clinical Guidelines for Stroke Management. Available online: https://informme.org.au/guidelines/living-clinical-guidelines-for-stroke-management (accessed on 10 August 2023).

77. Kennedy, P.; Garmon-Jones, L. Self-harm and suicide before and after spinal cord injury: A systematic review. *Spinal Cord* **2017**, *55*, 2–7. [CrossRef]
78. The Faculty of Intensive Care Medicine Guidelines for the Provision of Intensive Care Services. 2019. Available online: https://ficm.ac.uk/sites/ficm/files/documents/2021-10/gpics-v2.pdf (accessed on 10 August 2023).

Disclaimer/Publisher's Note: The statements, opinions and data contained in all publications are solely those of the individual author(s) and contributor(s) and not of MDPI and/or the editor(s). MDPI and/or the editor(s) disclaim responsibility for any injury to people or property resulting from any ideas, methods, instructions or products referred to in the content.

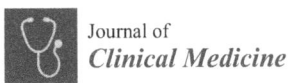

Article

Effects of Adaptations in an Interdisciplinary Follow-Up Clinic for People with Spinal Cord Injury in the Chronic Phase: A Prospective Cohort Study

Julia Tijsse Klasen [1,†], Tijn van Diemen [2,3,*,†], Nelleke G. Langerak [3] and Ilse J. W. van Nes [1,2]

1. Department of Rehabilitation Medicine, Radboud University Medical Center, 6525 GA Nijmegen, The Netherlands; julia.tijsseklasen@ru.nl (J.T.K.); i.vannes@maartenskliniek.nl (I.J.W.v.N.)
2. Department of Spinal Cord Injury Rehabilitation, Sint Maartenskliniek, 6500 GM Nijmegen, The Netherlands
3. Department of Research, Sint Maartenskliniek, 6500 GM Nijmegen, The Netherlands; n.langerak@maartenskliniek.nl
* Correspondence: t.vandiemen@maartenskliniek.nl; Tel.: +31-24-3659598
† These authors contributed equally to this work.

Abstract: People with spinal cord injury (SCI) often experience secondary health conditions (SHCs), which are addressed during interdisciplinary follow-up clinics. We adapted the design of our clinic, by introducing a questionnaire concerning functioning and SHCs, additional measurements of blood pressure and saturation, and participants were seen by either a specialized nurse or rehabilitation physician. In this study, we investigated the effects of these adaptations and the experienced satisfaction of the participants. The results showed an increased number of recommendations in the adapted design, compared to the initial design. Further, the nature of the recommendations shifted from somatic issues to recommendations regarding psychosocial functioning and regarding (the use of) devices. The added measurements revealed an average high systolic blood pressure, which led to more referrals to the general practitioner. The clinical weight and pulmonary functions stayed stable over time. The current adaptations in design expanded and optimized the number and nature of recommendations regarding SHCs to participants. The questionnaire helps the participant to prepare for the clinic and the professionals to tailor their recommendations, resulting in highly satisfied participants.

Keywords: spinal cord injuries; follow-up care; ambulatory care; prevention; interdisciplinary; secondary health conditions

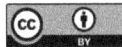

1. Introduction

A spinal cord injury (SCI) is damage to the bundle of nerves and nerve fibers that sends and receives signals from the brain. The spinal cord extends from the lower part of the brain down through the lower back [1]. This damage can cause temporary or permanent changes in feeling, movement, strength and body functions below the site of the injury [2]. Along with such an injury, people with SCI could also have secondary health conditions (SHCs) such as bladder and bowel problems, respiratory issues and skin issues [3].

These SHCs occur in both the physical and mental domains and might cause an additional burden and restrictions in participation [4–6]. In a large study examining the occurrence of SHCs, an average of eight different SHCs were found, for each person with an SCI [5]. Both physical and mental SHCs can influence quality of life and participation and lead to increased medical consumption with higher costs [3,7–10]. In an effort to reduce medical costs and because of the scarcity of health professionals, the Dutch government encourages various vulnerable groups to rely on formal and informal caregivers in order to enable them to live longer independently [11].

For primary-care professionals, providing care for people with an SCI can be challenging, especially when there is a lack of sufficient knowledge about this relatively rare disorder, which has an annual incidence of 40–80 cases per million [12]. Physicians in the rehabilitation centers specialized in SCI possess expertise, but they are no longer primarily responsible for medical care in the home situation [13].

In the Netherland s, there is a guideline in accordance with the Dutch and Flemish Spinal Cord Association [14], which emphasizes the need for interdisciplinary (bi-)annual follow-up care for people with SCI, focused on the prevention, monitoring and treatment of SHCs and to support the informal and primary caregivers.

In 2005, an interdisciplinary follow-up clinic for people with SCI was established at the Sint Maartenskliniek, the Netherlands. The main goal of this interdisciplinary follow-up clinic was to promote healthy aging of people with SCI. This goal is met by giving recommendations to the participants and the primary healthcare providers on how to prevent new SHCs or to control existing SHCs. This follow-up clinic is organized in a carrousel model, in which a participant visits five different disciplines within one appointment at the rehabilitation center. The therapeutic content of this follow-up clinic was investigated in an explorative retrospective study based on data between January 2012 and October 2020. That study showed that an interdisciplinary follow-up clinic can result in a wide and extensive range of recommendations for participants of these clinics [15]. Further, that same study recommended screening for SHCs prior to the interdisciplinary follow-up clinics, to be sure to cover all possible SHCs and tailoring the recommendations to improve healthcare [15].

In October 2020, based on these recommendations [15], adaptations were made in the design of the interdisciplinary follow-up clinic at Sint Maartenskliniek. To help participants of the interdisciplinary follow-up clinic think about all the possible changes and health problems and to prepare the team, a questionnaire was sent to the participants prior to their appointment, concerning the physical, mental and social wellbeing, as well as questions about practical aspects (e.g., use and state of assistive devices). The second adaptation to the interdisciplinary follow-up clinic was to add the measurement of blood pressure, oxygen saturation and heart rate during the visit. Further, the visit to the physician and the specialized nurse were combined and carried out by only one of the two disciplines. This was more efficient, since the participants experienced substantial overlap between the two professions in the initial follow-up clinic. Lastly, the satisfaction of the participants with the setup of the clinic was investigated. With these adaptations in the protocol, the professionals of the team gained more information about the participants, which was thought to result in better and more personalized recommendations after the follow-up visit.

The aim of this study was to investigate the impact of the changes made to the interdisciplinary follow-up clinic by (1) determining whether there was a change in the number and nature of recommendations given to participants with SCI between their visit to the initial interdisciplinary follow-up clinic and their more recent visit with the adapted design; (2) investigating the value of the physical outcomes; (3) investigating the value of the newly introduced questionnaire prior to the clinic; and (4) investigating the satisfaction of the participants with the adapted design and the given recommendations.

We hypothesized that the adapted follow-up care design, with more collected information, will contribute to more personalized recommendations leading to prevention of SHCs in the future and participants being more satisfied with their follow-up care.

2. Materials and Methods

Design and setting: This is a prospective cohort follow-up study of participants attending an interdisciplinary follow-up clinic for people with SCI conducted at the Sint Maartenskliniek in Nijmegen, one of the eight specialized SCI rehabilitation centers in the Netherlands. Participants were actively identified from electronic patient files.

Participants: People were eligible for this study if they were 18 years or older, had a diagnosis of SCI and visited one of the interdisciplinary follow-up clinics between October 2020 and October 2022. In general, people with SCI were considered for participation in the interdisciplinary follow-up clinic when they had a motor complete SCI, were wheelchair users, or had other complex physical conditions which might benefit from an interdisciplinary approach [15].

Procedure: After being invited to the interdisciplinary follow-up clinic, an electronic questionnaire was sent to the participant three weeks before the actual visit. If there was no e-mail address available or the participant preferred a paper version, this was sent by mail. Participants were asked to complete and return the questionnaire via mail or send the paper version back, so that the information could be up-loaded to the electronic patient file. All members of the interdisciplinary follow-up clinic had access to the completed questionnaire in order to prepare themselves for the clinic. On the interdisciplinary follow-up clinic day, five participants came to the Sint Maartenskliniek, where they started at the same time and visited five stations consisting of a rehabilitation physician or a specialized nurse, a physiotherapist, an occupational therapist, a psychologist or social worker and a nurse in a random order. At the end of the interdisciplinary follow-up clinic, the participants were asked for permission to use their anonymized data for research purposes. Further, they were asked to rate their satisfaction regarding the adapted interdisciplinary follow-up clinic. After the interdisciplinary follow-up clinic, the team members had a debriefing where all the recommendations to the participants were gathered and classified by one of the team members to one of the categories as determined and described in a previous retrospective study [15]. These recommendations were communicated to the participants by phone; their general practitioner and other involved healthcare professionals received a letter, including all recommendations and findings.

In line with the previous study [15], the nature of the recommendations was divided into four domains: preventative to be applied at home, treatment at the SCI department of Sint Maartenskliniek (internal treatment), treatment in a hospital or by a primary healthcare professional (external treatment), or (medication) prescription. In each of these four domains, the recommendations were divided into thirteen categories including pain, spasm, skin problems, bowel control problems, bladder control problems, lung problems, all other intercurrent physical/medical problems, splints, devices, social problems, psychological problems, seating advice and functioning.

The data were collected using Castor EDC (version 2022.1.0.3) (EU HQ, Amsterdam, The Netherlands).

Outcome measures: Data were based on demographic and SCI characteristics, a questionnaire completed by the participants prior to the interdisciplinary follow-up clinic visit, physical assessments during the clinic, a list of recommendations from the clinicians, and a questionnaire about participants' satisfaction with the set-up of the adapted interdisciplinary follow-up clinic.

Data collected from the participants' medical records included demographic characteristics, time since injury, level of SCI, completeness of SCI and cause of SCI.

The questionnaire was a combination of different outcome measures. This included some validated outcome measures, the Spinal Cord Injury Secondary Conditions Scale (SCI-SCS), International Spinal Cord Injury Quality of Life basic dataset (QoL-BDS), the Patient Health Questionnaire-2 (PHQ-2) and the Generalized Anxiety Disorder-2 (GAD-2). The selection of the validated measures was in close collaboration with all Dutch specialized SCI rehabilitation centers. While this took place during the inclusion period, some measures were added during the process of data collection. Further, the questionnaire consisted of some self-developed structured questions to gather information about current functioning.

The SCI-SCS [16] consists of 16 items, each addressing one health condition. Participants rate on a 4-point scale how much each health problem affected their activities and independence in the last three months, ranging from 0, not a problem, to 3, significant or chronic problem, resulting in a score between 0 and 48 [16]. Two extra questions were added to the SCI-SCS regarding sleeping problems [17] and weight problems. The response categories were the same.

The International Spinal Cord Injury Quality of Life basic dataset (QoL-BDS) consists of four questions regarding satisfaction with quality of life as a whole, with physical health, psychological health and with social life. Each question is rated on a 0–10 numeric rating scale. The total score is the average of the four items resulting in a range of 0–10 [18].

The PHQ-2 is the two item version of the original PHQ-9 [19]. The first two questions of the original scale were used to screen for basic symptoms of a depressive disorder according to the Diagnostic and Statistical Manual of Mental Disorders, 4th Edition [20]. The two questions are scored on a scale ranging from 0, not at all, to 3, nearly every day, resulting in a range of 0–6 [21].

The GAD-2 is the short screening version of the GAD-7 [22]. The first two questions of the original scale are used to screen for the basic symptoms of generalized anxiety and are scored on a scale ranging from 0, not at all, to 3, nearly every day, resulting in a combined total range of 0–6 [23].

The self-developed structured questionnaire started with seven questions focusing on information about the current functioning and the use of assistive devices. This was followed by eight questions about changes in physical functioning in daily life. An example of a question is the following: Since your last visit to the rehabilitation clinic, has there been any change in your walking, standing, or transfers? A total of eleven questions investigated changes in participation and social activities. An example of a question is the following: Since your last visit to the rehabilitation center, are there any problems with respect to leisure time or hobbies?

The physical assessment conducted by the nurse included clinical weight, blood pressure, oxygen saturation, heart rate and other physical signs, e.g., prevalence of pressure injuries and wounds. Assessments conducted by the physiotherapist included pulmonary function (forced vital capacity (FVC), peak expiratory flow (PEF), forced expiratory volume in 1 s (FEV_1)).

After the follow-up clinic visit, participants were asked to complete a questionnaire about their satisfaction with the set-up of the adapted interdisciplinary follow-up clinic. They were asked to what extent their expectations were met and whether their questions were answered. Answers were scored on a numeric rating scale, ranging from 0, very unsatisfied/not at all, to 10, very satisfied/completely.

Statistical analyses: Descriptive statistics were performed for all collected variables. Continuous data were presented as mean values with standard deviations and ranges (minimum–maximum). Categorical data were presented using counts and percentages.

When applicable, the gathered data included participants' last visit to the initial design (recommendations and some physical measurements), which were compared to the data of their first visit with the adapted design. The change in the number of recommendations given to the participants per domain and per category were analyzed using paired sample t tests. Due to repetitive measurements, a level of significance of $p < 0.001$ was used.

For calculating (sub)scale scores of the validated measures, missing items were replaced with the mean score of that scale if the total extent of missing items was less than 20%, otherwise the (sub)scale was considered missing [24].

To determine the relationships between the total amount of problems identified by the participants (based on the validated outcome measures of the questionnaire completed prior to the follow-up clinic visit) and the total number of recommendations provided by the professionals, Pearson product-moment correlation coefficients were calculated. p-values less than 0.05 were considered statistically significant. Correlations up to 0.3 were considered as weak, between 0.3 and 0.5 as moderate and above 0.5 as strong [25].

All analyses were conducted using SPSS for Windows (version 27) (IBM Corp, Armonk, NY, USA).

3. Results

3.1. Background

A total of 204 participants visited one of the 52 adapted interdisciplinary follow-up clinics between October 2020 and October 2022. Nine participants did not give consent and were excluded from the study.

Of the 195 participants, 56 did not visit the initial interdisciplinary follow-up clinic [15], and therefore, they were excluded from the analysis regarding the comparison between the two designs. The characteristics of the 195 and 139 participants are shown in Table 1.

Table 1. Characteristics of the participants of the interdisciplinary follow-up clinic.

Characteristics	All Participants (N = 195)	Participants in Both Designs (N = 139)
	n (%)/Mean (SD), Range	n (%)/Mean (SD), Range
Sex female/male	51 (26)/144 (74)	38 (27)/101 (73)
Age (years)	55.6 (14.0), 18–92	56.4 (13.4), 24–92
Time since injury (years)	20.9 (14.8), 2–67	23.8 (14.0), 5–67
Spinal cord injury characteristics		
Cause		
Traumatic	143 (73)	108 (78)
Vascular	12 (6)	8 (6)
Infection	16 (8)	9 (7)
Oncology	11 (6)	5 (4)
Other non-traumatic	8 (4)	6 (4)
Other/unknown	5 (3)	3 (2)
Height		
Cervical	67 (34)	50 (36)
Thoracic	113 (58)	80 (58)
Lumbar	15 (8)	9 (6)
Completeness		
AIS A	127 (65)	96 (69)
AIS B	24 (12)	13 (9)
AIS C	24 (12)	17 (12)
AIS D	18 (9)	11 (8)
Unknown/missing [#]	2 (1)	2 (1)

[#] Some participants acquired the SCI many years ago, before standardized measuring of level and completeness, resulting in two missing AIS scores.

3.2. Recommendations

For the 139 participants that visited both designs, a total of 523 recommendations were given in the initial design and 628 recommendations in the adapted design. This resulted in a significant increase in the average number of recommendations from 3.7 to 4.6 per participant. Figure 1 shows the total number of recommendations given to the 139 participants at both follow-up clinics in each of the four domains. Most recommendations were preventive in nature and could be applied at home, with 45% ($n = 234$) of the total number of recommendations in the initial design increasing to 66% ($n = 417$) in the adapted design ($p < 0.001$). A decrease in the number of recommendations was made regarding external treatment, which went from 24% ($n = 124$) in the initial design to 10% ($n = 62$) in the adapted design.

Table 2 shows the distribution of the recommendations per domain over the different categories for the initial and the adapted interdisciplinary follow-up clinic.

Most of the recommendations in the initial design ($n = 523$) were related to medical intercurrent (27%), while in the adapted design ($n = 628$), most recommendations were related to devices (19%), closely followed by functioning (18%). An increase in the number of recommendations was observed regarding social and psychological problems, preventive at home, which went from 2% and 2.5% in the initial design to 6% and 5% in the adapted design ($p < 0.001$), respectively.

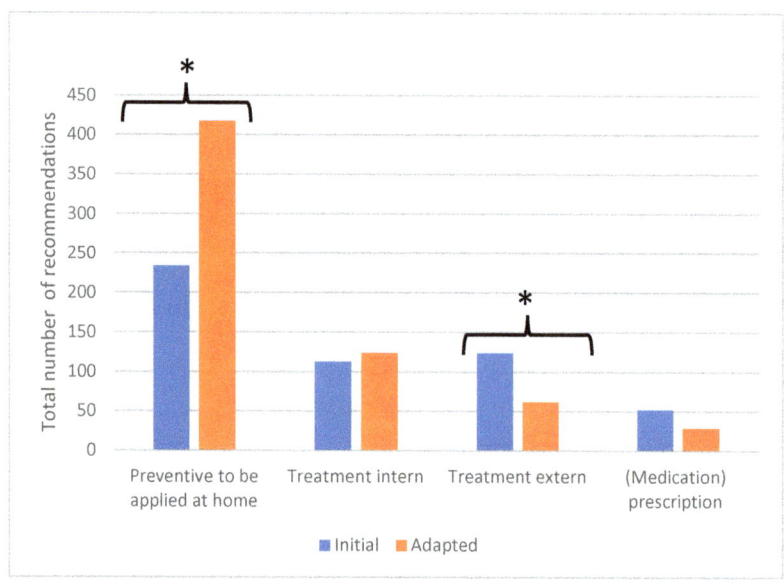

Figure 1. Total number of recommendations in four domains given in both designs of the follow-up clinic. (N = 139, * $p < 0.001$ according to a paired samples t-test).

Table 2. Total number of recommendations given in the initial (n = 523) and the adapted (n = 628) design of the follow-up clinic.

Recommendations	Preventive to Be Applied at Home		Internal Treatment		External Treatment		(Medication) Prescription		Total (%)	
	Initial	Adapted	Initial	Adapted	Initial	Adapted	Initial	Adapted	Initial	Adapted
Medical intercurrent	61	35	17	4	49	14 *	12	9	139 (27)	62 (10) *
Skin problems	14	24	3	6	2	2	3	0	22 (4)	32 (5)
Spasm	9	6	4	2	0	1	4	6	17 (3)	15 (2)
Pain	11	12	12	3	6	6	6	3	35 (7)	24 (4)
Bladder problems	28	19	2	0	25	6 *	5	1	60 (12)	27 (4) *
Bowel problems	24	16	3	4	1	1	8	4	36 (7)	25 (4)
Lung problems	10	42 *	2	4	1	5	0	2	13 (3)	53 (8) *
Functioning	35	73 *	18	22	10	14	1	1	64 (12)	110 (18)
Social	6	27 *	3	10	2	0	0	0	11 (2)	37 (6) *
Psychological	5	23 *	2	5	6	3	0	0	13 (3)	31 (5)
Devices	18	79 *	23	32	19	5	9	3	69 (13)	119 (19) *
Splints	1	12	6	7	3	1	4	0	14 (3)	15 (2)
Seating advice	12	49 *	18	25	0	4	0	0	30 (6)	78 (124) *

(N = 139, * $p < 0.001$ according to a paired samples t-test).

Over the four domains there was an increase in the number of recommendations regarding lung problems, social problems, devices and seating advice, while recommendations about medical intercurrent and bladder control problems decreased.

3.3. Physical Assessments

Outcomes of the physical assessments of the 139 participants who visited both designs of the follow-up clinic are shown in Table 3. Not every physical outcome was measured consistently during the follow-up clinic, which resulted in some missing data.

Table 3. Conducted measurements of the participants who visited both designs.

Measurements	N	Initial Design n (%)/Mean (SD), Range	N	Adapted Design n (%)/Mean (SD), Range
Pressure injuries or wounds present	136	30 (22)	139	42 (30)
Weight in kg	105	76.9 (8.9), 32.6–116.0	128	81.2 (16.4), 33.8–132.6
FVC, % of predicted value	101	72.9 (23.7)	86	67.4 (21)
PEF, % of predicted value	102	66.5 (22.7)	85	65.7 (30)
FEV_1, % of predicted value	101	73.0 (23.1)	85	67.8 (23.1)
Oxygen saturation in SpO2%			133	97.5 (1.9)
Systolic/diastolic blood pressure in mm Hg			137	136/80 (26/13)
Pulse rate in beats per minute			136	74 (14.9)

The total number and percentage of pressure injuries or wounds present remained consistent as well as the measurements of pulmonary functions, even though these functions were measured in fewer participants, 102 in the initial design and 86 in the adapted design. Due to COVID-19 regulations applied during part of the measurement period, only participants who were expected to be at high risk for pulmonary deterioration were measured.

The added cardiopulmonary measurements In the adapted design showed, on average, an oxygen saturation within the normal range (95–100%).

Concerning the systolic blood pressure, 55 participants who had taken part in both designs had a systolic pressure of $\geq$140 mm Hg, of which, 28 had a systolic pressure of $\geq$160 mm Hg. Of these 28 participants, 20 had a complete SCI (AIS A) and 11 had a level of SCI of Th6 or above. The average age and weight among these 28 participants were, respectively, 65 years (SD = 11.9) and 82.1 kg (SD = 15.9). The highest systolic pressure measured by a participant was 220 mm Hg.

The average heart rate of 74 BPM (SD = 14.9) was within the normal range (60–100 BPM).

3.4. Questionnaire

Table 4 shows the scores of the validated outcome measures completed prior to the interdisciplinary follow-up clinic.

Table 4. Mean scores on the validated scales used in the assessment and their correlation with the total number of recommendations.

Measurements	N	Mean (SD), Range	Correlation with Total Recommendations
SCI-SCS (16 items, range 0–48)	176	13.2 (7.3), 0–41	0.37 **
QoL-BDS total (4 items, range 0–10)	136	6.9 (1.5), 0–10	−0.12
QoL-BDS life as whole (range 0–10)	137	7.0 (1.7), 0–10	−0.13
QoL-BDS physical health (range 0–10)	136	6.4 (1.9), 0–10	−0.19 *
QoL-BDS psychological health (range 0–10)	136	7.1 (1.8), 0–10	−0.07
QoL-BDS social life (range 0–10)	136	7.1 (1.8), 0–6	−0.02
PHQ-2 (2 items, range 0–6)	175	0.91 (1.2), 0–6	0.08
GAD-2 (2 items, range 0–6)	103	0.91 (1.3)/0–5	0.21 *

Abbreviations: SCI-SCS, spinal cord injury secondary condition scale; QoL-BDS, international quality of life basic data set; PHQ-2, Patient Health Questionnaire-2; GAD-2, Generalized Anxiety Disorder-2. * $p < 0.01$, ** $p < 0.05$.

The score distribution on the separate questions of the SCI-SCS, including the two added questions regarding sleep problems and weight problems, is shown in Figure 2. On average, every participant indicated at least mild problems with six different SHCs on the original SCI-SCS and seven on all 18 questions used in this study. The SHCs reported by more than half of the participants as at least a mild problem were muscle spasms, joint and muscle pain, bowel dysfunction, chronic neuropathic pain, sleep problems, bladder dysfunction and urinary tract infections.

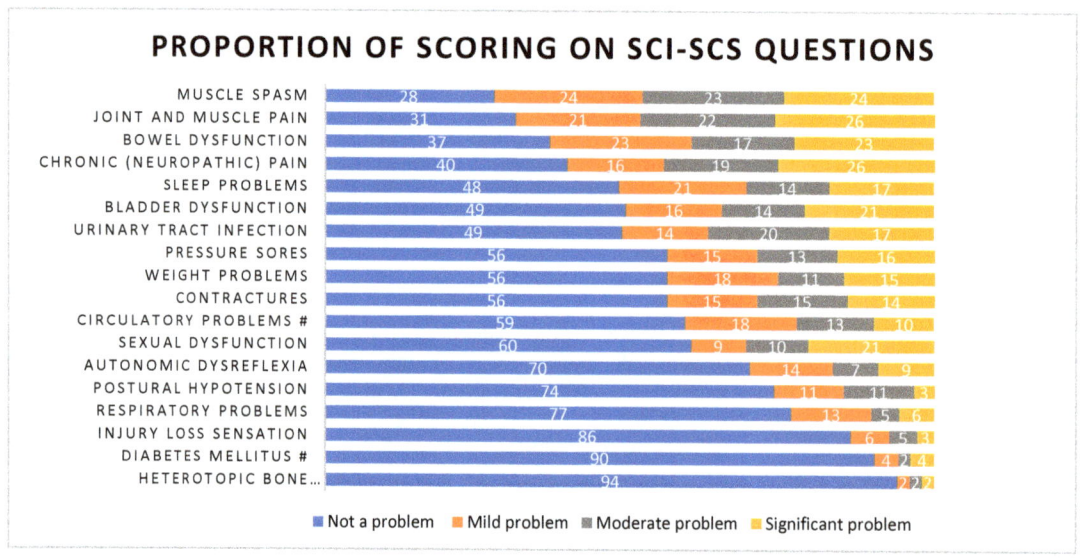

Figure 2. Proportions (%) of scorings on the separate questions of the Spinal Cord Injury Secondary Condition Scale. N = 176. Abbreviations: SCI-SCS, Spinal cord injury secondary condition scale. # N = 103 because the questions were added later.

The mean scores on the four Qol-BDS questions range between 6.4 (for physical health) and 7.1 (for psychological and social life).

With regard to PHQ-2 and GAD-2, a total of 30% and 29% participants scored two or higher, respectively, indicative of problems with depressive mood or anxiety [26,27].

A moderate association was found between the total number of recommendations and the SCI-SCS, and weak but significant associations were found with quality of life associated with physical health and the anxiety score of the GAD-2.

In the questionnaire, 87 of 180 participants indicated that they were receiving therapy in their home environment. Of those, eighty-five visited a physiotherapist, seven an occupational therapist, four a psychologist, two a social worker and two another healthcare professional. Of the eight questions regarding changes in physical functioning since their last visit, the participants on average answered positively on 1.4 (SD = 1.6, range 0–6) questions. On average, the participants positively answered 3.9 (SD = 2.2, range 0–11) out of eleven questions regarding changes in their participation and social activities. Note that part of the study period was during substantial social restrictions due to the COVID-19 pandemic.

3.5. Satisfaction with Adapted Design

A total of 191 participants completed the three questions after the interdisciplinary follow-up clinics. They indicated their satisfaction with the set-up of the adapted clinic as 8.8/10 on average. In addition, when asked to what extent their expectations were met and their questions were answered, they scored 8.9/10 and 9.0/10, respectively.

4. Discussion

The objective of this study was to investigate the value of adaptations to the design of an interdisciplinary follow-up clinic for people with SCI, by studying the change in the number and nature of recommendations, the value of physical measurements, the value of a questionnaire completed prior to the clinic and the participants' satisfaction with the adapted follow-up clinic.

Based on 139 participants who visited both designs of the interdisciplinary follow-up clinics, there was a significant increase in the average number of recommendations per participant. The increase in recommendations is related to more recommendations regarding devices and functioning, especially those that are preventive in nature. This increase could indicate an effect of the addition of the questionnaire, because this questionnaire draws attention to problems with facilities and devices, as well as psychosocial issues. In these three categories, there is an increase in the number of recommendations given to the participants. In general, when visiting health care providers, people tend to focus on somatic and physical discomfort, rather than mental or social issues [28]. Nevertheless, problems regarding social relationships and financial strain could contribute to the mental health burden of people with SCI [29]. Given these results, one could argue that the questionnaire ensures that problems regarding devices and psychosocial aspects become more insightful and thus easier to discuss. Because of the wide range of topics in the questionnaire, the participant might be primed to ask certain questions more easily during their visit to the interdisciplinary follow-up clinic, however, this might also result in decreased attention to issues of other categories.

The shift in nature of the recommendations may be due to the change in the clinic design, where the participant is now seeing either a rehabilitation physician or a specialized nurse but not both, resulting in less time to discuss all physical aspects related to the SCI. Constant attention for all physical and mental SHCs is essential for comprehensive follow-up care for all people with SCI. The decrease in the number of recommendations regarding bladder control needs further consideration and development of interdisciplinary follow-up clinics.

The decrease in the number of recommendations regarding intercurrent medical issues could be due to the changed method of registering the recommendations of the follow-up clinic. Although the same domains and categories were used in both studies, in the adapted design, the recommendations were classified by one of the team members during the debriefing, while in the initial design, the researcher had to subdivide the recommendations retrospectively from the letters to the general practitioner. This new method of registering may provide clearer categorization for recommendations as opposed to being classified as intercurrent medical issues.

People with SCI, particularly those with a high level of SCI, tend to have lower blood pressure in general and are more likely to have episodes of orthostatic hypotension [30]. However, the participants in this study had an, on average, high, mainly systolic blood pressure. The high systolic blood pressure might be caused by the so-called "white-coat-effect". As a British study mentions, this effect should not be overlooked, and with certain systolic pressures, it might be necessary to carry out an ambulatory, repetitive measurement, in order to gain a more realistic view of one's blood pressure [31]. Other factors can contribute as well, such as stress or the discomfort of getting to the follow-up clinic, especially for participants with higher spinal cord lesions. Also, the natural changes in blood pressure that can occur during the day, which more often occurs in people with SCI, could be an explanation for these findings [32]. The last contributing factor could be the fact that screening for high blood pressure does not take place adequately in people with SCI in general. When a physician is lacking sufficient knowledge about SCI, this might result in the delayed diagnosis and treatment of secondary health conditions, the so called doctor's delay. The findings in this study show that a one-time measurement during a participants' visit does not properly represent these possible patterns of blood pressure. All these contributing factors argue in favor of performing ambulatory/repeated blood pressure measurements, in order to distinguish between a one-time high systolic blood pressure or a structural problem. For this reason, more participants were referred to their general practitioner for regular check-ups.

Due to coronavirus, the measurement of the pulmonary function was restricted during part of the inclusion period. During these restrictions, only participants who were at risk for deterioration of their pulmonary function were measured. Despite these restrictions, there was no significant difference in the outcomes of the pulmonary function of the participants in the adapted design, consistent with previous findings from the retrospective study. This is consistent with retrospective findings of the initial design of the interdisciplinary follow-up clinic [15]. Notwithstanding the fact that pulmonary function remained stable over time, it is important for the wellbeing of the participants and to prevent deterioration to consistently monitor and conduct these measurements in order to give adequate recommendations with regard to their pulmonary function.

The total number of recommendations given to the participants shows a moderate positive correlation with the total score on the SCI-SCS. The more impact participants experience from different SHCs, the more recommendations they received during the interdisciplinary follow-up clinic. For the other validated scales, there was only a weak correlation; although for the QoL-BDS question regarding their physical health and the anxiety scale, the correlations were significant. The lack of a strong association between these scales and the total number of recommendations does not diminish their value. They might help provide the team members with a more comprehensive understanding of the participant's situation, which could further assist in tailoring the recommendations.

On the extended SCI-SCS (18 items), the participants indicated that they have problems with an average of seven different SHCs at the time of the interdisciplinary follow-up clinic. This is comparable with a large cross-sectional study in the Netherlands regarding SHCs, although the instruments used differ [5]. The average amount of SHCs on the original SCI-SCS (16 items) is the same as found in the validation and in another study with the SCI-SCS [16,33]. The distribution of the scoring on the different SCI-SCS questions is somewhat different between the different studies [8,16,33,34]. The differences found between the studies might be due to differences in the inclusion criteria, the time since injury and age of the participants investigated. The additional questions about sleep and weight problems appear valuable as almost half or more than half of the participants indicate weight problems or sleeping problems, respectively.

The scores on the QoL-BDS are very similar to the scores in an international clinometric study of the QoL-BDS [18]. Part of the inclusion period of the current study was during substantial social restrictions due to the COVID 19 pandemic, many participants stated that their score on the QoL-BDS social life was lower at that time than normal. Nevertheless, the average score on the QoL-BDS social life is comparable data from an international study gathered before the pandemic.

On the total PHQ-2 in this sample, 70% of the participants scored 0 or 1 indicating that there likely was no depressive mood problem [26]. This 70% which are not likely to have mood problems is still 10% less than a non-depressed community based sample [21].

The participants' satisfaction scored very high on average, which shows that participants considered this follow-up clinic of added value. These findings are consistent with previous research [35]. Participants saw value in the follow-up clinic and as a way to answer their questions regarding their SCI and to prevent or follow up on SHCs. The time invested in completing the questionnaire most participants was not a big investment, as supported by the very high ratings concerning satisfaction with the set-up of the interdisciplinary follow-up clinic.

The willingness to participate in health-benefitting behavior also needs to be taken into account [7]. Besides increasing and optimizing the number of recommendations, participants need to understand these recommendations. Further, they need to be willing to take action to follow these recommendations. In the future, this could be evaluated in the biannual visits to the follow-up clinic.

Limitations: In this study, only the participants that responded to the invitation were included. During the inclusion period, more than the 204 participants reported in this study were invited for an interdisciplinary follow-up clinic. We do not know how many did not keep appointments, nor if the participants in this study might be a subgroup and therefore form some bias. Nevertheless, in this study, every person who participated in the follow-up clinic and gave consent was included in the study which makes the results well generalizable.

The current study used the classification for the recommendations as used in a previous retrospective study, to make a comparison possible. Thus, the choice of not all subjective SHCs indicated in the questionnaire could directly be linked to a specific recommendation, nor were there separate categories for the recommendation regarding the extra conducted measurements.

There might be a possibility that the questionnaire is answered differently by participants with different educational levels. We did not ask for this, so we were not able to control for that.

Lastly, during the debriefing of the follow-up clinic, the outcomes of the recommendations were not noted by the same person every time. This could have led to one person classifying a certain recommendation in a different category than someone else.

5. Conclusions

This study shows that adding a questionnaire prior to an interdisciplinary follow-up clinic for participants with SCI helps to increase the number of recommendations regarding SHCs. This questionnaire seems to prompt participants to think about the subjects important to discuss with the team and provides specific information to the professionals. Further, the extra physical measurements reveal, on average, high systolic blood pressure, which needs extra attention in future research. This addition seems valuable for indicating potential risks. Participants of the adapted design of the interdisciplinary follow-up clinic were very satisfied with this and about the way their questions were answered.

By continuing to evaluate and optimize this interdisciplinary follow-up clinic and giving personalized recommendations, we aim to improve daily life of participants of these clinics, to ultimately prevent or solve SHCs and to support them with aging in a healthy way. This is especially important to reverse the decrease in the number of recommendations regarding bladder problems. Future research could focus more on the preventive value of the interdisciplinary follow-up clinic by comparing the people with SCI that do not attend interdisciplinary follow-up clinics with a matched group of those who do and follow both groups over time. In addition, information about educational level could be collected. Further, we need more studies on the evolvement of blood pressure and how this can be measured best for people with SCI.

Author Contributions: Conceptualization, T.v.D. and I.J.W.v.N.; methodology, T.v.D. and I.J.W.v.N.; validation, J.T.K. and T.v.D.; formal analysis, J.T.K. and T.v.D.; investigation, T.v.D.; resources, I.J.W.v.N.; data curation, J.T.K. and T.v.D.; writing—original draft preparation, J.T.K. and T.v.D.; writing—review and editing, J.T.K., T.v.D., N.G.L. and I.J.W.v.N.; visualization, J.T.K. and T.v.D.; supervision, N.G.L. and I.J.W.v.N.; project administration, T.v.D.. All authors have read and agreed to the published version of the manuscript.

Funding: This research received no external funding.

Institutional Review Board Statement: The Medical Ethics Committee of the University Medical Center Radboud declared that this study (prospective cohort study with anonymized data) did not need formal ethical approval under the Dutch law regulating medical research in human beings (reference number: 2021-7379). In accordance with local requirements, the Medical Ethics Committee of the Sint Maartenskliniek approved the conduct of this study in their center (reference number: 1006). This study was conducted in accordance with the Helsinki declaration.

Informed Consent Statement: Informed consent was obtained from all subjects involved in the study.

Data Availability Statement: The data presented in this study are available on request from the corresponding author.

Acknowledgments: We would like to thank Susan Charlifue for her effort to check the language and readability of this manuscript.

Conflicts of Interest: The authors declare no conflict of interest.

References

1. NIH Spinal Cord Injury. Available online: https://www.ninds.nih.gov/health-information/disorders/spinal-cord-injury#:~:text=A%20spinal%20cord%20injury (accessed on 30 January 2023).
2. Eckert, M.J.; Martin, M.J. Trauma: Spinal Cord Injury. *Surg. Clin. N. Am.* **2017**, *97*, 1031–1045. [CrossRef]
3. Sezer, N.; Akkuş, S.; Uğurlu, F.G. Chronic Complications of Spinal Cord Injury. *World J. Orthop.* **2015**, *6*, 24–33. [CrossRef]
4. Battalio, S.L.; Jensen, M.P.; Molton, I.R. Secondary Health Conditions and Social Role Satisfaction in Adults with Long-Term Physical Disability. *Health Psychol.* **2019**, *38*, 445–454. [CrossRef]
5. Bloemen-Vrencken, J.H.A.; Post, M.W.M.; Hendriks, J.M.S.; de Reus, E.C.E.; de Witte, L.P. Health Problems of Persons with Spinal Cord Injury Living in the Netherlands. *Disabil. Rehabil.* **2005**, *27*, 1381–1389. [CrossRef] [PubMed]
6. Jensen, M.P.; Truitt, A.R.; Schomer, K.G.; Yorkston, K.M.; Baylor, C.; Molton, I.R. Frequency and Age Effects of Secondary Health Conditions in Individuals with Spinal Cord Injury: A Scoping Review. *Spinal Cord* **2013**, *51*, 882–892. [CrossRef] [PubMed]
7. Mashola, M.K.; Mothabeng, D.J. Associations between Health Behaviour, Secondary Health Conditions and Quality of Life in People with Spinal Cord Injury. *Afr. J. Disabil.* **2019**, *8*, 1–9. [CrossRef] [PubMed]
8. Callaway, L.; Barclay, L.; Mcdonald, R.; Farnworth, L.; Casey, J. Secondary Health Conditions Experienced by People with Spinal Cord Injury within Community Living: Implications for a National Disability Insurance Scheme. *Aust. Occup. Ther. J.* **2015**, *62*, 246–254. [CrossRef] [PubMed]
9. DiPiro, N.D.; Murday, D.; Corley, E.H.; Krause, J.S. Prevalence of Chronic Health Conditions and Hospital Utilization in Adults with Spinal Cord Injury: An Analysis of Self-Report and South Carolina Administrative Billing Data. *Spinal Cord* **2019**, *57*, 33–40. [CrossRef] [PubMed]
10. Cao, Y.; Krause, J.S. The Association between Secondary Health Conditions and Indirect Costs after Spinal Cord Injury. *Spinal Cord* **2021**, *59*, 306–310. [CrossRef]
11. Van der Ham, L.; Den Draak, M.; Mensink, W.; Schyns, P.; Van den Berg, E. *De Wmo 2015 in Praktijk [The Social Support Act 2015 in Practice]*; Sociaal en Cultureel Planbureau: The Hague, The Netherlands, 2018.
12. Chhabra, H.S. (Ed.) *ISCoS Text Book on Comprehensive Management of Spinal Cord Injuries*; Wolters Kluwer: New Delhi, India, 2015; ISBN 978-9351294405.
13. Cox, R.J.; Amsters, D.I.; Pershouse, K.J. The Need for a Multidisciplinary Outreach Service for People with Spinal Cord Injury Living in the Community. *Clin. Rehabil.* **2001**, *15*, 600–606. [CrossRef]
14. Federatie Medische Specialisten Dwarsleasierevalidatie; Nazorg Bij Dwarslaesierevalidatie. Available online: https://richtlijnendatabase.nl/richtlijn/dwarslaesierevalidatie/nazorg_na_dwarslaesierevalidatie.html (accessed on 13 October 2023).
15. Van Diemen, T.; Verberne, D.P.J.; Koomen, P.S.J.; Bongers-Janssen, H.M.H.; van Nes, I.J.W. Interdisciplinary Follow-up Clinic for People with Spinal Cord Injury: A Retrospective Study of a Carousel Model. *Spinal Cord Ser. Cases* **2021**, *7*, 86. [CrossRef] [PubMed]
16. Kalpakjian, C.Z.; Scelza, W.M.; Forchheimer, M.B.; Toussaint, L.L. Preliminary Reliability and Validity of a Spinal Cord Injury Secondary Conditions Scale. *J. Spinal Cord Med.* **2007**, *30*, 131–139. [CrossRef] [PubMed]
17. Buzzell, A.; Camargos, K.C.; Chamberlain, J.D.; Eriks-Hoogland, I.; Hug, K.; Jordan, X.; Schubert, M.; Brinkhof, M.W.G. Self-Reports of Treatment for Secondary Health Conditions: Results from a Longitudinal Community Survey in Spinal Cord Injury. *Spinal Cord* **2021**, *59*, 389–397. [CrossRef] [PubMed]
18. Post, M.W.M.; Forchheimer, M.B.; Charlifue, S.; D'Andréa Greve, J.M.; New, P.W.; Tate, D.G. Reproducibility of the International Spinal Cord Injury Quality of Life Basic Data Set: An International Psychometric Study. *Spinal Cord* **2019**, *57*, 992–998. [CrossRef]
19. Kroenke, K.; Spitzer, R.L.; Williams, J.B.W. The PHQ-9: Validity of a Brief Depression Severity Measure. *J. Gen. Intern. Med.* **2001**, *16*, 606–613. [CrossRef]
20. American Psychiatric Association. *Diagnostic Criteria from DSM-IV*; American Psychiatric Press Inc.: Washington, DC, USA, 1994.
21. Kroenke, K.; Spitzer, R.L.; Williams, J.B.W.; Kroenke, K. The Patient Health Questionnaire-2 of a Two-Item Screener Validity Depression. *Med. Care* **2015**, *41*, 1284–1292. [CrossRef]
22. Spitzer, R.L.; Kroenke, K.; Williams, J.W.; Löwe, B. A Brief Measure for Assessing Generalized Anxiety Disorder: The GAD-7. *Arch. Intern. Med.* **2006**, *166*, 1092–1097. [CrossRef]
23. Seo, J.G.; Park, S.P. Validation of the Generalized Anxiety Disorder-7 (GAD-7) and GAD-2 in Patients with Migraine. *J. Headache Pain* **2015**, *16*, 97. [CrossRef]
24. Goretzko, D.; Heumann, C.; Bühner, M. Investigating Parallel Analysis in the Context of Missing Data: A Simulation Study Comparing Six Missing Data Methods. *Educ. Psychol. Meas.* **2020**, *80*, 756–774. [CrossRef]
25. Cohen, J. *Statistical Power Analysis for the Behavioral Sciences*; Lawrence Erlbaum Associates: New York, NY, USA, 1988; Volume 2, ISBN 0805802835.

26. Levis, B.; Sun, Y.; He, C.; Wu, Y.; Krishnan, A.; Bhandari, P.M.; Neupane, D.; Imran, M.; Brehaut, E.; Negeri, Z.; et al. Accuracy of the PHQ-2 Alone and in Combination with the PHQ-9 for Screening to Detect Major Depression: Systematic Review and Meta-Analysis. *JAMA—J. Am. Med. Assoc.* **2020**, *323*, 2290–2300. [CrossRef]
27. Duff, J.; Grant, L.C.; Coker, J.; Monden, K.R. Anxiety in Response to Sustaining Spinal Cord Injuries and Disorders: When Should Clinicians Be Concerned? *Arch. Phys. Med. Rehabil.* **2023**, *in press*. [CrossRef] [PubMed]
28. Bjørland, E.; Brekke, M. What Do Patients Bring up in Consultations? An Observational Study in General Practice. *Scand. J. Prim. Health Care* **2015**, *33*, 206–211. [CrossRef] [PubMed]
29. Piatt, J.A.; Nagata, S.; Zahl, M.; Li, J.; Rosenbluth, J.P. Problematic Secondary Health Conditions among Adults with Spinal Cord Injury and Its Impact on Social Participation and Daily Life. *J. Spinal Cord Med.* **2016**, *39*, 693–698. [CrossRef] [PubMed]
30. Claydon, V.E.; Steeves, J.D.; Krassioukov, A. Orthostatic Hypotension Following Spinal Cord Injury: Understanding Clinical Pathophysiology. *Spinal Cord* **2006**, *44*, 341–351. [CrossRef] [PubMed]
31. Thomas, O.; Shipman, K.E.; Day, K.; Thomas, M.; Martin, U.; Dasgupta, I. Prevalence and Determinants of White Coat Effect in a Large UK Hypertension Clinic Population. *J. Hum. Hypertens.* **2016**, *30*, 386–391. [CrossRef] [PubMed]
32. Goh, M.Y.; Millard, M.S.; Wong, E.C.K.; Berlowitz, D.J.; Graco, M.; Schembri, R.M.; Brown, D.J.; Frauman, A.G.; O'Callaghan, C.J. Comparison of Diurnal Blood Pressure and Urine Production between People with and without Chronic Spinal Cord Injury. *Spinal Cord* **2018**, *56*, 847–855. [CrossRef]
33. New, P.W. Secondary Conditions in a Community Sample of People with Spinal Cord Damage. *J. Spinal Cord Med.* **2016**, *39*, 665–670. [CrossRef]
34. Jørgensen, V.; von Rosen, P.; Butler Forslund, E. Considerations on the Psychometric Properties and Validity of the Spinal Cord Injury Secondary Conditons Scale. *Spinal Cord* **2021**, *59*, 894–901. [CrossRef]
35. Spreyermann, R.; Lüthi, H.; Michel, F.; Baumberger, M.E.; Wirz, M.; Mäder, M. Long-Term Follow-up of Patients with Spinal Cord Injury with a New ICF-Based Tool. *Spinal Cord* **2011**, *49*, 230–235. [CrossRef]

Disclaimer/Publisher's Note: The statements, opinions and data contained in all publications are solely those of the individual author(s) and contributor(s) and not of MDPI and/or the editor(s). MDPI and/or the editor(s) disclaim responsibility for any injury to people or property resulting from any ideas, methods, instructions or products referred to in the content.

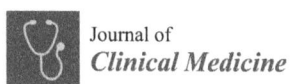 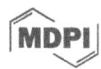

Article

Heart Rate Variability Biofeedback in Adults with a Spinal Cord Injury: A Laboratory Framework and Case Series

Jacob Schoffl [1,2,*], Mohit Arora [1,2], Ilaria Pozzato [1,2], Candice McBain [1,2], Dianah Rodrigues [1,2], Elham Vafa [1,2,3], James Middleton [1,2], Glen M. Davis [3], Sylvia Maria Gustin [4,5], John Bourke [1,2], Annette Kifley [1,2], Andrei V. Krassioukov [6], Ian D. Cameron [1,2] and Ashley Craig [1,2]

1. John Walsh Centre Rehabilitation Research, Northern Sydney Local Health District, Sydney, NSW 2065, Australia; mohit.arora@sydney.edu.au (M.A.); ilaria.pozzato@sydney.edu.au (I.P.); candice.mcbain@sydney.edu.au (C.M.); d.rodrigues@sydney.edu.au (D.R.); elham.vafa@sydney.edu.au (E.V.); james.middleton@sydney.edu.au (J.M.); johnny.bourke@sydney.edu.au (J.B.); annette.kifley@sydney.edu.au (A.K.); ian.cameron@sydney.edu.au (I.D.C.); a.craig@sydney.edu.au (A.C.)
2. The Kolling Institute, Faculty of Medicine and Health, The University of Sydney, Sydney, NSW 2065, Australia
3. School of Health Sciences, Faculty of Medicine and Health, The University of Sydney, Sydney, NSW 2050, Australia; glen.davis@sydney.edu.au
4. NeuroRecovery Research Hub, University of New South Wales, Sydney, NSW 2052, Australia; s.gustin@unsw.edu.au
5. The Centre for Pain IMPACT, Neuroscience Research Australia, Sydney, NSW 2052, Australia
6. ICORD, Faculty of Medicine, University of British Columbia, Vancouver, BC V6T 1Z4, Canada; andrei.krassioukov@vch.ca
* Correspondence: jacob.schoffl@sydney.edu.au

Abstract: Heart rate variability biofeedback (HRV-F) is a neurocardiac self-regulation therapy that aims to regulate cardiac autonomic nervous system activity and improve cardiac balance. Despite benefits in various clinical populations, no study has reported the effects of HRV-F in adults with a spinal cord injury (SCI). This article provides an overview of a neuropsychophysiological laboratory framework and reports the impact of an HRV-F training program on two adults with chronic SCI (T1 AIS A and T3 AIS C) with different degrees of remaining cardiac autonomic function. The HRV-F intervention involved 10 weeks of face-to-face and telehealth sessions with daily HRV-F home practice. Physiological (HRV, blood pressure variability (BPV), baroreflex sensitivity (BRS)), and self-reported assessments (Fatigue Severity Scale, Generalised Anxiety Disorder Scale, Patient Health Questionnaire, Appraisal of Disability and Participation Scale, EuroQol Visual Analogue Scale) were conducted at baseline and 10 weeks. Participants also completed weekly diaries capturing mood, anxiety, pain, sleep quality, fatigue, and adverse events. Results showed some improvement in HRV, BPV, and BRS. Additionally, participants self-reported some improvements in mood, fatigue, pain, quality of life, and self-perception. A 10-week HRV-F intervention was feasible in two participants with chronic SCI, warranting further investigation into its autonomic and psychosocial effects.

Keywords: autonomic nervous system; psychophysiology; biofeedback; heart rate; spinal cord injuries; case reports

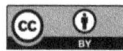

1. Introduction

Spinal cord injury (SCI) is a chronic condition requiring substantial rehabilitation and personal adjustment [1]. In addition to the loss of motor and sensory function resulting in disability, autonomic nervous system (ANS) disruption is prevalent following an SCI [2,3]. The ANS is the part of the nervous system responsible for maintaining a homeostatic state by eliciting fine control over the body's internal functions, including the heart, lungs, vasculature, bowel, bladder, and reproductive organs [4]. Following an SCI, neural pathways in the ANS, particularly sympathetic pathways in high-level injuries, are often disrupted, affecting the functioning of innervated organs [5]. Disruption of autonomic function is a significant contributor to severe cardiovascular complications, such as autonomic dysreflexia and postural hypotension, as well as secondary health conditions, including fatigue, psychological disorders, and cognitive impairment [2,3,5–9]. These conditions negatively impact on the quality of life (QoL) and social participation of those living with SCI and can contribute to a substantial financial burden [10,11]. Hence, interventions focusing on improving autonomic function can potentially improve health and QoL for individuals with SCI.

Heart rate variability biofeedback (HRV-F) is a self-regulation intervention that has shown effectiveness in improving cardiac autonomic function and physical and mental health in able-bodied populations [12]. Heart rate variability (HRV) is a cardiac autonomic marker reflecting changes in time intervals between beat-to-beat cycles of the heart, which can provide insights about overall health and a person's ability to self-regulate [13,14]. Higher HRV is associated with better cardiovascular health, reduced stress, greater emotional regulation, and better cognitive function [13,15]. In those with an SCI, HRV is reduced and is associated with increased fatigue [9]. HRV-F aims to maximise HRV through paced breathing at an individual's resonant frequency. Resonant frequency (e.g., 6 breaths/minute) refers to the respiration rate that synchronises the body's natural cardiovascular oscillations (i.e., heart rate and blood pressure), generating large amplitude cardiac oscillations and maximising HRV [16,17]. Enhancing HRV through this training has yielded various benefits, such as improved blood pressure regulation, pulmonary function, cognitive function, emotional regulation, physical performance, and reduced somatic symptoms like pain and fatigue [12]. These beneficial effects have been observed in non-neurological populations, such as in individuals with asthma [18], and populations with neurological conditions, such as individuals who have experienced an acute stroke [19], fibromyalgia [20], or a traumatic brain injury [21], using similar HRV-F protocols with different time periods (2 weeks to 3 months).

One of the primary mechanisms behind HRV-F and its beneficial health effects is the increase in baroreflex sensitivity (BRS) [16]. The baroreflex is responsible for maintaining blood pressure homeostasis by modulating both the heart rate (vagal component) and total peripheral vascular resistance (sympathetic component) [22]. The term BRS identifies the effectiveness of the baroreflex in detecting and compensating for changes in blood pressure [23] and commonly refers to its vagal component (i.e., the cardiac–vagal baroreflex function) [24]. The baroreflex is stimulated during resonant frequency breathing as paced respiration induces heart rate and blood pressure oscillations that must be regulated to maintain a stable BP. Biofeedback, using signals such as respiration and heart rate/HRV, empowers individuals to control their physiology during this breathing to maximise cardiorespiratory (respiration and heart rate) and cardiovascular (heart rate and blood pressure) resonant properties [25,26]. By achieving resonance regularly, it is believed that baroreflex sensitivity can be trained and enhanced.

While HRV-F may potentially improve rehabilitation outcomes and QoL following a SCI, there is a lack of evidence concerning the effectiveness of HRV-F in adults with SCI. This study presents preliminary data from the first two participants in a pilot study of HRV-F intervention for people with SCI. To evaluate autonomic and neural function in adults with an SCI following an HRV-F intervention, The Neuropsychophysiological Laboratory for People With Spinal Cord Injury was established, and an assessment protocol was developed [27]. This paper has two primary aims: (A) to present a thorough overview of our laboratory framework and (B) to present the preliminary results of two participants who participated in the pilot phase of a future randomised controlled trial.

2. Materials and Methods

A laboratory framework and pilot data from two adults with chronic SCI related to investigating the effectiveness of HRV-F are presented. These participants were part of the pilot phase of a randomised controlled trial prospectively registered with the Australian and New Zealand Clinical Trial Registry (ACTRN12621000870853), with the trial protocol published elsewhere [27]. Written informed consent was provided before they participated in the study. A COVID-19 safety protocol was adhered to during the trial.

2.1. Laboratory Framework

The Neuropsychophysiological Laboratory for People With Spinal Cord Injury was established in 2021. The laboratory has a range of specialised technology to comprehensively assess autonomic and neural function in adults with SCI. These include transcranial Doppler (for evaluating cerebral blood flow), electroencephalography (for assessing brain electrical activity), electrocardiography (ECG, for assessing cardiac electrical and vagal activity), non-invasive blood pressure (NIBP, for measuring blood pressure fluctuations and sympathetic adrenergic activity), electrooculography (for assessing the corneo-retinal potential), skin conductance (for assessing arousal and sympathetic sudomotor activity), body surface temperature (for monitoring thermal changes), functional near infra-red spectroscopy (for capturing changes in haemoglobin concentration), and respiration (for capturing patterns of respiration). This equipment captures physiological responses and provides valuable insights into autonomic regulation (i.e., vagal and sympathetic activity) and overall health. Figure 1 provides a detailed overview of the laboratory's equipment architecture and how data are collected during physiological assessments.

2.2. Case Series

Participants were recruited from the community via an SCI Unit database, SCI consumer newsletters, newspaper advertisements, referrals from outpatient physicians, and flyers distributed in hospital and wheelchair sports facilities. Inclusion criteria were as follows: (i) 18–80 years of age; (ii) English speaking; (iii) sustained an SCI of any level from traumatic or non-traumatic cause with either complete or incomplete lesions; and (iv) at least 12 months post-injury. Neurological level of injury and AIS were determined using the International Standards for Neurological Classification of Spinal Cord Injury (ISNCSCI). The exclusion criteria were as follows: (i) evidence of severe cognitive impairment (i.e., moderate to severe traumatic brain injury or dementia); (ii) evidence of psychiatric disorder (e.g., bipolar disorder or psychoses or severe depressive disorder), as determined by medical history or psychological screening (e.g., PHQ-9); (iii) taking β-blockers.

2.2.1. Study Design

This case series presents the pilot pre-post data of two adults with chronic SCI who received a 10-week HRV-F intervention.

2.2.2. Assessment and Outcome Measures

Both participants were assessed at baseline (Day 0) and post-intervention (Week 10). The assessment comprises two parts: (i) self-reported and (ii) physiological assessment.

Participants completed a self-reported questionnaire via a secure web platform (REDCap (2023), V12.5.8, Vanderbilt University). This included questions about demographic and injury characteristics and psychosocial outcomes such as mood, anxiety, secondary health conditions, appraisal of injury, pain, fatigue, and QoL (see Supplementary Table S1 for more details).

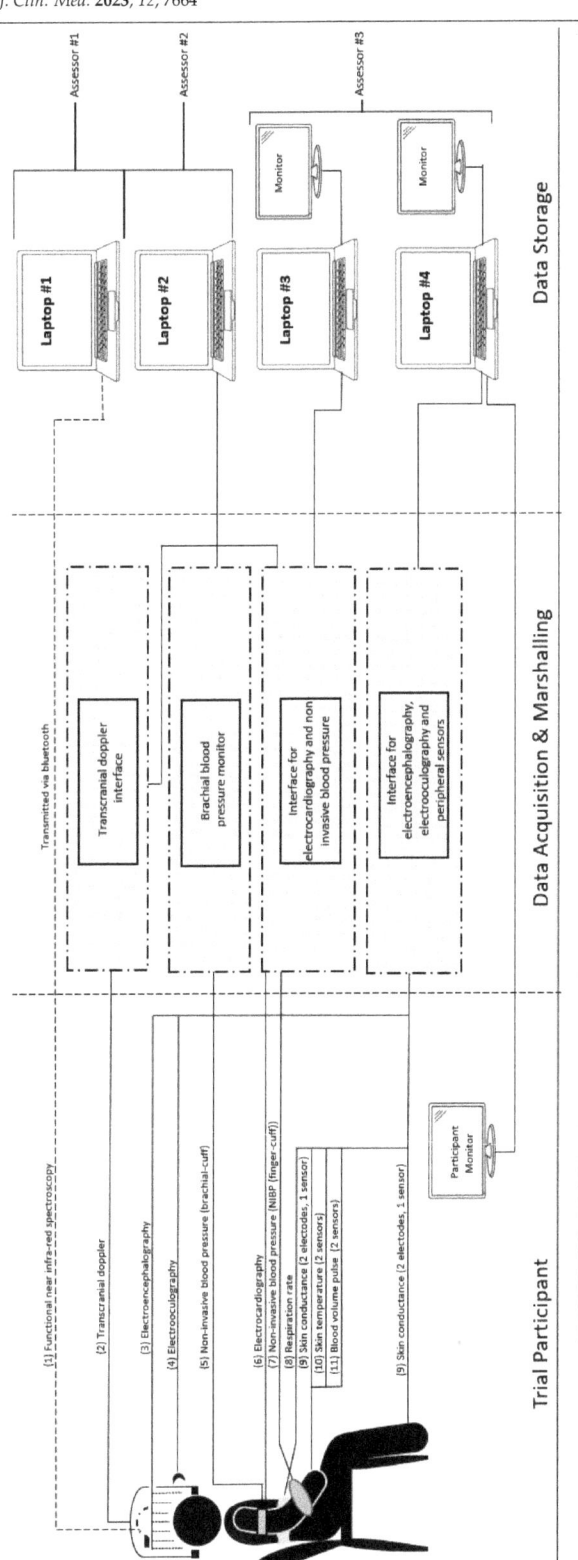

Figure 1. System architecture for the physiological assessment protocol and the laboratory's equipment.

The physiological assessment comprised a 5-stage physiological assessment protocol (29-min). ECG and NIBP (finger and brachial) were continuously collected during the assessment and used to calculate HRV, blood pressure variability (BPV), and baroreflex sensitivity (BRS). A minimum of five minutes of data were recorded for each stage, according to the minimum standard requirements specified in HRV guidelines [28]. The five stages are shown below:

(i) A resting condition, preceded by two minutes of habituation.
(ii) A mental stressor task (i.e., Stroop test). The Stroop test is a widely used cognitive stressor [29,30].
(iii) A recovery period.
(iv) A paced breathing task. This involved participants following a pacer, presented on a monitor display, to regulate their breathing to 6 breaths per minute. The inhalation–exhalation ratio was 1:1, with nil breath holds during this task.
(v) A second recovery period.

To minimise the effect of factors known to affect HRV, before the physiological assessment, participants were instructed to adhere to the following guidelines: regular sleep routine, no caffeine/alcohol/exercise/smoking, or large meals at least 2 h before. The assessment was conducted between 9 a.m. and 1 p.m. in a quiet, semi-darkened laboratory at a constant temperature of 23–24 degrees Celsius. Participants were also asked to empty their bladder/bowel immediately before the assessment and remained seated in their wheelchairs for the duration of the whole assessment (approximately 3 h).

2.2.3. Intervention

The 10-week intervention involved six weekly face-to-face sessions conducted in the laboratory lasting between 2 and 3 h per session and four weekly telehealth sessions (via phone call) lasting between 15 and 30 min. Table 1 provides an overview of the HRV-F program. The program was focussed on HRV-F, where participants performed slow diaphragmatic breathing at their optimal resonant frequency, using biofeedback technology to synchronise their respiration and heart signals [23]. The resonant frequency assessment was based on a protocol described elsewhere [31,32]. This involved assessing several respiration rates (5–8 breaths/minute) and identifying which frequency maximised HRV measures and synchronisation between heart rate and respiration oscillations. Further details regarding the resonant frequency assessment criteria may be found in Supplementary Table S2.

In addition to the 10 weekly HRV-F sessions, the participants were asked to practise HRV-F at home twice daily for 20 min [33]. HRV-F home practice was conducted independently by the participants (no clinicians) using equipment provided to them during the laboratory sessions. Participants were provided with a Polar H10 Heart Rate Monitor (Polar Electro Oy, Kempele, Finland) to record heart rate/HRV signals to guide biofeedback training. This was paired with an HRV feedback application on the participant's smartphone (Figure 2), with the respiration pacer set to the participant's resonant frequency. The telehealth sessions were used to check in with the participant and to troubleshoot any issues the participant may have with the home practice. Telehealth sessions were separate from home practice and no HRV-F practice was performed during these telehealth sessions.

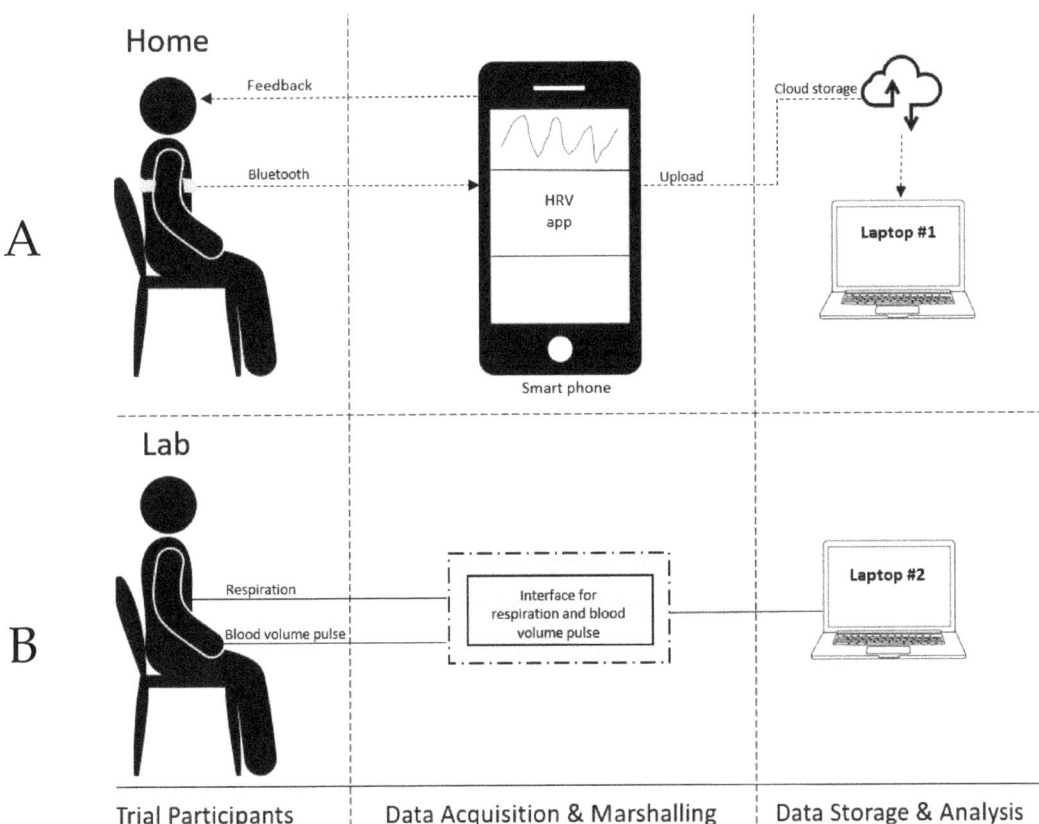

Figure 2. System architecture for the biofeedback intervention. (**A**): Set-up for home practice. (**B**): Set-up for laboratory. The same laboratory set-up is used for the resonant frequency assessment and the in-lab biofeedback practice. HRV: Heart rate variability.

Table 1. An overview of the intervention program.

Week	Contents and Visit Type
1	Introduction (laboratory) • Psychoeducation: What is HRV-F, physiological links between mind/body, diaphragmatic breathing • Familiarisation with biofeedback and home training equipment • Resonant frequency breathing (RFB) assessment
2	Mindful breathing (laboratory) • Education: Using RFB in everyday contexts • Mindful breathing • HRV-F practice
3	Visualisation strategies (laboratory) • Education: Visualisation and mental rehearsal exercises • HRV-F practice
4	Debrief (phone call) • Debrief and reflect upon the past three weeks • Troubleshoot any homework issues

Table 1. *Cont.*

Week	Contents and Visit Type
5	Mindfulness (laboratory) • Mindfulness strategies and techniques • RFB reassessment • HRV-F practice
6–8	Debrief (phone call) • Debrief and reflect upon the previous week • Troubleshoot any homework issues
9	Goal setting (laboratory) • Goal setting and flow state • RFB reassessment • HRV-F practice
10	Overview (laboratory) • Overview of the program • Where to from now? RFB beyond the program • HRV-F practice

2.2.4. Analyses

Self-Reported Outcomes

Self-reported questionnaires were completed via REDCap. These values were exported and tabulated. These outcomes were compared to normative data from other studies to reference whether the change in outcome was significant (see Table 2).

Physiological Outcomes

Kubios HRV Premium Analysis software (Version 3.5.0, Department of Applied Physics, University of Kuopio, Kuopio, Finland) was used for ECG signal preprocessing and HRV analysis in the time and frequency domain. Root mean square of successive differences (RMSSD), a time-domain measure of variability between consecutive beats, was used as a measure of cardiac vagal activity [14]. Frequency domain measures included low frequency (HRV-LF; 0.04–0.15 Hz) and high-frequency (HRV-HF; 0.15–0.4 Hz) power. HRV-LF power reflects a combination of sympathetic and parasympathetic activity upon the sinoatrial node and is suggested to reflect the cardiac-vagal baroreflex function [16]. HRV-HF power is another index of cardiac vagal activity correlated with RMSSD [14], with lower values associated with stress and anxiety [14].

Systolic blood pressure (SBP) signals were analysed using a custom-written program (MATLAB R2021b, MathWorks, Portola Valley, MA, USA) to calculate beat-to-beat BPV [34]. SBP low-frequency power (SBP-LF [0.04–0.15 Hz]) was used as a non-invasive estimate of the sympathetic control of vasculature [35].

Cardiovagal BRS was assessed using the sequence method [36] in a custom-written MATLAB program. The sequence method identifies sequences of >3 consecutive beats where a progressive shortening/lengthening of beat-to-beat intervals occurs as a function of progressive increasing/decreasing SBP. BRS gain was calculated as the average of the transfer function of these sequences. Baroreflex effectiveness index (BEI) was calculated as the number of identified sequences divided by the total number of systolic-only identified sequences (where a sequence of progressive increases/decreases in systolic BP occur without concurrent shortening/lengthening of heart beats).

Table 2. Psychosocial measures at baseline and 10-week assessments. Normative values from other studies are presented for reference.

	P1		P2		Normative Values		
	0 w	10 w	0 w	10 w	Population	Mean	SD
GAD-7	1	4	0	0	* SCI population (n = 465) [37]	3.86	4.34
PHQ9	8	8	0	2	* SCI population (n = 116) [38]	5.23	7.451
FSS	6	5	1.89	2.89	Chronic SCI—no cognitive impairment (n = 53) [39]	3.55	1.35
EQ-VAS	60	76	75	81	General Danish population (n = 1012) [40]	82.43	15.89
ADAPSS—SF	19	16	27	19	* SCI population (n = 256) [41]	16.32	6.84
ISCIPDS—Pain intensity	8	8	5	2	Chronic SCI—Non-neuropathic pain (n = 290) [42]	5.67	2.28
ISCIPDS—Activities	7	4	2	0	Chronic SCI—Non-neuropathic pain (n = 290) [42]	3.73	3.17
ISCIPDS—Mood	7	3	1	0	Chronic SCI—Non-neuropathic pain (n = 290) [42]	3.16	3.11
ISCIPDS—Sleep	5	6	5	1	Chronic SCI—Non-neuropathic pain (n = 290) [42]	3.64	3.41

ADAPSS-SF: Appraisal of Disability and Participation Scale- short form; EQVAS: EuroQol Visual Analog Scale; FSS: Fatigue Severity Scale; GADS: Generalised Anxiety Disorder Scale; ISCIPDS: International Spinal Cord Injury Pain Basic Data Set; P1: Participant 1; P2; Participant 2; PHQ9: Patient Health Questionnaire; 0 w: Baseline assessment; 10 w: 10-week assessment. Higher scores on GAD-7, PHQ-9, FSS, and ISCIPDS–pain intensity scales correspond to greater anxiety, depression, fatigue, and pain intensity, respectively. Lower scores on the ADAPSS-SF indicate a more positive appraisal of injury. Higher scores on the ISCIPDS-activities, ISCIPDS-mood, and ISCIPDS-sleep scales indicate a greater interference caused by pain in these aspects of life. Higher scores on the EQ-VAS indicate an improved quality of life. * SCI population is comprised of different injury levels and time since injury.

Further details regarding HRV, BPV, and BRS analyses may be found in Supplementary Table S1. HRV, BPV, and BRS analyses are presented for the resting condition, Stroop test, and paced breathing events to reflect changes in autonomic function during these tasks. Recovery data can be found in Supplementary Table S3.

3. Results

3.1. Case Presentations

Participant #1 (P1), aged 58 years, had a non-traumatic SCI (T1 AIS A), and was 3 years post-injury. P1 self-reported no previous mental health concerns, a vocational education, minimal alcohol consumption (1–2 drinks/3 months), no consumption of illicit drugs, and mobilised in a motorised wheelchair. Their medications included amitriptyline (25 mg/day), pregabalin (125 mg/morning, 75 mg/3 p.m., 75 mg/evening), and tylenol (3 × 1000 mg/day).

Participant #2 (P2), aged 54 years, had a non-traumatic SCI (T3 AIS C), and was over 25 years post-injury. P2 reported no previous mental health concerns, a vocational education, minimal alcohol consumption (1–2 drinks/3 months), no consumption of illicit drugs or any medications, and mobilised in a manual wheelchair.

3.2. Psychosocial Measures

Table 2 reports the psychosocial measures from the baseline and 10-week assessments. Normative data from other studies have been provided for reference. The EQ-VAS, ADAPSS-SF, and ISCIPDS indicated improvements in participants' quality of life, appraisal of injury, and pain interference. A decrease in fatigue for P1 and increase in fatigue for P2 were evident from FSS. A slight increase in anxiety, as shown by the GAD7 was seen for P1, with no change for P1 and an increase in depression for P2 was indicated by the PHQ9; although their scores were not clinically significant, remaining below 10.

3.3. Physiological

3.3.1. HRV, BPV, and BRS

Table 3 reports HRV, BPV, and BRS measures from the baseline and 10-week physiological assessments. Normative data from populations with SCI and able-bodied populations have been provided for reference. Due to the heterogeneity in acquiring and processing physiological data, comparing data from different studies should be performed with caution. P1 demonstrated little change in RMSSD during all events and an increase in HRV-HF at the 10-week assessment during the Stroop (ratio: 2.64) and paced breathing tasks (ratio: 3.07). HRV-LF only increased during the paced-breathing task (ratio: 2.10). Diastolic BP increased across all events (+4 to 9 mmHg), and systolic BP increased in the resting condition (+12 mmHg) and Stroop task (+21 mmHg) but not in the paced breathing task (−1 mmHg). SBP-LF decreased during the resting condition and Stroop task but increased during paced breathing (+1.05 mmHg^2). BRS gain decreased slightly in the resting condition (−0.07 ms/mmHg) and Stroop task (−0.17 ms/mmHg), but increased during the paced breathing task (+0.4 ms/mmHg). BEI ratio saw improvements during the Stroop (+0.03) and paced breathing tasks (+0.13).

P2 demonstrated increases from baseline to 10-week assessment in RMSSD, HRV-LF, and HRV-HF across all physiological events, except for HRV-HF paced breathing (ratio: 0.997). Changes from baseline to 10-weeks in the the resting condition were: RMSSD (ratio: 1.94), LF power (ratio: 4.33), and HF power (ratio: 2.16). The changes in the Stroop task were: RMSSD (ratio: 2.41), LF power (ratio: 6.75), HF power (ratio: 9.24). Changes that occurred during the paced breathing task were: RMSSD (ratio: 1.67) and LF power (ratio: 6.68). Systolic BP decreased slightly during the resting condition (−2 mmHg) but increased during the Stroop (+19 mmHg) and paced breathing tasks (+10 mmHg). Diastolic BP increased during the resting condition (+7 mmHg), slightly decreased during the Stroop task (−2 mmHg), and did not change during the paced breathing task. SBP-LF power decreased for all events. BRS gain increased during resting (+0.94 ms/mmHg) and the paced breathing task (+0.1 ms/mmHg) and decreased during the Stroop task (−1.82 ms/mmHg). BEI ratio improved across all events (resting: +0.3, Stroop: +0.25, paced breathing: +0.38).

Figure 3 displays the power spectrum (HRV-LF and HRV-HF bands) at baseline and 10 weeks for both participants during paced breathing. During this condition, a peak around 0.1 Hz within the HRV-LF band is desirable as it indicates effective cardiorespiratory resonance and enhanced baroreflex function [16]. Both P1 and P2 demonstrated significant increases in this peak.

Table 3. Heart rate variability, blood pressure variability and baroreflex sensitivity measures for baseline and 10-week assessment.

	Baseline			10-Weeks			Normative Values under Resting Conditions	
	HRV							
	R	S	PB	R	S	PB	Mean (SD)	Population
P1								
RMSSD (ms)	7.28	3.86	4.69	5.13	4.36	6.96	29.8 (24.3)	Chronic SCI T3 and above (n = 21) [43]
HRV-LF (ms^2)	116.19	8.82	60.45	40.07	7.22	127.08	285.4 (325.5)	
HRV-HF (ms^2)	38.61	3.97	5.46	25.6	10.50	16.74	513.4 (879.4)	
P2								
RMSSD (ms)	20.82	23.51	18.66	40.49	56.64	31.11	29.8 (24.3)	
HRV-LF (ms^2)	349.43	318.00	254.21	1512.98	2146.35	1698.77	285.4 (325.5)	
HRV-HF (ms^2)	186.92	201.84	131.75	403.69	1865.93	131.3	513.4 (879.4)	

Table 3. Cont.

	Baseline			10-Weeks			Normative Values under Resting Conditions	
	HRV							
	R	S	PB	R	S	PB	Mean (SD)	Population
	BPV							
	R	S	PB	R	S	PB	Mean (SD)	Population
P1								
BP (mmHg)	101/57	98/52	106/53	113/61	119/61	105/58	126.8 (7.0)/66.2 (4.1)	Chronic thoracic SCI (n = 12) [44]
SBP-LF (mmHg^2)	5.02	2.54	2.73	4.88	2.43	3.77	17.32 (7.7)	
P2								
BP (mmHg)	111/69	107/71	105/73	109/76	126/69	115/73	126.8 (7.0)/66.2 (4.1)	
SBP-LF (mmHg^2)	6.65	7.64	12.22	5.05	5.83	11.13	17.32 (7.7)	
	BRS							
	R	S	PB	R	S	PB	Mean (SD)	Population
P1								
BRS gain (ms/mmHg)	5.08	4.38	5.02	5.01	4.21	5.42	10.65 (3.2)	Chronic thoracic SCI (n = 12) [44]
BEI [ratio]	0.21	0.04	0.10	0.13	0.07	0.23	0.7 (0.1)	AB (n = 35) [45]
P2								
BRS gain (ms/mmHg)	7.15	9.00	7.93	8.09	7.18	8.03	10.65 (3.2)	Chronic thoracic SCI (n = 12) [44]
BEI [ratio]	0.32	0.45	0.39	0.62	0.70	0.77	0.7 (0.1)	AB (n = 35) [45]

BP: Brachial blood pressure; BEI: Baroreflex Effectiveness Index; BRS gain: Vagal Baroreflex Sensitivity; HRV: Heart rate variability; HRV-HF: HRV high-frequency power; HRV-LF: HRV low-frequency power; AB: Able-bodied population; PB: Paced breathing; P1: Participant 1; P2: Participant 2; R: Resting condition; RMSSD: Root mean square of successive differences; S: Stroop test; SBP-LF: Systolic low-frequency power.

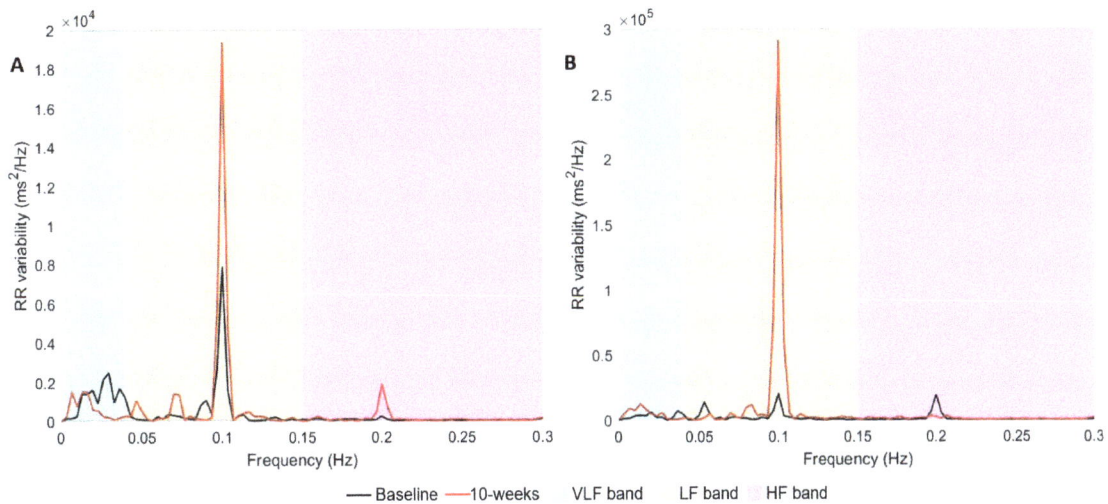

Figure 3. Heart rate variability power spectrum during paced breathing for Participant 1 (A) and Participant 2 (B) at baseline and 10 weeks post HRV-F. VLF band: very-low frequency band (0–0.04 Hz); LF band: low-frequency band (0.04–0.15 Hz); HF band: high-frequency band (>0.15 Hz); RR variability: variation in time period between beat-to-beat intervals of the heart.

3.3.2. HRV-F Results

Both participants had an initial resonant frequency of 6 breaths/minute with an inhalation–exhalation ratio of 4 s:6 s. Over the intervention, this ratio was slightly modified in both participants (increased inhalation period) according to patient comfort and fatigue levels. Supplementary Figure S1 provides data for each individual's baseline resonant frequency assessment.

P1 practised HRV-F at home for approximately 34 h over the 10 weeks with an adherence rate of twice daily HRV-F of 76% (102 out of 134 biofeedback sessions). P2 practised HRV-F at home for approximately 24 h with an adherence rate of 54% (72/134).

3.3.3. Self-Reported Weekly Diaries

Over the 10 weeks, small trends were noted in the participants' weekly diaries. Both participants trended towards a slight improvement in mood. P1 trended towards a slight decrease in anxiety and pain, whereas P2 trended towards a slightly larger decrease in anxiety and pain. Both participants trended towards reduced sleep quality.

Over the course of the intervention, both participants reported several life and adverse events. Life events included hospitalisation of family members, issues with pets, and housing rearrangements which were reported to affect adherence to the twice-daily HRV-F home practice. Adverse events included fatigue, difficulty sleeping, and low energy. Whilst these did not occur during HRV-F home practice, they may have been directly related to the intervention.

Despite these events, both participants reported enhanced body awareness, improved pain management, and a better ability to manage stress. P1 also reported increased confidence and independence in the community. For example, being able to take public transport independently for the first time since their injury.

4. Discussion

This case series demonstrated preliminary evidence for the effect of a 10-week HRV-F intervention in two adults with chronic T1 AIS A and T3 AIS C injuries, respectively. While we only present two cases, and therefore any conclusions are limited in terms of generalising to the larger population, our findings showed that HRV-F was associated with changes in cardiac autonomic regulation, appraisal of injury, and health-related QoL for these two adults with chronic non-traumatic SCI.

4.1. Cardiovascular Changes

Cardiac autonomic regulation improved to varying extents for each individual. Given many factors influence cardiac autonomic regulation, including seasonal variation and circadian rhythm, it is difficult to identify which factors are responsible for this. We hypothesise that the varying degrees of remaining cardiac autonomic control for each participant may have played a significant role in this. The greatest improvement was shown by P2, who had a lower-level incomplete injury and would be expected to have a greater preservation of cardiac innervation compared to P1. P2 showed increases in HRV and BEI measures across all conditions. These improvements are not unexpected, given that similar outcomes have been found in both healthy, able-bodied individuals and diverse disease populations [12,46]. Preservation of cardiac autonomic innervation should be explored further as a possible determinant of how individuals with SCI respond to HRV-F.

In contrast, P1 saw a decrease in some HRV measures during the resting condition and Stroop tasks (Resting condition: RMSSD, HRV-LF, HRV-HF. Stroop: HRV-LF), which differs from the previous literature and the hypothesised effect of HRV-F [46]. These findings need clarification with a larger sample with more diverse injury characteristics and may be confounded by concurrent medical and psychosocial factors. Factors such as level of injury, time since injury, completeness of injury, amount of exercise, and medication use differed between participants and may also contribute to the disparity between these participants. Beyond being a marker of cardiac function, HRV is negatively associated with psychosocial factors such as stress and anxiety [13]. Life events experienced by P1, such as family concerns and the hospitalisation of family members, may increase stress and decrease HRV [47].

Nevertheless, P1 demonstrated increases in most HRV and BRS measures, such as RMSSD, HRV-LF, HRV-HF, and BEI, during the paced breathing task. This task appears to provide optimal conditions for cardiorespiratory and cardiovascular resonance and maximise HRV/autonomic changes [48]. Figure 3 depicts the increase in HRV power for both participants during the paced breathing task, represented as a single peak within the HRV-LF region, at the 0.1 Hz frequency (corresponding to 6 breaths/minute). Around this frequency range, it is known that the baroreflex reaches resonance with respiration, a phenomenon referred to as 'baroreflex resonance' [16]. Whilst it is difficult to control for confounders in a case series design, these observed changes may likely be vagally mediated [14] and suggest the potential for HRV-F to improve cardiac autonomic regulation, especially under optimal conditions such as paced breathing [49]. However, it is important to acknowledge that various factors may also have contributed to this change, such as environmental factors (i.e., seasonal changes, circadian rhythm) and technical factors (i.e., participants learning to follow the pacer correctly).

Blood pressure changes (absolute values) between tasks trended towards a physiological response that would be expected in a healthy population. This was reflected in an increase in the value in response to a cognitive stressor (Stroop task) and a decrease in response to paced breathing. Blood pressure is typically reduced in the SCI population due to several factors, including a reduced vasomotor tone and reduced vascular muscle pump, which becomes more evident in higher-level injuries [3]. Poor blood pressure management contributes to complications such as orthostatic hypotension [3]. A larger sample is needed to validate these findings and investigate the effect that HRV-F may have on the occurrence of these complications.

SBP-LF provides a measure of vascular sympathetic activity [44]. In an able-bodied population, lower blood pressure variability is desirable as it leads to a more stable BP and reduced adverse cardiovascular events [50]. In contrast, lower SBP-LF in an SCI population has previously been shown to mirror reduced sympathetic activity and potentially more significant disruption of autonomic control [35,44]. Recently, Lucci and colleagues showed that a cutoff of <2 mmHg of SBP-LF could be used to identify adults with an autonomic complete SCI [34]. Whilst both participants in the current case series possessed autonomic incomplete injuries (cutoff > 2 mmHg^2), they had different degrees of cardiac autonomic control. Minimal change in SBP-LF was observed for P1 whereas a reduction was noted for P2. Many factors could be responsible for these changes and it is not possible to conclude these changes were the result of HRV-F. Further investigation is needed to evaluate ideal SBP-LF values in a population with SCI and the impact that HRV-F has on blood pressure variability. It may be that for incomplete lower-level lesions, a lower SBP-LF is desirable whereas higher SBP-LF may be appropriate for complete higher-level lesions.

4.2. Psychosocial Changes

Previous studies have highlighted that as little as 2–4 weeks of HRV-F effectively improves psychological health in various populations [46]. In this case series, minimal change was noted in the psychological measures for anxiety and depressive mood. Whilst the n = 2 case series limits our ability to draw conclusions, this may be due to participants scoring low-to-mild levels of depressive mood and anxiety at baseline. It has been previously shown that biofeedback can be more effective for those with psychopathology [51]. We hypothesise that certain sub-groups of the SCI population with psychological problems would see more significant improvements in mood following HRV-F. By identifying groups that respond positively to HRV-F, personalised treatment plans and better patient outcomes can be achieved.

By contrast, improvements were shown in other psychosocial measures, including appraisal and quality of life. These findings are aligned with P1's self-report of improved independence in the community, independently taking public transport for the first time since their injury. Improved quality of life following HRV-F has been found in other populations, including adults with obesity and chronic neck and shoulder pain [46]. In contrast, there is minimal literature exploring the effect of HRV-F on the appraisal of injury. Positive appraisal of injury is necessary for positive adjustment following an SCI and contributes to greater quality of life [1]. Given that HRV-F is known to improve emotional regulation and promote prosocial states [52], it may be that emotions surrounding an individual's injury are better regulated, providing a more positive outlook on the injury. Additionally, given that helpful social relationships are essential for positive adjustment following injury [1], HRV-F may promote prosocial behaviours, which contribute to the positive appraisal of injury following an SCI.

Pain is often difficult to treat and poses a significant barrier to participation for many adults with an SCI [53]. Currently, it is minimally responsive to existing non-pharmacological treatments [54]. Therefore, new non-pharmacological treatments need to be explored. In this study, HRV-F was associated with a reduction in pain intensity and the impact that pain has on daily life. These were consistent with the self-reported notes, whereby both participants reported an improved awareness of pain.

"...say I've got a headache, or I am my headache, it's kind of like I am my pain. It characterises who I am and how much I'm able to do in a day and being able to separate it as something separate to be managed has allowed me to be more productive during the day and to kind of ground myself and do more, be more active, be more independent." Comment received from P1.

In addition, greater cardiac vagal activity, as measured by HRV-RMSSD and HRV-HF power, has been linked with reduced pain [55]. Similarly, HRV-F has been shown to reduce measures of pain in chronic disease populations, such as fibromyalgia and chronic shoulder and neck pain [46]. Pain may be associated with changes in the ANS, and stable improvements in pain may occur by improving cardiac vagal control via HRV-F. The reduction in sleep quality reported by both participants during the 10 weeks was unexpected and will hopefully be clarified by additional follow-up and a larger sample size.

4.3. Considerations for Future Research

For future investigations exploring HRV-F, dosage is a key consideration. Participants were encouraged in the current case series to perform 20 min of HRV-F home practice twice daily, which was often difficult for them to achieve. Nevertheless, some benefits were still achieved by both participants. In a review of studies with chronic disease populations, Fournie and colleagues found improvements from HRV-F in as little as 4 weeks, and with home practice for as little as 15 min a day [46]. Our findings indicate that some reorganisation in the cardiac ANS can occur in as little as 10 weeks, however, it may only be apparent under controlled physiological conditions (e.g., slow/paced breathing). Whilst P1 completed more sessions of HRV-F home practice than P2, greater cardiac autonomic benefits were noted by P2. Therefore, the optimal dosage of HRV-F for certain benefits needs clarification, as does the impact of the injury aetiology, level of injury, degree of remaining cardiac autonomic control, psychosocial status, and time since injury.

Another consideration is the role of inhalation–exhalation ratios. It is established that a longer exhalation increases vagal efferent activity, resulting in a greater parasympathetic response [56]. Previous studies have found that a lower ratio is associated with greater relaxation and less stress [57]. In able-bodied populations, dominant sympathetic activity tends to be an important consideration. This is generally opposite to the state found in a SCI population with high-level lesions. Therefore, customisation of this ratio for each individual may be essential to realise further benefits, and future studies should investigate how these ratios affect HRV-F outcomes.

4.4. Limitations

There are several limitations to this study. Firstly, this case series included two participants only, limiting our ability to draw conclusions and generalise findings to the broader SCI population. The current study is not intended to be robust enough to reflect a proof-of-concept for the effectiveness of HRV-F. Rather, it is essentially a pilot phase, which highlights that HRV-F is a feasible intervention and has the potential to provide therapeutic and possibly diverse benefits to two participants with different SCI characteristics. This suggests that it is worth pursuing in a larger randomised controlled trial. Given the heterogeneity of a population with SCI, a larger sample size with a greater representation of SCI characteristics, such as time since injury, level of injury, aetiology of injury, and completeness of injury, is warranted for more generalisable results. Another area for improvement is the need for standardisation of home biofeedback practice. Whilst participants were instructed to perform HRV-F in a seated position with eyes open, various other factors such as circadian rhythm, meals/caffeine consumption, and amount of exercise and sleep could influence HRV results. However, placing additional restrictions would arguably impact adherence to HRV-F practice. Furthermore, using the Elite HRV app, we were unable to verify if participants followed the visual respiration pacing correctly during their home practice. Lalanza and colleagues recommended using respirometers for this issue; however, these can be costly [58]. Furthermore, respiration rate is known to influence HRV in a SCI population [59], which may confound HRV results. Whilst we did not restrict respiration rate during the assessment, a paced breathing task was added to the assessment protocol to control this.

5. Conclusions

A 10-week HRV-F intervention was shown to be feasible in two participants with chronic non-traumatic SCI with different injury characteristics. Varying degrees of change were found between participants, with notable changes in cardiac autonomic regulation, health-related quality of life, and perception of injury. Further research using a larger sample size with greater heterogeneity in SCI characteristics and a more extended follow-up period is required to understand the effectiveness of this intervention on adults with chronic SCI. These results provide initial support for a 10-week HRV-F intervention to be further investigated as to its autonomic and psychosocial effects on adults with chronic SCI.

Supplementary Materials: The following supporting information can be downloaded at: https://www.mdpi.com/article/10.3390/jcm12247664/s1, Table S1: Description of presented measures; Table S2: Criteria for the resonant frequency assessment; Table S3: HRV, BPV and BRS outcomes for all physiological events; Figure S1: Baseline resonant frequency assessments for P1 and P2. References [60–66] are cited in the Supplementary Materials.

Author Contributions: Conceptualization, J.S., M.A., I.P., C.M., D.R., E.V., J.M., G.M.D. and A.C.; Data curation, J.S., M.A., I.P., C.M., D.R. and E.V.; Formal analysis, J.S., M.A., I.P. and A.C.; Funding acquisition, J.M. and A.C.; Investigation, J.S., M.A., I.P., C.M., D.R., E.V. and A.C.; Methodology, J.S., M.A., I.P., C.M., D.R., E.V., J.M., G.M.D., S.M.G., J.B., A.K., A.V.K., I.D.C. and A.C.; Project administration, J.S., M.A., I.P., C.M., D.R., E.V., J.M., G.M.D. and A.C.; Resources, J.S., M.A., I.P., C.M., J.M., G.M.D., J.B., A.K., A.V.K., I.D.C. and A.C.; Software, J.S. and I.P.; Supervision, M.A., I.P., J.M., A.V.K., I.D.C. and A.C.; Validation, J.S., M.A., I.P., D.R., J.M., S.M.G., A.K., A.V.K. and A.C.; Visualization, J.S., M.A., I.P., J.M., G.M.D. and A.C.; Writing—original draft, J.S.; Writing—review and editing, J.S., M.A., I.P., C.M., D.R., E.V., J.M., G.M.D., S.M.G., J.B., A.K., A.V.K., I.D.C. and A.C. All authors have read and agreed to the published version of the manuscript.

Funding: This research was funded by the NSW Ministry of Health, Australia (Grant number: H21-125024) via Spinal Cord Injury Research Grants Program 2019/20 and The University of Sydney, Australia (IRMA ID: 207165).

Institutional Review Board Statement: The study was conducted in accordance with the National Health and Medical Research Council's National Statement on Ethical Conduct in Human Research (2007) and the Note for Guidance on Good Clinical Practice (CPMP/ICH-135/95). The larger trial was approved by the Northern Sydney Local Health District Human Research Ethics Committee (2020/ETH02554, 2 December 2020).

Informed Consent Statement: Informed consent was obtained from all subjects involved in the study. Written informed consent has been obtained from the patients to publish this paper.

Data Availability Statement: The data presented in this study are available on request from the corresponding author. The data are not publicly available to ensure participant privacy.

Acknowledgments: We would like to thank the NSW Ministry of Health, Australia and The University of Sydney, Australia for the funding for this study. We would also like to thank Ali Gholamrezaei for his assistance in data analysis and Rowan Hayes for his assistance in the architecture figures.

Conflicts of Interest: The authors declare no conflict of interest.

References

1. Craig, A.; Tran, Y.; Middleton, J. Theory of adjustment following severe neurological injury: Vidence supporting the Spinal Cord Injury Adjustment Model. In *Horizons in Neuroscience Research*; Costa, A., Villalba, E., Eds.; Nova Science Publishers: New York, NY, USA, 2017; pp. 117–139.
2. Sezer, N.; Akkuş, S.; Uğurlu, F.G. Chronic complications of spinal cord injury. *World J. Orthop.* **2015**, *6*, 24–33. [CrossRef]
3. Hou, S.; Rabchevsky, A.G. Autonomic consequences of spinal cord injury. *Compr. Physiol.* **2011**, *4*, 1419–1453. [CrossRef]
4. Karemaker, J.M. An introduction into autonomic nervous function. *Physiol. Meas.* **2017**, *38*, R89–R118. [CrossRef]
5. Teasell, R.W.; Arnold, J.M.; Krassioukov, A.; Delaney, G.A. Cardiovascular consequences of loss of supraspinal control of the sympathetic nervous system after spinal cord injury. *Arch. Phys. Med. Rehabil.* **2000**, *81*, 506–516. [CrossRef]
6. Fossey, M.P.M.; Balthazaar, S.J.T.; Squair, J.W.; Williams, A.M.; Poormasjedi-Meibod, M.-S.; Nightingale, T.E.; Erskine, E.; Hayes, B.; Ahmadian, M.; Jackson, G.S.; et al. Spinal cord injury impairs cardiac function due to impaired bulbospinal sympathetic control. *Nat. Commun.* **2022**, *13*, 1382. [CrossRef]
7. Sandalic, D.; Craig, A.; Tran, Y.; Arora, M.; Pozzato, I.; McBain, C.; Tonkin, H.; Simpson, G.; Gopinath, B.; Kaur, J.; et al. Cognitive impairment in individuals with spinal cord injury: Findings of a systematic review with robust variance and network meta-analyses. *Neurology* **2022**, *99*, e1779–e1790. [CrossRef]
8. Singh, V.; Mitra, S. Psychophysiological impact of spinal cord injury: Depression, coping and heart rate variability. *J. Spinal Cord Med.* **2023**, *46*, 441–449. [CrossRef]
9. Rodrigues, D.; Tran, Y.; Guest, R.; Middleton, J.; Craig, A. Influence of neurological lesion level on heart rate variability and fatigue in adults with spinal cord injury. *Spinal Cord* **2016**, *54*, 292–297. [CrossRef]
10. Charlifue, S.; Gerhart, K. Community integration in spinal cord injury of long duration. *NeuroRehabilitation* **2004**, *19*, 91–101. [CrossRef] [PubMed]
11. Cao, Y.; Krause, J.S. Estimation of indirect costs based on employment and earnings changes after spinal cord injury: An observational study. *Spinal Cord* **2020**, *58*, 908–913. [CrossRef]
12. Lehrer, P.; Kaur, K.; Sharma, A.; Shah, K.; Huseby, R.; Bhavsar, J.; Sgobba, P.; Zhang, Y. Heart rate variability biofeedback improves emotional and physical health and performance: A systematic review and meta analysis. *Appl. Psychophysiol. Biofeedback* **2020**, *45*, 109–129. [CrossRef]
13. Thayer, J.F.; Åhs, F.; Fredrikson, M.; Sollers, J.J.; Wager, T.D. A meta-analysis of heart rate variability and neuroimaging studies: Implications for heart rate variability as a marker of stress and health. *Neurosci. Biobehav. Rev.* **2012**, *36*, 747–756. [CrossRef]
14. Shaffer, F.; McCraty, R.; Zerr, C.L. A healthy heart is not a metronome: An integrative review of the heart's anatomy and heart rate variability. *Front. Psychol.* **2014**, *5*, 1040. [CrossRef]
15. Forte, G.; Favieri, F.; Casagrande, M. Heart Rate Variability and Cognitive Function: A Systematic Review. *Front. Neurosci.* **2019**, *13*, 710. [CrossRef]
16. Sevoz-Couche, C.; Laborde, S. Heart rate variability and slow-paced breathing: When coherence meets resonance. *Neurosci. Biobehav. Rev.* **2022**, *135*, 104576. [CrossRef]
17. Lehrer, P.M.; Gevirtz, R. Heart rate variability biofeedback: How and why does it work? *Front. Psychol.* **2014**, *5*, 756. [CrossRef]
18. Lehrer, P.M.; Vaschillo, E.; Vaschillo, B.; Lu, S.E.; Scardella, A.; Siddique, M.; Habib, R.H. Biofeedback treatment for asthma. *Chest* **2004**, *126*, 352–361. [CrossRef]
19. Chang, W.-L.; Lee, J.-T.; Li, C.-R.; Davis, A.H.T.; Yang, C.-C.; Chen, Y.-J. Effects of heart rate variability biofeedback in patients with acute ischemic stroke: A randomized controlled trial. *Biol. Res. Nurs.* **2020**, *22*, 34–44. [CrossRef]
20. Hassett, A.L.; Radvanski, D.C.; Vaschillo, E.G.; Vaschillo, B.; Sigal, L.H.; Karavidas, M.K.; Buyske, S.; Lehrer, P.M. A pilot study of the efficacy of heart rate variability (HRV) biofeedback in patients with fibromyalgia. *Appl. Psychophysiol. Biofeedback* **2007**, *32*, 1–10. [CrossRef]

21. Wearne, T.A.; Logan, J.A.; Trimmer, E.M.; Wilson, E.; Filipcikova, M.; Kornfeld, E.; Rushby, J.A.; McDonald, S. Regulating emotion following severe traumatic brain injury: A randomized controlled trial of heart-rate variability biofeedback training. *Brain Inj.* **2021**, *35*, 1390–1401. [CrossRef]
22. Phillips, A.A.; Krassioukov, A.V.; Ainslie, P.N.; Warburton, D.E. Baroreflex function after spinal cord injury. *J. Neurotrauma* **2012**, *29*, 2431–2445. [CrossRef]
23. Lehrer, P. How does heart rate variability biofeedback work? Resonance, the baroreflex, and other mechanisms. *Biofeedback* **2013**, *41*, 26–31. [CrossRef]
24. Schrezenmaier, C.; Singer, W.; Swift, N.M.; Sletten, D.; Tanabe, J.; Low, P.A. Adrenergic and vagal baroreflex sensitivity in autonomic failure. *Arch. Neurol.* **2007**, *64*, 381–386. [CrossRef]
25. Frank, D.L.; Khorshid, L.; Kiffer, J.F.; Moravec, C.S.; McKee, M.G. Biofeedback in medicine: Who, when, why and how? *Ment. Health Fam. Med.* **2010**, *7*, 85–91. [PubMed]
26. Laborde, S.; Allen, M.S.; Borges, U.; Iskra, M.; Zammit, N.; You, M.; Hosang, T.; Mosley, E.; Dosseville, F. Psychophysiological effects of slow-paced breathing at six cycles per minute with or without heart rate variability biofeedback. *Psychophysiology* **2022**, *59*, e13952. [CrossRef]
27. Craig, A.; Pozzato, I.; Arora, M.; Middleton, J.; Rodrigues, D.; McBain, C.; Tran, Y.; Davis, G.M.; Gopinath, B.; Kifley, A.; et al. A neuro-cardiac self-regulation therapy to improve autonomic and neural function after SCI: A randomized controlled trial protocol. *BMC Neurol.* **2021**, *21*, 329. [CrossRef]
28. Task Force of the European Society of Cardiology the North American Society of Pacing Electrophysiology. Heart rate variability. *Circulation* **1996**, *93*, 1043–1065. [CrossRef]
29. Treisman, A.; Fearnley, S. The Stroop test: Selective attention to colours and words. *Nature* **1969**, *222*, 437–439. [CrossRef]
30. Tulen, J.H.; Moleman, P.; van Steenis, H.G.; Boomsma, F. Characterization of stress reactions to the Stroop color word test. *Pharmacol. Biochem. Behav.* **1989**, *32*, 9–15. [CrossRef]
31. Shaffer, F.; Meehan, Z.M. A practical guide to resonance frequency assessment for heart rate variability biofeedback. *Front. Neurosci.* **2020**, *14*, 570400. [CrossRef]
32. Lehrer, P.; Vaschillo, B.; Zucker, T.; Graves, J.; Katsamanis, M.; Aviles, M.; Wamboldt, F. Protocol for heart rate variability biofeedback training. *Biofeedback* **2013**, *41*, 98–109. [CrossRef]
33. Lehrer, P.M.; Vaschillo, E.; Vaschillo, B.; Lu, S.E.; Eckberg, D.L.; Edelberg, R.; Shih, W.J.; Lin, Y.; Kuusela, T.A.; Tahvanainen, K.U.; et al. Heart rate variability biofeedback increases baroreflex gain and peak expiratory flow. *Psychosom. Med.* **2003**, *65*, 796–805. [CrossRef]
34. Gholamrezaei, A.; Van Diest, I.; Aziz, Q.; Vlaeyen, J.W.S.; Van Oudenhove, L. Influence of inspiratory threshold load on cardiovascular responses to controlled breathing at 0.1 Hz. *Psychophysiology* **2019**, *56*, e13447. [CrossRef]
35. Lucci, V.E.M.; Inskip, J.A.; McGrath, M.S.; Ruiz, I.; Lee, R.; Kwon, B.K.; Claydon, V.E. Longitudinal assessment of autonomic function during the acute phase of spinal cord injury: Use of low-frequency blood pressure variability as a quantitative measure of autonomic function. *J. Neurotrauma* **2021**, *38*, 309–321. [CrossRef]
36. Bertinieri, G.; di Rienzo, M.; Cavallazzi, A.; Ferrari, A.U.; Pedotti, A.; Mancia, G. A new approach to analysis of the arterial baroreflex. *J. Hypertens. Suppl.* **1985**, *3*, S79–S81. [PubMed]
37. Kisala, P.A.; Tulsky, D.S.; Kalpakjian, C.Z.; Heinemann, A.W.; Pohlig, R.T.; Carle, A.; Choi, S.W. Measuring anxiety after spinal cord injury: Development and psychometric characteristics of the SCI-QOL anxiety item bank and linkage with GAD-7. *J. Spinal Cord Med.* **2015**, *38*, 315–325. [CrossRef]
38. Poritz, J.M.P.; Mignogna, J.; Christie, A.J.; Holmes, S.A.; Ames, H. The patient health questionnaire depression screener in spinal cord injury. *J. Spinal Cord Med.* **2018**, *41*, 238–244. [CrossRef]
39. Craig, A.; Guest, R.; Tran, Y.; Middleton, J. Cognitive impairment and mood states after spinal cord injury. *J. Neurotrauma* **2016**, *34*, 1156–1163. [CrossRef]
40. Jensen, M.B.; Jensen, C.E.; Gudex, C.; Pedersen, K.M.; Sørensen, S.S.; Ehlers, L.H. Danish population health measured by the EQ-5D-5L. *Scand. J. Public. Health* **2023**, *51*, 241–249. [CrossRef]
41. McDonald, S.; Goldberg, L.; Mickens, M.; Ellwood, M.; Mutchler, B.; Perrin, P. Appraisals of DisAbility Primary and Secondary Scale-Short Form (ADAPSS-sf): Psychometrics and association with mental health among U.S. military veterans with spinal cord injury. *Rehabil. Psychol.* **2018**, *63*, 372. [CrossRef]
42. Felix, E.R.; Cardenas, D.D.; Bryce, T.N.; Charlifue, S.; Lee, T.K.; MacIntyre, B.; Mulroy, S.; Taylor, H. Prevalence and impact of neuropathic and nonneuropathic pain in chronic spinal cord injury. *Arch. Phys. Med. Rehabil.* **2022**, *103*, 729–737. [CrossRef] [PubMed]
43. Schoffl, J.; Pozzato, I.; Rodrigues, D.; Arora, M.; Craig, A. Pulse rate variability: An alternative to heart rate variability in adults with spinal cord injury. *Psychophysiology* **2023**, *60*, e14356. [CrossRef]
44. Claydon, V.E.; Krassioukov, A.V. Clinical correlates of frequency analyses of cardiovascular control after spinal cord injury. *Am. J. Physiol. Heart Circ. Physiol.* **2008**, *294*, H668–H678. [CrossRef] [PubMed]
45. Gholamrezaei, A.; Van Diest, I.; Aziz, Q.; Vlaeyen, J.W.S.; Van Oudenhove, L. Psychophysiological responses to various slow, deep breathing techniques. *Psychophysiology* **2021**, *58*, e13712. [CrossRef] [PubMed]
46. Fournie, C.; Chouchou, F.; Dalleau, G.; Caderby, T.; Cabrera, Q.; Verkindt, C. Heart rate variability biofeedback in chronic disease management: A systematic review. *Complement. Ther. Med.* **2021**, *60*, 102750. [CrossRef] [PubMed]

47. Kim, H.G.; Cheon, E.J.; Bai, D.S.; Lee, Y.H.; Koo, B.H. Stress and heart rate variability: A meta-analysis and review of the literature. *Psychiatry Investig.* **2018**, *15*, 235–245. [CrossRef] [PubMed]
48. Six Dijkstra, M.; Soer, R.; Bieleman, A.; McCraty, R.; Oosterveld, F.; Gross, D.; Reneman, M. Exploring a 1-minute paced deep-breathing measurement of heart rate variability as part of a workers' health assessment. *Appl. Psychophysiol. Biofeedback* **2019**, *44*, 83–96. [CrossRef] [PubMed]
49. Zaccaro, A.; Piarulli, A.; Laurino, M.; Garbella, E.; Menicucci, D.; Neri, B.; Gemignani, A. How breath-control can change your life: A systematic review on psycho-physiological correlates of slow breathing. *Front. Hum. Neurosci.* **2018**, *12*, 353. [CrossRef]
50. Stevens, S.L.; Wood, S.; Koshiaris, C.; Law, K.; Glasziou, P.; Stevens, R.J.; McManus, R.J. Blood pressure variability and cardiovascular disease: Systematic review and meta-analysis. *BMJ* **2016**, *354*, i4098. [CrossRef]
51. Drexler, A.; Mur, E.; Gunther, V. Efficacy of an EMG-biofeedback therapy in fibromyalgia patients. A comparative study of patients with and without abnormality in (MMPI) psychological scales. *Clin. Exp. Rheumatol.* **2002**, *20*, 677–682. [PubMed]
52. Schumann, A.; de la Cruz, F.; Köhler, S.; Brotte, L.; Bär, K.-J. The influence of heart rate variability biofeedback on cardiac regulation and functional brain connectivity. *Front. Neurosci.* **2021**, *15*, 691988. [CrossRef] [PubMed]
53. Siddall, P.; Loeser, J. Pain following spinal cord injury. *Spinal Cord* **2001**, *39*, 63–73. [CrossRef] [PubMed]
54. Boldt, I.; Eriks-Hoogland, I.; Brinkhof, M.W.G.; de Bie, R.; Joggi, D.; von Elm, E. Non-pharmacological interventions for chronic pain in people with spinal cord injury. *Cochrane Database Syst. Rev.* **2014**, *11*, CD009177. [CrossRef] [PubMed]
55. Forte, G.; Troisi, G.; Pazzaglia, M.; Pascalis, V.; Casagrande, M. Heart rate variability and pain: A systematic review. *Brain Sci.* **2022**, *12*, 153. [CrossRef] [PubMed]
56. Russo, M.A.; Santarelli, D.M.; O'Rourke, D. The physiological effects of slow breathing in the healthy human. *Breathe* **2017**, *13*, 298–309. [CrossRef] [PubMed]
57. Komori, T. The relaxation effect of prolonged expiratory breathing. *Ment. Illn.* **2018**, *10*, 7669. [CrossRef] [PubMed]
58. Lalanza, J.F.; Lorente, S.; Bullich, R.; García, C.; Losilla, J.-M.; Capdevila, L. Methods for heart rate variability biofeedback (HRVB): A systematic review and guidelines. *Appl. Psychophysiol. Biofeedback* **2023**, *48*, 275–297. [CrossRef]
59. Solinsky, R.; Schleifer, G.D.; Draghici, A.E.; Hamner, J.W.; Taylor, J.A. Methodologic implications for rehabilitation research: Differences in heart rate variability introduced by respiration. *PM&R* **2022**, *14*, 1483–1489. [CrossRef]
60. Spitzer, R.L.; Kroenke, K.; Williams, J.B.; Löwe, B. A brief measure for assessing generalized anxiety disorder: The GAD-7. *Arch. Intern. Med.* **2006**, *166*, 1092–1097. [CrossRef]
61. Kroenke, K.; Spitzer, R.L.; Williams, J.B.W. The PHQ-9. *J. Gen. Intern. Med.* **2001**, *16*, 606–613. [CrossRef]
62. Krupp, L.B.; LaRocca, N.G.; Muir-Nash, J.; Steinberg, A.D. The fatigue severity scale. Application to patients with multiple sclerosis and patients with lupus erythematosus. *Arch. Neurol.* **1989**, *46*, 1121–1123. [CrossRef] [PubMed]
63. Cheng, L.J.; Tan, R.L.-Y.; Luo, N. Measurement properties of the EQ VAS around the globe: A systematic review and meta-regression analysis. *Value Health* **2021**, *24*, 1223–1233. [CrossRef]
64. Garin, O.; Ayuso-Mateos, J.L.; Almansa, J.; Nieto, M.; Chatterji, S.; Vilagut, G.; Alonso, J.; Cieza, A.; Svetskova, O.; Burger, H.; et al. Validation of the "World Health Organization Disability Assessment Schedule, WHODAS-2" in patients with chronic diseases. *Health Qual. Life Outcomes* **2010**, *8*, 51. [CrossRef] [PubMed]
65. Middleton, J.W.; Tran, Y.; Lo, C.; Craig, A. Reexamining the validity and dimensionality of the Moorong Self-Efficacy Scale: Improving its clinical utility. *Arch. Phys. Med. Rehabil.* **2016**, *97*, 2130–2136. [CrossRef] [PubMed]
66. Widerström-Noga, E.; Biering-Sørensen, F.; Bryce, T.N.; Cardenas, D.D.; Finnerup, N.B.; Jensen, M.P.; Richards, J.S.; Siddall, P.J. The International Spinal Cord Injury Pain Basic Data Set (version 2.0). *Spinal Cord* **2014**, *52*, 282–286. [CrossRef]

Disclaimer/Publisher's Note: The statements, opinions and data contained in all publications are solely those of the individual author(s) and contributor(s) and not of MDPI and/or the editor(s). MDPI and/or the editor(s) disclaim responsibility for any injury to people or property resulting from any ideas, methods, instructions or products referred to in the content.

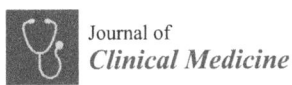

Article

Activity-Based Therapy for Mobility, Function and Quality of Life after Spinal Cord Injuries—A Mixed-Methods Case Series

Camila Quel de Oliveira [1,2,*], Anita Bundy [1,3], James W. Middleton [4], Kathryn Refshauge [1], Kris Rogers [5] and Glen M. Davis [1]

1. Sydney School of Health Sciences, Faculty of Medicine and Health, The University of Sydney, Sydney, NSW 2006, Australia; anita.bundy@sydney.edu.au (A.B.); kathryn.refshauge@sydney.edu.au (K.R.); glen.davis@sydney.edu.au (G.M.D.)
2. Discipline of Physiotherapy, Graduate School of Health, Faculty of Health, University of Technology Sydney, Ultimo, NSW 2007, Australia
3. Department of Occupational Therapy, Colorado State University, Fort Collins, CO 80524, USA
4. John Walsh Center for Rehabilitation Research, Kolling Institute, Northern Sydney Local Health District and Sydney Medical School Northern, The University of Sydney, Sydney, NSW 2006, Australia; james.middleton@sydney.edu.au
5. Graduate School of Health, Faculty of Health, University of Technology Sydney, Ultimo, NSW 2007, Australia; kris.rogers@uts.edu.au
* Correspondence: camila.queldeoliveira@uts.edu.au

Abstract: (1) Background: Despite inconclusive evidence on the benefits of activity-based therapies (ABTs) in people with spinal cord injuries, implementation has occurred in clinics worldwide in response to consumers' requests. We explored the clinical changes and participants' perceptions from engaging in an ABT program in the community. (2) Methods: This mixed-methods study involved a pragmatic observational multiple-baseline design and an evaluation of participants' perceptions. Fifteen participants were included. Outcome measures were balance in sitting using the Seated Reach Distance test, mobility using the Modified Rivermead Mobility Index and quality of life using the Quality of Life Index SCI version pre- and post-participation in an ABT community-based program. Linear mixed models and logistic regressions were used to analyse the effects of intervention. Semi-structured interviews explored participants' perceptions using inductive thematic analysis. (3) Results: There was an increase of 9% in the standardised reach distance (95% CI 2–16) for sitting balance, 1.33 points (95% CI: 0.81–1.85) in mobility and 1.9 points (0.17–2.1) in quality of life. Two themes emerged from the interviews: (1) reduced impact of disability and an increased sense of life as before, and (2) the program was superior to usual rehabilitation. No adverse events related to the intervention were observed. (4) Conclusion: ABT delivered in the community improved clinical outcomes in people with a chronic SCI. High levels of satisfaction with the program were reported.

Keywords: spinal cord injuries; exercise; rehabilitation; activity-based therapies; recovery; physical activity

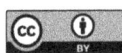

1. Introduction

Over the past 30 years, evidence has grown related to spinal cord plasticity, repair and regeneration. However, in many countries, the concept of an irreparable, "hard-wired" spinal cord still guides rehabilitation after a spinal cord injury (SCI) [1]. In general, physical rehabilitation has focused solely on teaching patients how to achieve independence in day-to-day functioning by using compensatory techniques and assistive devices to overcome significant neurological deficits [2,3].

Animal studies have suggested that repeated sensory stimulation and intense exercise can elicit neuroplastic changes to the spinal cord and brain [4–8]. In humans, functional recovery may occur when appropriate levels of sensory stimulation associated with repetitive exercise for the areas above and below the damaged spinal cord are employed [1,9].

Neuroplasticity and recovery of function, therefore, seem to be possible in people with SCI, but how to optimise recovery and achieve clinically worthwhile changes in mobility, independence and quality of life remains unclear [9].

Exercises that target systems below the level of injury (muscle, bone and circulation) are crucial to improve health outcomes and prevent complications due to paralysis after SCI [10–12]. New interventions aiming not only to facilitate tasks using compensatory strategies but also focused on functional improvements through neurological recovery have been termed "Activity-Based Therapies" (ABT), and numerous programs have emerged with the aim to assist people with SCI to achieve their maximal potential for recovery [1,9,13,14].

To date, ABT interventions have been most frequently investigated for their efficacy and effectiveness using single training modalities, such as locomotor training, functional electrical stimulation (FES) or robotics [15]. Two community-based randomised controlled trials (RCTs) that compared multimodal ABT to no-intervention or self-selected exercises found greater improvements in the ABT group for neurological function and walking capacity but had inconclusive results for independence and general mobility [16,17]. In contrast, another RCT compared a 12-week multimodal ABT intervention to usual care during inpatient rehabilitation, showing no differences in neurological recovery and functional or behavioural outcomes between groups [18].

Previous studies have highlighted the gap between research findings and clinical practice. There is an increasing demand for evidence-based clinical practice; however, most evidence-based recommendations for clinical interventions are derived from highly controlled efficacy trials [19]. The highly controlled nature of randomised controlled trials is important to draw causal inferences; however, their focus on internal validity often reduces external relevance and generalisability, limiting implementation into clinical practice. Hence, there is a need for more studies to be conducted in settings where community constraints are prioritised over optimal conditions, including the testing of the feasibility of interventions in real-world settings [20].

Despite ambiguous evidence in support of multimodal ABT, consumer interest has encouraged many rehabilitation centres to implement ABT programs for people with SCI worldwide. However, it remains unclear what changes can be expected when ABT is provided to people with SCI living in the community, in terms of health outcomes as well as consumer satisfaction. In this study, we sought to investigate functional changes of people with SCI when following an ABT program delivered in a community setting. Hence, the objectives were: (i) to identify potential changes in mobility, functional outcomes and quality of life in people with SCI after an ABT intervention, and (ii) to examine participants' satisfaction with ABT.

2. Materials and Methods

2.1. Study Design

We conducted an exploratory mixed-methods case series using an observational multiple-baseline single case design combined with a qualitative component. We followed participants who participated in an ABT program, using a 4-week qualification period of weekly baseline measurements to assess the stability of the primary outcomes, followed by a period of at least 4 weeks of the ABT intervention, where participants were assessed every second week. Due to the observational nature of this study, and the fact that it was conducted in a "real-world" community exercise setting, participants engaged with the program for varying frequencies and durations. Eight weeks after finishing the program, participants were reassessed to evaluate for any post-intervention changes. In addition, we conducted follow-up semi-structured interviews 1 week after the intervention period to evaluate participants' experiences and perspectives.

2.2. Participants

Participants were paying clients from the NeuroMoves ABT program, a community outreach initiative of Spinal Cord Injuries Australia (SCIA). We invited adults who had sustained SCI (at any injury level below C2 and of any lesion severity) and had contacted SCIA to enrol in the NeuroMoves ABT program at The University of Sydney, Australia, to participate. All participants were new to ABT and provided written consent following thorough client–therapist discussions. This study was approved by The University of Sydney Human Research Ethics Committee (HREC 2012/477).

All participants needed to have a minimum total score of 2 points on the Modified Rivermead Mobility Index (MRMI) and medical permission to participate in an intensive exercise program. Participants were excluded if they were ventilator-dependent; had other associated neurological diseases; had complications such as severe urinary tract infections, pressure ulcers or osteoporosis in the lower limbs; or were diagnosed by a medical practitioner with any other health condition that could contraindicate participation in an exercise program. Participants who attended the program for a minimum of 8 weeks, were fluent in English and provided consent were asked to participate in an audio-recorded interview.

2.3. ABT Program

Exercise programs were individually tailored by a physiotherapist or accredited exercise physiologist according to the person's goals and functional abilities. The intervention involved three key elements: (i) task-specific training, (ii) weight-bearing tasks and (iii) whole-body muscle strengthening. This approach included training in different positions such as sitting on the edge of the bed, 4-point kneeling, kneeling, standing with partial or full body weight, body-weight-supported treadmill training, active-assisted exercises, resistance training, neuromuscular electrical stimulation and balance and coordination tasks. All exercises were performed out of the wheelchair, incorporating whole-body movements. (Refer to Appendix A for a detailed description of the exercise components.) Participants were encouraged to perform all exercises to their maximum capacity with 1 to 5 min for recovery, if required, between exercises. The length of intervention varied from 4 to 24 weeks with a frequency of 2 to 4 times per week. Each session was 2 h long.

2.4. Outcome Measures

Our primary outcomes were balance in sitting, mobility and quality of life. For balance in sitting, we used the Seated Reach Distance test (SRD) as described by Boswell-Ruys [21]. The greatest reach distance in each direction (forward, lateral left and right, diagonal left and right) was recorded in centimetres and then divided by the arm length to constitute a normalised score. Thus, the score can be interpreted as the percentage of the arm length that the individual was able to reach in each direction. A final score was obtained by calculating the mean score of all directions. The Modified Rivermead Mobility Index (MRMI) was used to assess mobility. The scoring for each task is based on a scale from 0 (unable to perform the task) to 5 (performs the task independently) and reflects the amount of assistance necessary to perform each task [22]. The Quality of Life Index (QoLI) SCI version measures satisfaction within four quality of life domains: health and functioning, psychological/spiritual, social and economic, and family. The maximum score is 30; higher scores reflect better quality of life [23,24].

Our secondary outcomes were independence during activities of daily living using the Spinal Cord Independence Measure version III (SCIM) [25], participation using the Community Integration Questionnaire (CIQ) [26], and satisfaction with life using the Satisfaction with Life Scale (SWLS) [27]. Adverse events, defined as any untoward medical occurrence that does not necessarily have a causal relationship with the intervention, were monitored and recorded [28]. During the multiple-baseline 4-week period, we assessed the primary outcomes weekly (same day of the week and time of day). After completing the multiple-baseline assessment period, we evaluated participants at the start and end of the intervention period, and at 8-week follow-up for primary and secondary outcomes. In addition, the primary outcomes were assessed at 2-week intervals during the intervention period.

2.5. Interviews

We conducted a semi-structured interview (Appendix B) with individuals who completed at least 8 weeks of the ABT intervention in the week of or 1 week following the participants' final assessment to capture their overall perceptions of, and satisfaction with, the program. The interview included questions about participants' opinions and beliefs about ABT, any perceived changes resulting from the program and the logistics involved in participating in the ABT exercise program. All questions were open-ended; follow-up probes were used to gain a more in-depth understanding of participants' responses. Recordings of the interviews were transcribed verbatim by a professional transcriber. As part of the interview, participants also rated aspects of the program on a scale from 0 to 10, with 0 indicating "really bad" and 10 being "really great".

2.6. Data Analysis

Only participants who were exposed to the intervention were included in the data analysis. Statistical analyses of the primary outcomes were conducted independently of the primary author by a professional biostatistician who was otherwise not involved in the study (KRo). The analysis for the primary-outcome measures was conducted using R software version 4.1 packages lme4 and nlme [29]. For other analyses, the software IBM SPSS Statistics 22™ was utilised.

Primary-outcome measures: Linear mixed-model regression was used to assess changes in outcomes across baseline and intervention phases. We fitted a model with a random intercept for each participant (allowing for each participant to have a unique baseline starting measurement), and with (a) time included as a fixed effect (i.e., there was a common trajectory of the outcomes over time) and (b) time included as a random effect (i.e., each patient had their own trajectory in how the outcomes changed over time). We assessed whether there was an overall or individual trajectory by assessing measures of model fit using Akaike's Information Criteria (AIC) and Bayesian Information Criteria (BIC) and visually inspecting the predicted outcomes for each participant over time against the actual values.

Secondary-outcome measures: The effects of treatment on the secondary-outcome measures were assessed by paired-sample *t*-tests at the 5% confidence level.

Maintenance of effects: We obtained 8-week follow-up assessments for only 4 of the 13 participants. Due to the small sample size, the follow-up period was not included in the statistical analysis and data are presented individually.

2.7. Qualitative Analysis

Inductive thematic analysis of semi-structured interviews was used, as described by Braun and Clarke [30]. An open coding process was performed whereby all passages in each interview were examined line by line and coded to reflect the content. One of the interviews, judged by the first author to be particularly difficult to code, was reviewed in its entirety by a more experienced author (AB) and discussed until consensus was reached on the coding. The first author then recoded all the interviews, and the recoding was reviewed by the experienced author.

3. Results

3.1. Participants

Fifteen NeuroMoves clients expressed interest in participating in the study after contact from an SCIA staff member (not involved in the study) and met the inclusion criteria. All 15 participants completed a weekly assessment during 4 weeks of multiple-baseline data collection. Thirteen participants completed the intervention period, two having withdrawn for medical reasons or to engage in sports activities. Eight participants undertook the semi-structured interview. The flow of participants through the study, with reasons for dropping out, is shown in Figure 1.

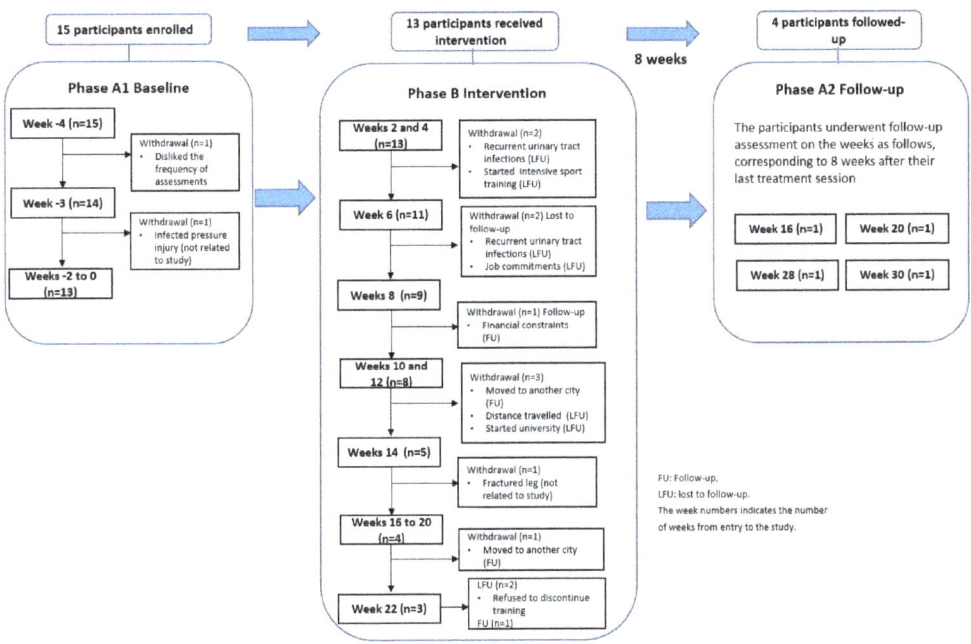

Figure 1. Flow of participants through the study with reasons for dropouts.

The characteristics of the 13 participants who completed the study and duration of their intervention are described in Table 1. The mean age of participants was 32.1 years (SD = 12.4), and the mean duration post-injury was 46.5 months (SD = 65.9).

Table 1. Participants characteristics and duration of intervention.

Participant	Age (Years)	Gender	Duration Post-Injury (mo)	Level of Injury	AIS Classification	Number of Sessions Attended	Number of Sessions per Week
1	22	M	26	C5	A	43	4
2	23	F	10	C5	A	45	2
3	37	F	6	T11	C	46	2
4	20	M	11	C4	B	42	2
5	54	M	15	C3	D	16	2
6	31	M	12	C4	B	70	3
7	20	F	6	L1	A	52	2
8	43	M	30	T4	B	45	2
9	23	F	212	T2	A	15	2
10	33	M	121	T12	B	14	2
11	56	M	135	T6	A	11	2
12	32	M	9	C5	B	19	2
13	23	M	12	T11	A	15	2

M: male, F: female; AIS: ASIA Impairment Scale; A: complete; B: sensory incomplete; C: motor incomplete (more than half of key muscle functions below level of injury have a muscle grade less than 3); D: motor incomplete (at least half of key muscle functions below level of injury have a muscle grade greater than 3). Participants in bold italic have completed the qualitative arm of this study.

We attempted to fit both random intercept and random intercept + slope models to all variables but were only able to do so for the quality of life outcome. Both measures of model fit indicated that the random-intercept-only model had the best fit. For MRMI and SRD, the models including a random effect of time did not converge, which indicated that they were a poor fit to the data. We, therefore, considered random intercept models with an overall trajectory for the three outcomes. See Appendix C, Table A1.

3.2. Sitting Balance

Visual inspection of the data reveals high variability on SRD scores at baseline. Overall, participants had similar SRD across baseline, and with good evidence of an increase of 0.09 (95% CI 0.02–0.16), meaning that participants could reach a further 9% of their arm length in sitting by the end of the intervention period. Figure 2 shows the individual SRD scores during the baseline and intervention periods.

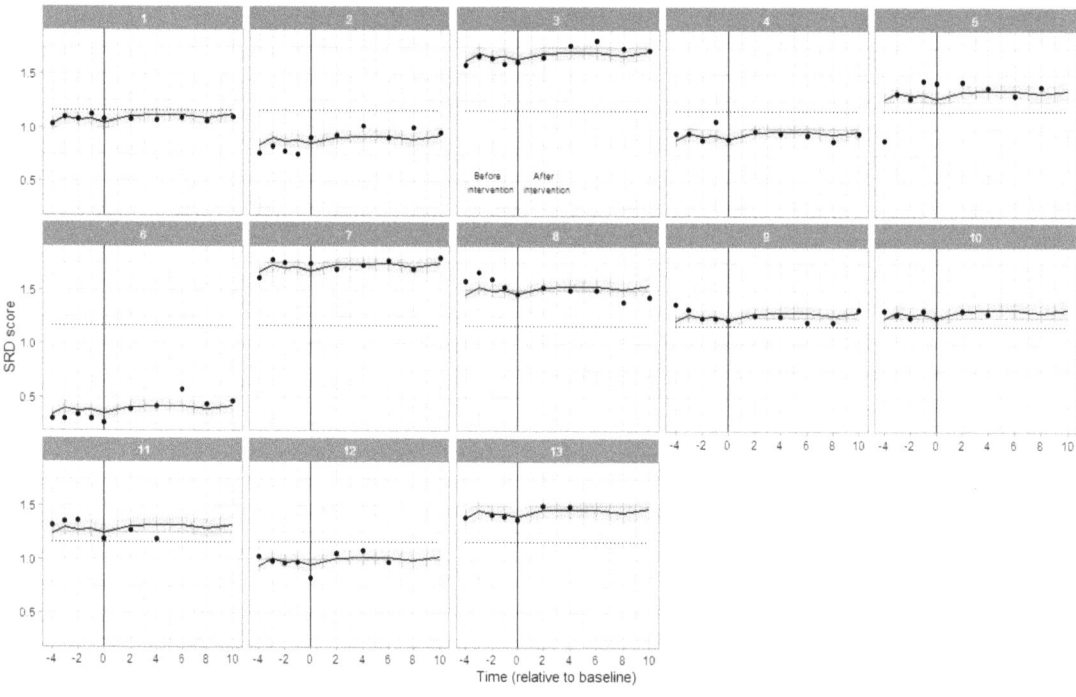

Figure 2. Seated Reach Distance (SRD) scores over time for each participant with estimated SRD from the linear mixed model and overall mean score. The participant number is indicated at the top of each graph. The vertical line denotes commencement of ABT intervention. Each dot represents an assessment timepoint.

3.3. Mobility

Visual inspection of the data demonstrates stability of scores during the baseline period for most participants, except for participants 3 and 13, who exhibited a slight positive slope during the baseline phase. There was a small but inconsistent shift in MRMI before the intervention period of 0.23 (95% CI: −0.22–0.68), and then the overall trajectory was for MRMI to steadily increase by 1.33 (95% CI: 0.81–1.85) points after intervention. There were no changes in mobility for participants 4, 9, 10 and 11 when compared to baseline. Figure 3 portrays the individual MRMI scores during the baseline and intervention periods.

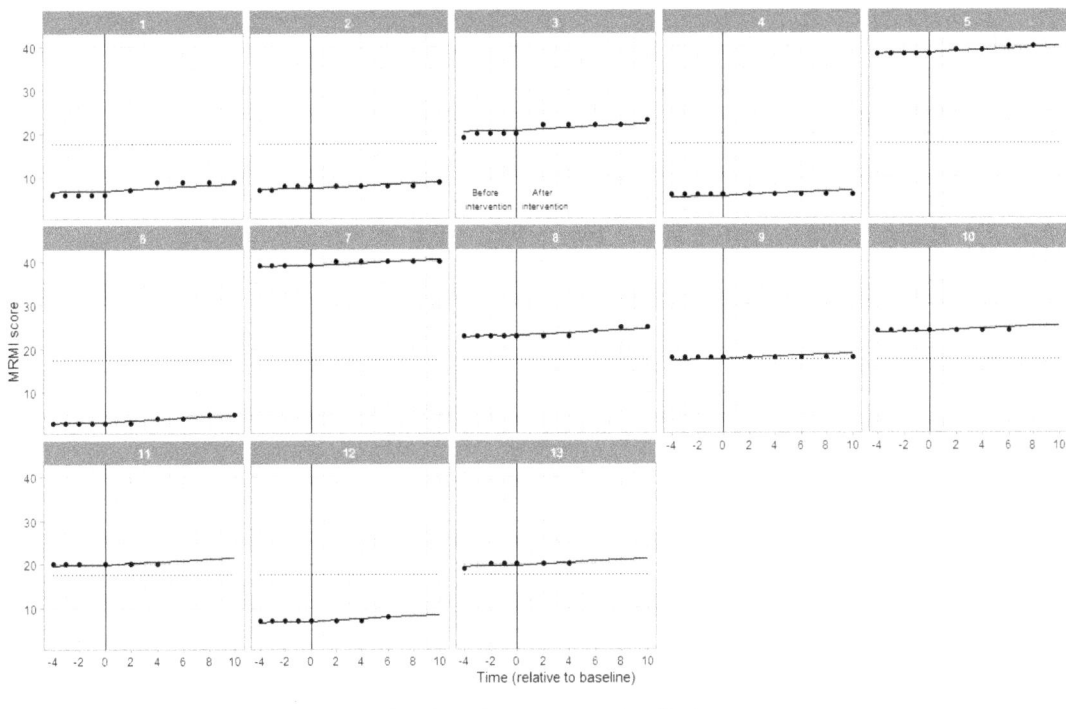

Figure 3. Modified Rivermead Mobility Index (MRMI) scores over time for each participant with estimated MRMI from the linear mixed model and overall mean score. The participant number is indicated at the top of each graph. The vertical line denotes commencement of ABT intervention. Each dot represents an assessment timepoint.

3.4. Quality of Life

Visual inspection demonstrates considerable variability in the quality of life scores at baseline. There was an overall increase in slope of 2.42 points (95% CI: 1.35–3.50) during baseline, and a smaller increase of 1.9 points (95% CI:0.17–2.1) by the end of the intervention phase. For most participants, the slope was positive during baseline, followed by an increase of small magnitude during the treatment period. The exception was participant 9, who showed a steep decline in quality of life during baseline followed by a slight positive change during the intervention period. Participant 5 also presented a negative change during intervention when compared to baseline. Figure 4 shows the individual quality of life scores during the baseline and intervention periods.

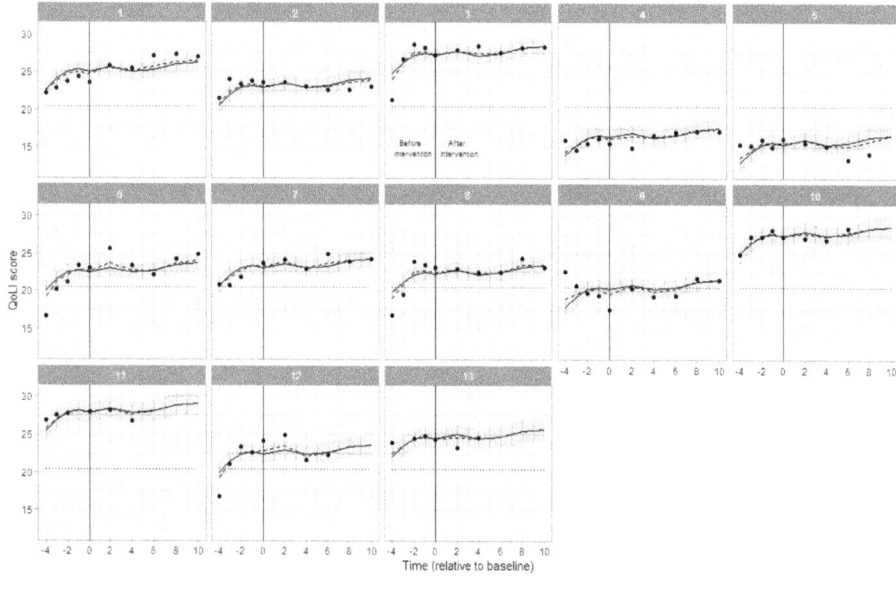

Figure 4. Quality of Life Index (QoLI) scores over time for each participant with estimated QoLI scores from the linear mixed model and overall mean score. The participant number is indicated at the top of each graph. The vertical line denotes commencement of ABT intervention. Each dot represents an assessment timepoint.

3.5. Secondary Outcomes

There were small positive changes in the SCIM with a mean change in score of 2.2 (95% CI: 0.3 to 4.2) points and in the CIQ of 1.7 (95% CI 0.3 to 3.1) points after participation in the ABT program. No significant changes were seen in the SWLS with a mean change in score of 2.0 (95% CI: −0.5 to 4.4) points, with the 95% confidence interval spanning zero (Appendix D).

3.6. Retention and Adherence

Attendance varied in duration from 4 to 22 weeks (average 12.6, SD = 6.94), with most participants (11/13) attending two sessions per week. Only four participants undertook the 8-week follow-up assessment. Most participants left the program due to health-related problems, such as urinary tract infections. Engagement in social activities such as sports, work, university and moving to another city were also reasons to discontinue participation. The reasons for loss to follow-up are presented in Figure 1.

3.7. Maintenance of Effects

Participants 1, 2, 5 and 7 underwent follow-up assessments. There was a further small improvement in quality of life of 1% and 6% for subjects 1 and 7. Participant 5 had no changes in quality of life at follow-up, while participant 2 declined by 7%. The changes in mobility were maintained for all participants. There was some stability in balance in sitting, with two participants (1 and 5) maintaining the changes and two participants (2 and 7) experiencing a slight decrease in the MRMI at follow-up of 4% and 5%, respectively. All participants continued to show some improvements in independence that ranged from 2% to 11%. Community integration continued to improve for participants 1 and 5 after cessation of intervention, by 7% and 18%, respectively, although the score returned to the baseline value for participant 7. Supplemental follow-up data for each subject is contained in Appendix E.

3.8. Adverse Events

No adverse events related to the intervention were observed. One participant discontinued involvement in the study during the baseline period due to infected pressure injuries, and three discontinued during the intervention period: two due to recurrent urinary tract infections and one due to a leg fracture.

3.9. Participants' Perceptions and Experiences

Analysis of the content of the interviews (n = 8) yielded two themes: (a) the impact that my disability has in my life has decreased (i.e., sense of life as before), and (b) the program is different from (superior to) usual rehabilitation. These themes revealed that all participants believed the program was beneficial and yielded physical and psychosocial gains. A summary of the themes and subthemes generated by the thematic analysis appears in Table 2.

Table 2. Themes and subthemes identified in the inductive thematic analysis.

1.	The impact that my disability has in my life has decreased (sense of life as before).
1.1	I am more independent and participate in life again.
1.2	I am more confident to do things by myself and to attempt new things.
1.3	The gains that I got from the program made my everyday life easier.
1.4	My improvements had a positive impact on my family and friends.
1.5	I feel part of a community again.
2.	**The program is different from usual rehabilitation**
2.1	I tried new things (exercises and equipment) including exercising out of the wheelchair.
2.2	The environment is uplifting and motivating.
2.3	The treatment is individually tailored and specialised to my injury and needs.
2.4	The amount of time and money invested was big, but it was worth it.
2.5	Negatives, of course, but they are minor.

3.9.1. Theme 1: The Impact That My Disability Has in My Life Has Decreased (Sense of Life as before)

Overall, participants enjoyed attending the program and reported that the positive experiences outweighed any negative aspects. Seven participants rated the program with a score of at least 8 out of 10; the eighth participant rated it between 6 and 7. All participants acknowledged the need for and importance of community-based rehabilitation programs; the majority indicated they would recommend it to anyone with an SCI. This general perspective is reflected in the following quotes:

> "The improvement is just unbelievable. So, for me, that's the best thing about it, and the bad thing about it is I can't do it more times than I do. I really enjoy it." (P8)

> "Before I wouldn't have gone out of the golf club, now I go out to the golf course and walk around a bit, and even around the restaurant after having dinner and a few drinks and staying around rather than just not doing any social activities at all." (P5)

All participants reported psychological and emotional gains, such as feeling more motivated and happier. Participation in the program led to increased confidence associated with greater independence and a willingness to attempt tasks and be involved in activities that they had previously considered impossible due to the injury.

> "It's not just the functional benefits. It's the psychological and emotional positives that come out of it. Feeling more confident and feeling better, having more independence. I think that's what most people want to gain after they've had an injury." (P2)

Combined physical and psychological gains made participants' everyday lives easier with less reliance on others for assistance or use of external aids and functioning more like before their injury.

> "I'm eating with whatever utensils I have. I can actually remove them from my lap to the table without any assistance... I can grab the remote, work the remote from the shelf in my

room onto my lap to access the TV if I want. . . .I found eating most types of food that I've had trouble with beforehand have been a lot easier, like holding something like a burger." (P1)

Participants reported that the program gave them access to a new community by providing an environment where they could socialise with others in similar situations. One participant compared it to being part of a sports team. Participants regained the opportunity to connect and socialise with a variety of people and not be treated as *"different"* or *"disabled"*. Talking to people in a similar situation allowed them to learn from each other and exchange experiences that helped to deal better with their injury.

3.9.2. Theme 2: The Program Is Different from (Superior to) Usual Rehabilitation

Participants used words to describe the program such as *"fun"*, *"unique"*, *"novel"* and *"exciting"* when making comparisons to the hospital system and conventional physiotherapy programs. They evaluated the ABT program as being superior due to the variety of equipment and exercises available, and the uplifting and encouraging environment.

Participants considered the exercise modalities and equipment used during sessions as novel and unique. Exercising out of the wheelchair in different body positions, including standing, was considered vital for their health and functional recovery. Even if their goals did not include standing or walking, being in the upright position and having the lower limbs stimulated to move seemed to have positive physical and psychological effects.

"For me, is all about getting out of my chair. When you are in the chair you are mainly just restricted to doing weights, maybe a bit of trunk. When you get out of the chair at least you can stretch your whole body. You use everything. You try different exercises. You not only work out what you have but just test out and try and work out things that are weaker or that you don't have." (P2)

Negative aspects of the program were reported; however, participants qualified that these were relatively minor. The distance travelled to get to the program was perceived as a negative. The time commitment and the cost were considered high. However, most participants considered the cost and time invested worthwhile, given the benefits. Other negative aspects were the different levels of skill and expertise amongst staff and the size of the exercise area, which sometimes became too busy, interfering with the quality of the sessions and making performance of certain exercises and the use of certain equipment impractical.

4. Discussion

To our knowledge this is the first multiple-baseline study to assess the potential effects of ABT in a "real-life" setting, while adding contextual details about participants' perceptions and experiences. Overall, we found that ABT led to small positive changes in sitting balance, mobility and quality of life in people with a chronic SCI. Furthermore, the qualitative analysis showed high levels of satisfaction and perceived benefits that surpassed what was identified by the outcome measures. However, the magnitude of change was small and possibly not clinically meaningful. The SCIM III was the only outcome measured in the current study that has previously been found to have a minimal clinically important difference in a population with SCI [31]. An increase of at least four points on the total SCIM during acute care/subacute rehabilitation is usually considered to equate to a small but worthwhile improvement, and an increase of 10 points to equate to a substantial improvement [32].

All participants in our study had undergone in-hospital rehabilitation programs and had been injured for at least six months. Therefore, they were not expected to experience further changes in their functional status due to the reduced potential for spontaneous recovery, especially for motor function, wherein the greatest rate of change occurs within the first three months post-injury [33]. Furthermore, most participants in our sample (n = 11/13) had a motor-complete injury (AIS A and B), which might have contributed to the small magnitude of the gains. Previous research [34-36] showed that individuals with motor-incomplete injuries (AIS C and D) experience greater benefits from ABT than individuals with motor-complete injuries (AIS A and B).

Regardless of the small changes in the outcome measures employed in this study, the perceived benefits reported by the participants were in many areas including independence and community participation, which corroborates a more recent qualitative study where ABT participants reported a perceived positive impact on physical, functional and psychosocial domains, leading to improved independence and quality of life. Furthermore, their participants believed that ABT had a key role in the evolving and lifelong recovery after SCI [37]. Overall, the analysis from the interviews showed that the perceived benefits were greater than the changes detected by the outcome measures. The discordance between patient-reported and performance-based tools could be due to an overestimation of the changes by the participants, which could be related to the (1) novelty effect, (2) lower expectation of rehabilitation outcome and (3) Hawthorne effect. Firstly, the novelty effect is defined as "the perceived usability of something on the account of newness" [38]. In our study, all participants were new to ABT, which could have resulted in a bias towards overestimation of benefits due to excitement with the opportunity to access the novel treatment. Secondly, the level of expectation could have affected the participants' perception of change. The lack of improvements experienced in the chronic phase after SCI could have accounted for a lowered expectation for recovery after that time and therefore resulted in an overestimation of perceived improvement, which means that even a subtle change will be perceived as important and significant [39]. Thirdly, the Hawthorne effect is a phenomenon where participants tend to report the effects of a treatment differently due to being aware of the nature and purpose of the study [40]. Our participants were informed about the nature and purpose of the study prior to enrolment, which could have led them to providing more positive perspectives and opinions about the training they received.

Most participants attended only two 2-h sessions per week, which could have contributed to the relatively small magnitude of the improvements identified by the standardised outcome measures. Other researchers have reported that ABT performed for 2 to 5 h per day at a frequency of three to five times per week produced benefits in participants with chronic SCI that included improved lower-limb muscle strength, balance, mobility, increased gait speed, symmetry and endurance [2,41,42]. Only two participants attended more than two sessions per week. When observing the individual data, the participants who attended the program at a higher frequency experienced greater improvements than individuals with similar injury characteristics who attended fewer sessions.

Previous research focused on assessing the effects of ABT interventions on outcomes related to lower limb mobility, such as walking, standing and balance [15,43–46]. Typically, ABT involves the practice of intense exercise, performed out of the wheelchair, in various body positions, mostly against gravity, which can positively impact other aspects of mobility and function, as well as enhance psychological outcomes, such as mood and self-image, promoting greater quality of life [47–50]. The fact that the ABT intervention in our study was delivered in a community setting is likely to have promoted social interactions that were beneficial for the participants' mental health, as identified in the interviews. Hence, it is important to investigate not only the effects of a multimodal ABT exercise program on functional outcomes related to physical abilities, but also its impact on psychological well-being, quality of life and community participation. Furthermore, due to the growing numbers of people with SCI seeking to participate in ABT programs in the community [51], it is necessary to assess this intervention when applied outside the research setting.

Cost, distance and time commitment are possible barriers for participation in ABT and should be considered when implementing ABT programs in the community, particularly given that evidence shows that high intensity and frequency seem to be determinants for the effectiveness of ABT [2,52–54]. Our findings support the necessity of ABT programs in the community to be delivered at high frequency per week for greatest benefits. One strategy to overcome the barriers while delivering an effective dose of ABT may be to deliver it in a block of high-frequency for short periods. Such an approach may facilitate adherence and reduce disruption of other community engagement activities.

Study Limitations

In this study, we evaluated the changes and participants' perceptions of a multimodal ABT intervention in a clinical setting that reflected the reality of a community-based clinic. Several limitations affect the generalisation of our findings, such as the clinical heterogeneity of participants, different lengths of exposure to the intervention, the fact that participants were paying to attend the program, loss to follow-up and the small sample size. We believe that the small sample size was driven largely by potential participants not being willing to wait for the four-week baseline assessments before starting the program. The high degree of variability in the number of weeks that the intervention was delivered was potentially caused by the reduced ability of participants to attend a long-term ABT program due to costs, distance to travel and difficulties fitting it in with other life demands.

Another limitation was the lack of stability of baseline measures for quality of life and Seated Reach Distance. Studies employing a multiple-baseline design can demonstrate if a significant change in behaviour has occurred as result of the intervention. However, strong conclusions can only be drawn when the baseline is neutral or in the opposite direction to an observed behaviour [55,56].

We were unable to assess maintenance of the changes from the ABT treatment, mainly due to the high number of participants lost to follow-up. Despite considerable variability in outcomes at the follow-up assessment across remaining participants, some maintenance of mobility was observed. Two of the three participants who completed the maximum intervention period of 22 weeks were unwilling to discontinue the ABT treatment due to concerns that an 8-week pause would cause deterioration, delay or hinder further progress in important benefits already achieved. These participants were free to continue to attend the NeuroMoves ABT program; thus, duration of outcomes could not be measured.

Lastly, the high satisfaction levels and perceived changes reported by participants in the present study may have been influenced by the fact that they enrolled in the ABT program independently, leading to participation bias. They were potentially more motivated, open to new interventions and have more financial resources than the general SCI population, potentially biasing the findings.

5. Conclusions

ABT delivered in the community can be beneficial and was well regarded by participants with a chronic SCI. Multimodal ABT programs, applied after in-patient rehabilitation, can maximise gains in the outcomes of quality of life, mobility, sitting balance, independence and community participation. However, the changes were of small magnitude, possibly due to the challenges in achieving the recommended therapeutic dosage in a community setting.

Author Contributions: Conceptualisation, all authors; methodology, G.M.D., J.W.M., A.B. and K.R. (Kathryn Refshauge); validation, all authors; formal analysis, C.Q.d.O., A.B. and K.R. (Kathryn Refshauge); investigation, C.Q.d.O.; resources, G.M.D. and Spinal Cord Injuries Australia; data curation, C.Q.d.O. and G.M.D.; writing—original draft, C.Q.d.O.; writing—review and editing, all authors; visualisation, K.R. (Kris Rogers).; supervision, G.M.D., K.R. (Kathryn Refshauge), J.W.M. and A.B.; project administration, C.Q.d.O. All authors have read and agreed to the published version of the manuscript.

Funding: The first author, Dr Camila Quel de Oliveira, was the recipient of a PhD scholarship provided by Spinal Cure Australia and Spinal Cord Injuries Australia (SCIA). SCIA is the provider of the NeuroMoves program.

Institutional Review Board Statement: This study was conducted in accordance with the Declaration of Helsinki and approved by The University of Sydney Human Research Ethics Committee (HREC 2012/477).

Informed Consent Statement: Informed consent was obtained from all subjects involved in this study. Written informed consent has been obtained from the patient(s) to publish this paper.

Data Availability Statement: Data are available upon contact with the corresponding author, Dr. Camila Quel de Oliveira. Email: camila.queldeoliveira@uts.edu.au.

Acknowledgments: The authors would like to thank all NeuroMoves staff and participants included in the study. The first author was the recipient of a PhD scholarship awarded by the University of Sydney on funding from Spinal Cord Injuries Australia. The present study was conducted at the NeuroMoves clinic at Lidcombe, Australia. NeuroMoves is a not-for-profit community activity-based therapy and exercise program operated by Spinal Cord Injuries Australia; however, the study was fully independent from day-to-day activities of the clinic.

Conflicts of Interest: The authors declare no conflict of interest. The funders (Spinal Cord Injuries Australia) had no role in the design of the study; in the collection, analyses or interpretation of data; in the writing of the manuscript; or in the decision to publish the results.

Appendix A. Key Elements of Multimodal ABT

- Active-assisted exercises: Performed on a plinth or mat in supine, prone or side-lying position. The therapist assisted the lower-limb movements through different ranges of motion, and when possible provided resistance. Participants were encouraged to attempt and visualise actively assisting or resisting the movement performed.
- Resistance training for upper and/or lower limbs: Used when a participant demonstrated voluntary motor control and consisted of concentric and eccentric exercises against gravity or adding external resistance, such as weights or resistance bands.
- Load bearing: Consists of activities on hands or elbows and/or feet or knees in contact with the ground, with some percentage of body weight supported through the extremities. While on hands and knees or in the kneeling position, the participant is encouraged to perform upper- and lower-body movements, in order to enhance trunk and pelvic control. Crawling and locomotion in the kneeling position were also performed.
- Standing with or without standing frames: Participants stand with the assistance of a frame and are encouraged to perform trunk and arm movements, or if able, to raise themselves into a standing position to load the lower extremities, using the parallel bars, and perform lower-limb movements, until fatigue.
- Partial body weight using antigravity board: Participants complete active and/or active-assisted squat exercises (unilateral or bilateral) while partially loading their lower extremities. Participants also perform exercises for postural control in a seated position with partial body weight borne through their lower limbs.
- Leg ergometry: Using a stationary exercise bicycle, the participants are seated with trunk support provided by a therapist, if necessary, and attempt to pedal the bike under his/her own power. If unable to do so, manual external assistance is provided to complete the movement.
- Electrically stimulated leg ergometry: While seated in their wheelchair or in a chair with back support, the gluteus maximus, hamstrings, quadriceps, triceps surae and tibialis anterior could be electrically stimulated by surface electrodes, according to the participant's needs to produce a cycling movement. Leg ergometry could also be conducted in a standing position with electrodes on the gluteus maximus, hamstrings, gastrocnemius, quadriceps and the tibialis anterior muscle groups with body-weight support and assistance of a robotic stepping device that simulates gait movements.
- Gait training or supported ambulation: Involves different forms of gait training, including body-weight-supported treadmill training with or without FES or manual external assistance, overground training with a frame with or without manual external assistance, or treadmill training without support, according to participants' locomotor capability. These activities sometimes required assistance from up to four therapists, depending on the participant's ability to control their trunk and lower limbs.
- Vibration training: The aim of this intervention is to promote sensory input putatively to alter muscle spindle sensitivity to stretch and modulate reflex alpha motoneuron

activation of muscle contractions. Exercises are performed with the feet in contact with an oscillatory platform in either a seated or standing position.
- Task-specific training: According to the participant's goals and abilities, this involves bed mobility, transfers, balance in sitting or standing, walking mobility and postural changes.

Appendix B. Semi-Structured Interview

(1) Tell me about your experiences during the period that you were in the ABT program?
   - I want to know the good things and the things that weren't good as well.
(2) Tell me about the benefits (changes) that you've got from the program?
   - Physically/Functionally?
   - Socially?
   - Emotionally/Psychologically/Well being?
   - Family/carers?
(3) What is your opinion about the program? Could you tell me on a scale from 0–10 your opinion about the program, being 0: really bad and 10: really great.
(4) What are your feelings about the program? How do you feel about it?
(5) Tell me about the logistics during the period that you were in the program?
   - Time
   - Transport
(6) Is there anything else that you would like to tell me?

Appendix C

Table A1. Model fit parameters (Akaike Information Criterion (AIC) and Bayesian Information Criterion (BIC)) for the main study outcomes (Quality of Life Index, SCI version (QoL), Modified Rivermead Mobility Index (MRMI) and Seated Reach Distance test (SRD)) with random intercept and random intercept and slope (time as random effect) models.

Outcome	Model	AIC	BIC
QoL	Random Intercept	475.8	476.9
	Random Intercept + Slope	477.8	479.5
MRMI	Random Intercept	325.3	326.4
	Random Intercept + Slope	*	*
SRD	Random Intercept	−154.3	−153.2
	Random Intercept + Slope	*	*

* Not estimable—model failed to converge.

Appendix D. Secondary Outcomes

Table A2. Changes in secondary-outcome measures.

Outcome Measure	Baseline Mean ± SD	Post-Intervention Mean ± SD	Change Score Mean ± SD	95% CI	t Value	p-Value	Effect Sizes (Cohen's d)
SCIM	46.7 ± 24.7	48.9 ± 25.9	2.2 ± 3.2	0.3 to 4.2	2.52	0.027 *	0.09 (very small)
CIQ	16.5 ± 3.9	18.2 ± 4.6	1.7 ± 2.3	0.3 to 3.1	2.62	0.023 *	0.41 (small)
SWLS	18.3 ± 4.9	20.3 ± 7.5	2 ± 4.1	−0.5 to 4.4	1.78	0.101	-

SCIM = Spinal Cord Independence Measure version III; CIQ = Community Integration Questionnaire; SWLS = Satisfaction With Life Scale; * denotes statistical significance.

Appendix E. Changes at Follow-Up

Table A3. Changes over time for the four participants that underwent all scheduled follow-up assessments.

Outcome Measures	Baseline	Post-Intervention	% Change from Baseline to Post-Intervention	Follow-Up	% Change from Post-Intervention to Follow-Up
Participant 1					
QoLI	23.3 ± 0.8	26.9	16	27.2	1
MRMI	6.8 ± 0.4	9.0	32	9.0	0
SRD	1.1 ± 0.0	1.2	10	1.2	1
SCIM	26.0	27.0	4	30	11
CIQ	14.5	15.8	9	18.6	18
SWLS	24.0	28.0	17	24.0	−14
Participant 2					
QoLI	23.3 ± 1.0	22.8	−2	21.3	−7
MRMI	7.6 ± 0.6	9.0	18	9.0	0
SRD	0.8 ± 0.1	1.0	23	0.9	−4
SCIM	25.0	28.0	12	30.0	7
CIQ	22.0	22.0	0	22.0	0
SWLS	19.0	23.0	21	17.0	26
Participant 5					
QoLI	16.6 ± 0.5	14.2	−15	14.2	0
MRMI	38 ± 0.0	40	5	40.0	0
SRD	1.3 ± 0.2	1.4	11	1.4	0
SCIM	71.0	73.0	3	79.0	8
CIQ	11.3	15.0	33	16.0	7
SWLS	17.0	12.0	−29	13.0	8
Participant 7					
QoLI	21.7 ± 1.4	23.3	8	24.7	6
MRMI	39.0 ± 0.0	40.0	3	40.0	0
SRD	1.7 ± 0.1	1.8	2	1.7	−5
SCIM	81.0	92.0	14	94.0	2
CIQ	16.4	22.0	34	16.5	−25
SWLS	26.0	28.0	8	29.0	4

References

1. Sadowsky, C.L.; McDonald, J.W. Activity-based restorative therapies: Concepts and applications in spinal cord injury-related neurorehabilitation. *Dev. Disabil. Res. Rev.* **2009**, *15*, 112–116. [CrossRef]
2. Behrman, A.L.; Bowden, M.G.; Nair, P.M. Neuroplasticity after spinal cord injury and training: An emerging paradigm shift in rehabilitation and walking recovery. *Phys. Ther.* **2006**, *86*, 1406–1425. [CrossRef]
3. Field-Fote, E.C.; Lindley, S.D.; Sherman, A.L. Locomotor training approaches for individuals with spinal cord injury: A preliminary report of walking-related outcomes. *J. Neurol. Phys. Ther.* **2005**, *29*, 127–137. [CrossRef]
4. Hutchinson, K.J.; Gomez-Pinilla, F.; Crowe, M.J.; Ying, Z.; Basso, D.M. Three exercise paradigms differentially improve sensory recovery after spinal cord contusion in rats. *Brain* **2004**, *127 Pt 6*, 1403–1414. [CrossRef]
5. Zholudeva, L.V.; Qiang, L.; Marchenko, V.; Dougherty, K.J.; Sakiyama-Elbert, S.E.; Lane, M.A. The Neuroplastic and Therapeutic Potential of Spinal Interneurons in the Injured Spinal Cord. *Trends Neurosci.* **2018**, *41*, 625–639. [CrossRef] [PubMed]
6. Gazula, V.R.; Roberts, M.; Luzzio, C.; Jawad, A.F.; Kalb, R.G. Effects of limb exercise after spinal cord injury on motor neuron dendrite structure. *J. Comp. Neurol.* **2004**, *476*, 130–145. [CrossRef] [PubMed]
7. Goldshmit, Y.; Lythgo, N.; Galea, M.P.; Turnley, A.M. Treadmill training after spinal cord hemisection in mice promotes axonal sprouting and synapse formation and improves motor recovery. *J. Neurotrauma* **2008**, *25*, 449–465. [CrossRef]
8. Walker, J.R.; Detloff, M.R. Plasticity in Cervical Motor Circuits following Spinal Cord Injury and Rehabilitation. *Biology* **2021**, *10*, 976. [CrossRef] [PubMed]
9. Backus, D.; Apple, D.L.H. Systematic Review of Activity-Based Interventions to Improve Neurological Outcomes after SCI January 1998–March 2009. In Disability Research Right to Know. (n.d.). Available online: http://www.bu.edu/drrk/research-syntheses/spinal-cord-injuries/activity-based-interventions (accessed on 29 August 2023).
10. Galea, M.P. Spinal cord injury and physical activity: Preservation of the body. *Spinal Cord* **2012**, *50*, 344–351. [CrossRef]
11. Atkins, K.D.; Bickel, C.S. Effects of functional electrical stimulation on muscle health after spinal cord injury. *Curr. Opin. Pharmacol.* **2021**, *60*, 226–231. [CrossRef]

12. Martin, R.; Sadowsky, C.; Obst, K.; Meyer, B.; McDonald, J. Functional electrical stimulation in spinal cord injury: From theory to practice. *Top. Spinal Cord Inj. Rehabil.* **2012**, *18*, 28–33. [CrossRef]
13. Dromerick, A.W.; Lum, P.S.; Hidler, J. Activity-based therapies. *NeuroRx* **2006**, *3*, 428–438. [CrossRef] [PubMed]
14. Harkema, S.; Behrman, A.; Barbeau, H. Evidence-based therapy for recovery of function after spinal cord injury. *Handb. Clin. Neurol.* **2012**, *109*, 259–274. [PubMed]
15. de Oliveira, C.Q.; Refshauge, K.; Middleton, J.; de Jong, L.; Davis, G.M. Effects of Activity-Based Therapy Interventions on Mobility, Independence, and Quality of Life for People with Spinal Cord Injuries: A Systematic Review and Meta-Analysis. *J. Neurotrauma* **2017**, *34*, 1726–1743. [CrossRef] [PubMed]
16. Harness, E.T.; Yozbatiran, N.; Cramer, S.C. Effects of intense exercise in chronic spinal cord injury. *Spinal Cord* **2008**, *46*, 733–737. [CrossRef] [PubMed]
17. Jones, M.L. Activity-based therapy for recovery of walking in individuals with chronic spinal cord injury: Results from a randomized clinical trial. *Arch. Phys. Med. Rehabil.* **2014**, *95*, 2239–2246.e2. [CrossRef]
18. Galea, M.P.; Dunlop, S.A.; Geraghty, T.; Davis, G.M.; Nunn, A.; Olenko, L. SCIPA Full-On: A Randomized Controlled Trial Comparing Intensive Whole-Body Exercise and Upper Body Exercise After Spinal Cord Injury. *Neurorehabil. Neural. Repair.* **2018**, *32*, 557–567. [CrossRef] [PubMed]
19. Glasgow, R.E.; Green, L.W.; Klesges, L.M.; Abrams, D.B.; Fisher, E.B.; Goldstein, M.G.; Hayman, L.L.; Ockene, J.K.; Orleans, C.T. External validity: We need to do more. *Ann. Behav. Med.* **2006**, *31*, 105–108. [CrossRef]
20. Green, L.W.; Glasgow, R.E. Evaluating the Relevance, Generalization, and Applicability of Research: Issues in External Validation and Translation Methodology. *Eval. Health Prof.* **2006**, *29*, 126–153. [CrossRef]
21. Boswell-Ruys, C.L.; Sturnieks, D.L.; Harvey, L.A.; Sherrington, C.; Middleton, J.W.; Lord, S.R. Validity and reliability of assessment tools for measuring unsupported sitting in people with a spinal cord injury. *Arch. Phys. Med. Rehabil.* **2009**, *90*, 1571–1577. [CrossRef]
22. Walsh, J.M.; Barrett, A.; Murray, D.; Ryan, J.; Moroney, J.; Shannon, M. The Modified Rivermead Mobility Index: Reliability and convergent validity in a mixed neurological population. *Disabil. Rehabil.* **2010**, *32*, 1133–1139. [CrossRef] [PubMed]
23. May, L.A.; Warren, S. Measuring quality of life of persons with spinal cord injury: External and structural validity. *Spinal Cord* **2002**, *40*, 341–350. [CrossRef]
24. May, L.A.; Warren, S. Measuring quality of life of persons with spinal cord injury: Substantive and structural validation. *Qual. Life Res.* **2001**, *10*, 503–515. [CrossRef] [PubMed]
25. Catz, A.; Itzkovich, M.; Tesio, L.; Biering-Sorensen, F.; Weeks, C.; Laramee, M.T.; Craven, B.C.; Tonack, M.; Hitzig, S.L.; Glaser, E.; et al. A multicenter international study on the Spinal Cord Independence Measure, version III: Rasch psychometric validation. *Spinal Cord* **2007**, *45*, 275–291. [CrossRef] [PubMed]
26. Kratz, A.L.; Chadd, E.; Jensen, M.P.; Kehn, M.; Kroll, T. An examination of the psychometric properties of the community integration questionnaire (CIQ) in spinal cord injury. *J. Spinal Cord Med.* **2015**, *38*, 446–455. [CrossRef] [PubMed]
27. Post, M.W.; van Leeuwen, C.M.; van Koppenhagen, C.F.; De Groot, S. Validity of the Life Satisfaction questions, the Life Satisfaction Questionnaire, and the Satisfaction With Life Scale in persons with spinal cord injury. *Arch. Phys. Med. Rehabil.* **2012**, *93*, 1832–1837. [CrossRef]
28. Health NSWG. *Safety Monitoring and Reporting for Clinical Trials Conducted in NSW Public Health Organisations*; Health NSWG: Sydney, NSW, Australia, 2017.
29. R Core Team. *R: A Language and Environment for Statistical Computing*; R Foundation for Statistical Computing: Vienna, Austria, 2016.
30. Clarke, V.; Braun, V.; Hayfield, N. Thematic analysis. Qualitative psychology: A practical guide to research methods. In *Qualitative Psychology: A Practical Guide to Research Methods*; Smith, J.A., Ed.; SAGE Publications: London, UK, 2015; pp. 222–248.
31. Wirth, B.; van Hedel, H.J.; Kometer, B.; Dietz, V.; Curt, A. Changes in activity after a complete spinal cord injury as measured by the Spinal Cord Independence Measure II (SCIM II). *Neurorehabil. Neural. Repair* **2008**, *22*, 279–287. [CrossRef]
32. Scivoletto, G.; Tamburella, F.; Laurenza, L.; Molinari, M. The spinal cord independence measure: How much change is clinically significant for spinal cord injury subjects. *Disabil. Rehabil.* **2013**, *35*, 1808–1813. [CrossRef]
33. Fawcett, J.; Curt, A.; Steeves, J.; Coleman, W.; Tuszynski, M.; Lammertse, D.; Bartlett, P.F.; Blight, A.R.; Dietz, V.; Ditunno, J.; et al. Guidelines for the conduct of clinical trials for spinal cord injury as developed by the iccp panel: Spontaneous recovery after spinal cord injury and statistical power needed for therapeutic clinical trials. *Spinal Cord* **2006**, *45*, 190–205. [CrossRef]
34. de Oliveira, C.Q.; Middleton, J.W.; Refhauge, K.; Davis, G.M. Activity-Based Therapy in a community Setting for independence, mobility, and sitting balance for people with spinal cord injuries. *J. Cent. Nerv. Syst. Dis.* **2019**, *11*, 1179573519841623. [CrossRef]
35. Jones, M.L.; Evans, N.; Tefertiller, C.; Backus, D.; Sweatman, M.; Tansey, K.; Morrison, S. Activity-based therapy for recovery of walking in chronic spinal cord injury: Results from a secondary analysis to determine responsiveness to therapy. *Arch. Phys. Med. Rehabil.* **2014**, *95*, 2247–2252. [CrossRef]
36. Dobkin, B.; Barbeau, H.; Deforge, D.; Ditunno, J.; Elashoff, R.; Apple, D.; Basso, M.; Behrman, A.; Fugate, L.; Harkema, S.; et al. The evolution of walking-related outcomes over the first 12 weeks of rehabilitation for incomplete traumatic spinal cord injury: The multicenter randomized Spinal Cord Injury Locomotor Trial. *Neurorehabilit. Neural Repair* **2007**, *21*, 25–35. [CrossRef] [PubMed]
37. Swaffield, E.; Cheung, L.; Khalili, A.; Lund, E.; Boileau, M.; Chechlacz, D.; Musselman, K.E.; Gauthier, C. Perspectives of people living with a spinal cord injury on activity-based therapy. *Disabil. Rehabil.* **2022**, *44*, 3632–3640. [CrossRef] [PubMed]

38. Rutten, I.; Van den Bogaert, L.; Geerts, D. From initial encounter with mid-air haptic feedback to repeated use: The role of the novelty effect in user experience. *IEEE Trans. Haptics* **2020**, *14*, 591–602. [CrossRef] [PubMed]
39. Groeneveld, I.F.; Goossens, P.H.; van Braak, I.; van der Pas, S.; Meesters, J.J.; Mishre, R.D.R.; Arwert, H.J.; Vlieland, T.P.V.; SCORE-Study Group. Patients' outcome expectations and their fulfilment in multidisciplinary stroke rehabilitation. *Ann. Phys. Rehabil. Med.* **2019**, *62*, 21–27. [CrossRef] [PubMed]
40. Bernstein, D.N.; Mahmood, B.; Ketonis, C.; Hammert, W.C. A comparison of PROMIS physical function and pain interference scores in patients with carpal tunnel syndrome: Research collection versus routine clinical collection. *HAND* **2020**, *15*, 771–775. [CrossRef]
41. Fritz, S.; Merlo-Rains, A.; Rivers, E.; Peters, D.M.; Goodman, A.; Watson, E.T.; Carmichael, B.M.; McClenaghan, B.A. An intensive intervention for improving gait, balance, and mobility in individuals with chronic incomplete spinal cord injury: A pilot study of activity tolerance and benefits. *Arch. Phys. Med. Rehabil.* **2011**, *92*, 1776–1784. [CrossRef]
42. Behrman, A.L.; Harkema, S.J. Physical rehabilitation as an agent for recovery after spinal cord injury. *Phys. Med. Rehabil. Clin. N. Am.* **2007**, *18*, 183–202. [CrossRef]
43. Padula, N.; Costa, M.; Batista, A.; Gaspar, R.; Motta, C.; Palma, G.; Torriani-Pasin, C. Long-term effects of an intensive interventional training program based on activities for individuals with spinal cord injury: A pilot study. *Physiother. Theory Pract.* **2015**, *31*, 568–574. [CrossRef]
44. Dobkin, B.; Apple, D.; Barbeau, H.; Basso, M.; Behrman, A.; Deforge, D.; Ditunno, J.; Dudley, G.; Elashoff, R.; Fugate, L.; et al. Weight-supported treadmill vs over-ground training for walking after acute incomplete SCI. *Neurology* **2006**, *66*, 484–493. [CrossRef]
45. Harkema, S.J.; Schmidt-Read, M.; Lorenz, D.J.; Edgerton, V.R.; Behrman, A.L. Balance and ambulation improvements in individuals with chronic incomplete spinal cord injury using locomotor training-based rehabilitation. *Arch. Phys. Med. Rehabil.* **2012**, *93*, 1508–1517. [CrossRef] [PubMed]
46. Backus, D.; Apple, D.; Hudson, L. Neural and functional outcomes after lower extremity and walking activity-based interventions for persons with spinal cord injury: A research synthesis. *Top. Spinal Cord Inj. Rehabil.* **2011**, *16*, 72.
47. Adams, M.M.; Hicks, A.L. Comparison of the effects of body-weight-supported treadmill training and tilt-table standing on spasticity in individuals with chronic spinal cord injury. *J. Spinal Cord Med.* **2011**, *34*, 488–494. [CrossRef]
48. Semerjian, T.; Montague, S.; Dominguez, J.; Davidian, A.; de Leon, R. Enhancement of quality of life and body satisfaction through the use of adapted exercise devices for individuals with spinal cord injuries. *Top. Spinal Cord Inj. Rehabil.* **2005**, *11*, 95–108. [CrossRef]
49. Sharif, H.; Gammage, K.; Chun, S.; Ditor, D. Effects of FES-Ambulation Training on Locomotor Function and Health-Related Quality of Life in Individuals With Spinal Cord Injury. *Top. Spinal Cord Inj. Rehabil.* **2014**, *20*, 58–69. [CrossRef] [PubMed]
50. Hitzig, S.; Craven, B.; Panjwani, A.; Kapadia, N.; Giangregorio, L.; Richards, K.; Masani, K.; Popovic, M. Randomized trial of functional electrical stimulation therapy for walking in incomplete spinal cord injury: Effects on quality of life and community participation. *Top. Spinal Cord Inj. Rehabil.* **2013**, *19*, 245–258. [CrossRef]
51. Harkema, S.J.; Schmidt-Read, M.; Behrman, A.L.; Bratta, A.; Sisto, S.A.; Edgerton, V.R. Establishing the NeuroRecovery Network: Multisite rehabilitation centers that provide activity-based therapies and assessments for neurologic disorders. *Arch. Phys. Med. Rehabil.* **2012**, *93*, 1498–1507. [CrossRef]
52. Edgerton, V.R.; Roy, R.R. Activity-Dependent Plasticity of Spinal Locomotion: Implications for Sensory Processing. *Exerc. Sport Sci. Rev.* **2009**, *37*, 171–178. [CrossRef]
53. Edgerton, V.R.; Tillakaratne, N.J.; Bigbee, A.J.; de Leon, R.D.; Roy, R.R. Plasticity of the spinal neural circuitry after injury. *Annu. Rev. Neurosci.* **2004**, *27*, 145–167. [CrossRef]
54. Roy, R.R.; Harkema, S.J.; Edgerton, V.R. Basic concepts of activity-based interventions for improved recovery of motor function after spinal cord injury. *Arch. Phys. Med. Rehabil.* **2012**, *93*, 1487–1497. [CrossRef]
55. Biglan, A.; Ary, D.; Wagenaar, A.C. The value of interrupted time-series experiments for community intervention research. *Prev. Sci.* **2000**, *1*, 31–49. [CrossRef] [PubMed]
56. Tate, R.L.; Perdices, M.; Rosenkoetter, U.; Shadish, W.; Vohra, S.; Barlow, D.H.; Horner, R.; Kazdin, A.; Kratochwill, T.; McDonald, S.; et al. The Single-Case Reporting Guideline In BEhavioural Interventions (SCRIBE) 2016 Statement. *Phys. Ther.* **2016**, *96*, e1–e10. [CrossRef] [PubMed]

Disclaimer/Publisher's Note: The statements, opinions and data contained in all publications are solely those of the individual author(s) and contributor(s) and not of MDPI and/or the editor(s). MDPI and/or the editor(s) disclaim responsibility for any injury to people or property resulting from any ideas, methods, instructions or products referred to in the content.

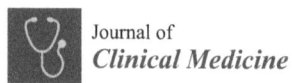

Article

Restoration of Over-Ground Walking via Non-Invasive Neuromodulation Therapy: A Single-Case Study

Monzurul Alam [1,*], Yan To Ling [1,2], Md Akhlasur Rahman [1,3], Arnold Yu Lok Wong [4], Hui Zhong [5], V. Reggie Edgerton [5,6,7] and Yong-Ping Zheng [1]

1. Department of Biomedical Engineering, The Hong Kong Polytechnic University, Hong Kong, China; jane.yt.ling@connect.polyu.hk (Y.T.L.); akhlas.physio@gmail.com (M.A.R.); yongping.zheng@polyu.edu.hk (Y.-P.Z.)
2. Centre for Developmental Neurobiology, Institute of Psychiatry, Psychology and Neuroscience, King's College London, London SE1 9NH, UK
3. Department of Physiotherapy, Centre for the Rehabilitation of the Paralysed, Savar Union 1343, Bangladesh
4. Department of Rehabilitation Sciences, The Hong Kong Polytechnic University, Hong Kong, China; arnold.wong@polyu.edu.hk
5. Rancho Research Institute, Rancho Los Amigos National Rehabilitation Center, Downey, CA 90242, USA; zhonghui731@gmail.com (H.Z.); vre@ucla.edu (V.R.E.)
6. Neurorestoration Center, University of Southern California, Los Angeles, CA 90089, USA
7. Department of Neurological Surgery, Keck School of Medicine, University of Southern California, Los Angeles, CA 90089, USA
* Correspondence: md.malam@connect.polyu.hk

Abstract: Spinal cord injuries (SCI) can result in sensory and motor dysfunctions, which were long considered permanent. Recent advancement in electrical neuromodulation has been proven to restore sensorimotor function in people with SCI. These stimulation protocols, however, were mostly invasive, expensive, and difficult to implement. In this study, transcutaneous electrical stimulation (tES) was used to restore over-ground walking of an individual with 21 years of chronic paralysis from a cervical SCI. After a total of 66 weeks of rehabilitation training with tES, which included standing, functional reaching, reclined sit-up, treadmill walking, and active biking, significant improvement in lower-limb volitional movements and overall light touch sensation were shown as measured by the International Standards for Neurological Classification of Spinal Cord Injury (ISNCSCI) score. By the end of the study, the participant could walk in a 4-m walking test with the aid of a walking frame and ankle–foot orthoses. The successful sensorimotor recovery of our study participant sheds light on the future of non-invasive neuromodulation treatment for SCI paralysis.

Keywords: chronic spinal cord injury; sensorimotor rehabilitation; transcutaneous electrical stimulation; neuromodulation; over-ground walking

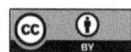

1. Introduction

A spinal cord injury (SCI) is an immediate, severe, disabling, and life-altering neurological impairment that has a significant adverse impact on patients, their families, and the healthcare system, as well as their physical, emotional, social, and occupational well-being [1–3]. Spinal cord injuries can cause severe damage to individuals, often leading to paralysis as they lose conscious control below the damaged area. SCI substantially impacts an individual's bodily functions, resulting in loss of sensation and limb control and poor bladder and bowel control [4,5]. Secondary issues include autonomic dysreflexia, cardiovascular disease, osteoporosis, spasticity, infections, and pressure ulcers [6]. Chronic pain is another common complication after SCI, affecting up to 80% of individuals with SCI [7]. It can be due to nerve damage, musculoskeletal imbalances, or psychological factors that worsen physical function and lower the quality of life for people with SCI [2]. People with SCI have been found to have a higher level of prevalence of depression and anxiety, ranging from 22% to 40% [8]. Emotional consequences after SCI have been widely reported; for example, 30% of individuals with SCI have a risk of developing a depressive disorder in the rehabilitation phase, and 27% of them show depression symptoms when living in the community [9]. It has been reported that the re-employment rate ranges from 14% to 44%, and social involvement in terms of an individual's social roles and interactions varies due to several factors, including the characteristics of the patient and the definition of employment [10]. Physical barriers can prevent people with SCI from participating in social activities and community events. Furthermore, SCI can limit a person's ability to work, which can have significant economic and social consequences. Unemployment and underemployment are common among people with SCI, which can affect their financial stability and social status [11]. Given the significant negative effects of SCI on individuals with SCI, caregivers, the healthcare system, and society, reversing paralysis in people with SCI is one of the highest priorities in treating these individuals.

Paralysis was long thought to be irreversible, but recent advances in spinal cord neuromodulation therapies have shown remarkable success in restoring movements and sensation to the paralyzed areas [12,13]. These successes have been achieved using an invasive method called epidural electrical stimulation, in which electrodes are implanted in the dura mater of the spinal cord. Although successful, the surgery involved in this treatment is expensive and can cause various complications and risks [14]. Non-invasive spinal cord neuromodulation, specifically transcutaneous electrical stimulation (tsDCS and tsPCS), uses transcutaneous electrical stimulation through the spinal cord and its peripheral nerves and is an effective treatment protocol for SCI and other neurological conditions. Successful applications have been demonstrated in the conditions of chronic pain [15], spasticity [16], respiratory problems [17], cardiovascular ischemia [18], neuropathic bladder [19], bowel dysfunction [20], and upper and lower limb function including fine motor function with digit function [21,22]. The impact of the possibility of regaining mobility could become even greater, realizing that the intervention can be developed for home use and is less challenging technologically and economically. Further reports amplify the impact of the non-invasive strategy used in this study [23,24].

In a previous report [25], we described how a chronic SCI individual with tetraplegia, who had been wheelchair-bound for the previous 21 years following a traumatic cervical cord injury in a car accident, regained volitional movements in bilateral leg muscles after 16 weeks of non-invasive spinal cord stimulation (tES) and activity-based physical training. The current report reveals the effects of an additional 44 weeks of tES and progressive physical training in helping the study participant walk independently.

2. Materials and Methods

2.1. Study Participant

Our study participant was a 48-year-old woman who was involved in a road traffic accident 21 years ago (cervical burst fracture) and sustained a C7 cervical cord injury resulting in Brown Séquard Syndrome. Although her bilateral distal upper limb muscles remained impaired and she could not fully flex her fingers, she was able to perform most of her upper limb tasks for moderate-intensity household and functional activities. Further, she had moderate trunk control, allowing her to sit on the edge of a bed with the support of her hands. However, her lower limb functions were severely limited following the injury. As a result, she had been wheelchair-bound since her injury. At the beginning of the study, she had very limited active movement in the right leg, while her left leg was completely paralyzed. In addition, moderate muscle spasm was noted in both legs, especially in the left leg. Some weak and altered sensation was retained in her saddle region, but no motor function was preserved in the bowel/bladder.

2.2. Stimulation Protocol

Two constant current stimulators (Model DS8R, Digitimer, UK) were utilized in this study to simultaneously stimulate the participant's T11 and L1 spinal segments (Figure 1a).

An arbitrary function generator (Model AFG1022, Tektronix, Inc., Beaverton, OR, USA) was used to generate a 9.4 kHz burst trigger at 20 to 30 Hz. From this trigger, each stimulator produced a biphasic tES (50 µs negative and 50 µs positive pulse currents with 1 µs inter-pulse interval). Two 3.2 cm diameter self-adhesive electrodes (ValuTrode, Axelgaard Manufacturing Co., Ltd., Fallbrook, CA, USA) were placed at the midline, immediately below the T11 and L1 spinous processes, to deliver tES currents at an intensity ranging from 20 mA to 120 mA. Two internally connected 6 × 9 cm² self-adhesive rectangular electrodes (Guangzhou Jetta Electronic Medical Device Manufacturing Co., Ltd., Guangzhou, China) were also attached to the skin above the iliac crests to act as a sink for the stimulation current.

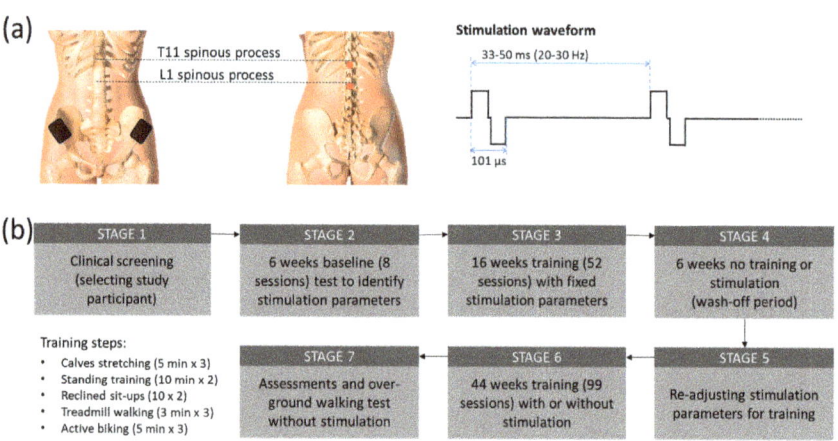

Figure 1. (**a**) Overall training methods and study procedures. After passing the clinical screening (STAGE 1), eight transcutaneous electrical stimulation (tES) sessions were conducted on the study participant on assisted standing and walking to determine the optimum stimulation parameters for training, followed by pre-training assessments (STAGE 2). A total of 16 weeks of physical training were then provided 3 times/week in conjunction with stimulation (tES). The training steps included a total of 15 min stretching of calves; 2 sets (7–10 times each) of unassisted sit-ups on a reclined position; 20, 15, and 9 min of assisted standing, biking, and treadmill walking. After 52 intensive training sessions (STAGE 3), functional reassessments were conducted to determine the participant's improvement. Following this, a 6-week break from the stimulation training was provided to examine the retainment of the participant's newly gained functional abilities (STAGE 4). Following the break, the stimulation parameters were re-adjusted for the new functionality of the participant (STAGE 5). Then, 44 weeks of discontinuous training with and without stimulation were provided to see the effect on motor learning (STAGE 6). Upon completion, final post-training assessments, including, for the first time, an overground walking test, were conducted (STAGE 7). (**b**) tES setup. (Left) Stimulation electrode placements in both anterior and posterior views. Two 3.2 cm diameter electrodes were placed at the midline, immediately below the T11 and L1 spinous processes. Two internally connected 6 × 9 cm² rectangular electrodes were also attached to the skin above the iliac crests. (Right) Stimulation waveform of biphasic pulses (50 µs positive and 50 µs negative pulse currents with 1 µs inter-pulse interval) delivered at 20–30 Hz stimulation frequency.

2.3. Study Procedure

After completing an initial screening for the subject's cardiac health for physical activity and a bone density evaluation by an independent physician, the participant was included in a non-invasive spinal cord stimulation called transcutaneous electrical stimulation (tES) trial. Figure 1b shows the overall outline of the study procedure. In a previous report [25], we reported the first part (STAGE 1–STAGE 4) of the study, where the study participant regained volitional leg movements and weight-bearing standing after 16 weeks of stimulation and physical training. In brief, after the baseline sensorimotor assessment using the International Standards for Neurological Classification of Spinal Cord Injury

(ISNCSCI), the participant attended eight baseline sessions for pre-training tests to identify the optimal tES parameters from lower limb motor evoked potentials for the physical training. The study participant subsequently attended 16 weeks of 2-h training sessions at an average of 3 times a week (the subject missed some sessions due to her schedule but attended at least 2 times per week. We also compensated for the missed sessions with additional sessions to maintain the average training constant). Each training session started with a set of three 5-min stretches (a total of 15 min), with a 2-min rest between sets. Each tES-assisted physical training session was divided into four parts in the following order: (1) a set of three 10-min standing and functional reaching (a total of 30 min), with a 3-min break between sets; (2) a set of two 7–10 sit-ups on a reclined chair; (3) a set of three 3 min of treadmill walking with 20–30% body-weight support (a total of 9 min) with a 3-min break between sets; and (4) a set of three 5-min forward and reverse biking (a total of 15 min), with a 3-min break interspersed between sets. Blood pressure was regularly checked between each training set. During the standing and functional reaching part, the participant was instructed to perform some trunk and lower body exercises, such as side and forward bending and/or squatting, depending on the physical condition on a given treatment date. The period of walking on the treadmill and load of biking exercise was increased gradually based on the participant's condition as the training progressed. Sometimes, the subject could not reach the expected training duration because of fatigue and other factors. The reduced duration was, however, normally within 30% of the expected. A final neurological assessment (ISNCSCI) was conducted at the end of the study to evaluate the post-treatment effect.

2.4. Standing and Functional Reaching Training with tES

Optimum tES was chosen based on the participant's comfort and reported ease of standing with the least physical support after multiple iterations over the first 6 weeks of the trial. The participant could sense the stimulation and provided verbal feedback during the process. The participant was unblinded to the parameter changes, and when the chosen tES parameters reached the optimum stimulation, the participant reported that she felt "more connected" to her paretic body parts; these parameters were used for stimulation for her standing training. The tES was delivered at 20 Hz at an intensity of 105 mA at the T11 level and 100 mA at the L1 level. Throughout the training period, the stimulation parameters were kept constant. Only the intensity was adjusted (± 10 mA) based on the participant's comfort. At the beginning of the training, manual support was given to the pelvis, knees, and feet. These supports were gradually lifted as the standing ability improved. After several initial training sessions, the participant was instructed to semi-squat from standing once she gained control over her knees. The same tES parameters were applied for the semi-squat training.

2.5. Reclined Sit-Ups with tES

After each standing session, our study participant was seated in a reclined wheelchair and completed 7 to 10 sit-ups. The same standing training tES parameters were used for the sit-ups exercise. Only the current intensity was adjusted to provide ease to do the task. The researcher verbally encouraged the study participant to complete all 10 sit-ups. An occasional break was given to allow her to catch breaths as needed. We increased the wheelchair backrest angle for the sit-ups once the study participant was able to complete all 10 sit-ups easily and regularly using the resistance training progression principle [26]. We evaluated the immediate response after the adjustment to ensure that the exercise would overload the target muscles without causing damage.

2.6. Treadmill Walking Training with tES

The tES was used to help our participant during body weight-assisted treadmill walking. During treadmill walking, two trainers assisted the participant's legs to move throughout the gait cycle (1.125 km/h), while another trainer emulated pelvis rotation.

Optimum stimulation parameters were chosen by the participant after multiple sessions throughout the first 6 weeks of the trial, using the same technique mentioned in the standing training. The tES was delivered at 30 Hz at an intensity of 90–110 mA at T11 and L1 levels. During the training session, the participant walked for up to three sets of 3 min on a moving treadmill belt with 20–30% body-weight support (a total of 9 min). A 2-min break was given between each walking training session. The stimulation parameters were kept constant throughout the walk.

2.7. Active Biking Training with tES

The tES was used to help our participant during forward and reverse biking. A motorized bike with passive and active operation options (MOTOmed viva2, RECK-Technik GmbH and Co. KG, Betzenweiler, Germany) was set on 10 cycles/min for 5 min for each session of forward and reverse biking with a 3-min rest time between each session. The study participant was encouraged to pedal at a speed higher than the preset biking speed while tES was delivered to her T11 and L1 spinal segments at 25 Hz. Following the assisted active biking exercise, another 2 min of passive biking (1-min forward and 1-min reverse) was given to relax the lower limb muscles.

2.8. Testing of Over-Ground Walking with and without tES

In the current study, tES was used to help the study participant regain volitional control of her paretic legs to restore over-ground walking. The participant was encouraged to move her legs voluntarily. At the early stage of the training, the tES current was delivered during the volitional activities. However, our study participant was able to move her legs nearly without the assistance of tES at the end of the 16-week training. By the end of the study, our study participant could ambulate over-ground with the assistance of a walker even without the tES. A 4-m walking test was conducted to evaluate her recovery from walking. Body kinematics and lower limb muscle activities were captured using an integrated motion capture system (Vicon Nexus, Vicon Motion Systems Ltd., Oxford, UK) and an 8-channel wireless electromyography EMG acquisition system (Trigno Avanti, ADInstruments, Otago, New Zealand). For EMG recording, four pairs of EMG electrodes were placed at the bilateral quadriceps muscle belly, tibialis anterior, hamstrings, and gastrocnemius. The EMG signal was digitized and saved on a computer at a sample rate of 2 kS/s for offline analysis. Videos were also shot with a digital camera during walking and juxtaposed with the kinematic data.

2.9. Data Analysis and Statistics

Gait and muscle dynamics were analyzed offline from the motion markers and EMG signals of lower-limb movements using a customized MATLAB script (MathWorks Inc., Natick, MA, USA). The difference between left and right leg gait performances was determined using paired t-tests. Statistical software (GraphPad Software Inc., La Jolla, CA, USA) was used for all statistical analyses. The significant level was set at 0.05.

3. Results

3.1. Improvement in Sensory and Motor Functions

Figure 2 shows the pre- and post-treatment ISNCSCI scores. Improvement in both light touch appreciation and manual muscle tests is shown as the shift in color from red to green. The ISNCSCI score on left-leg volitional movements increased from a grade of 0 to a grade of 9 ($p = 0.009$; two-tailed paired t-test), while right-leg motor function improved from grade 17 to 20 ($p = 0.071$, two-tailed paired t-test). It has been observed in various spinal neuromodulation applications that stimulation enhances not just motor activity but also sensory function in SCI individuals. In the present study, the overall light touch sensation also significantly improved from grade 71 to grade 77 ($p = 0.031$, two-tailed paired t-test). However, pin-prick discrimination did not change (grade 73 to 72, $p = 0.769$, two-tailed paired t-test) after the tES therapy.

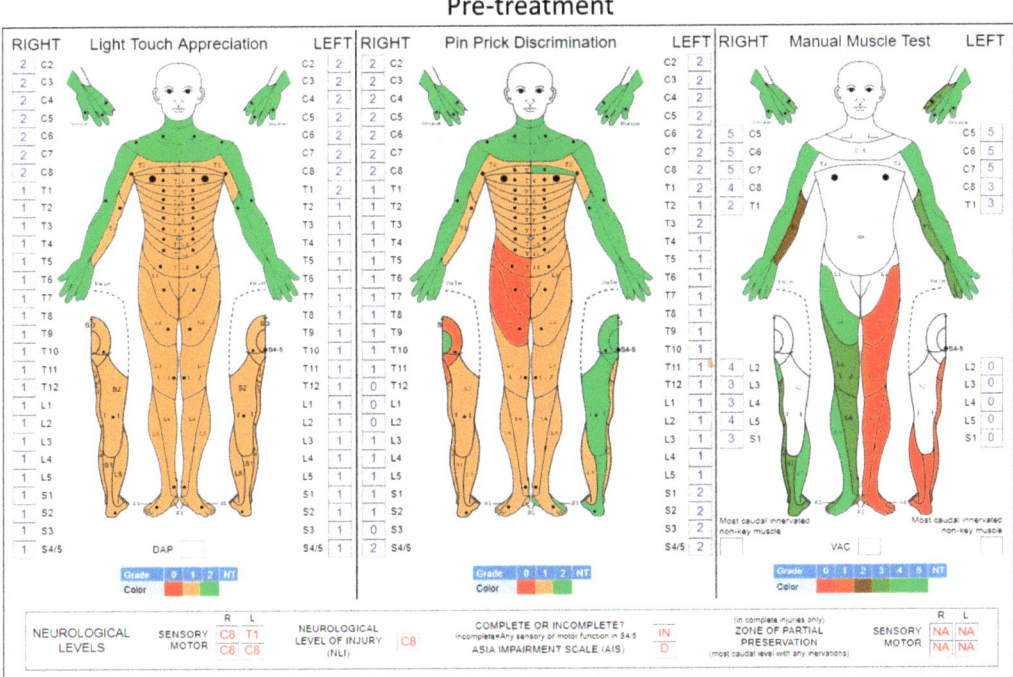
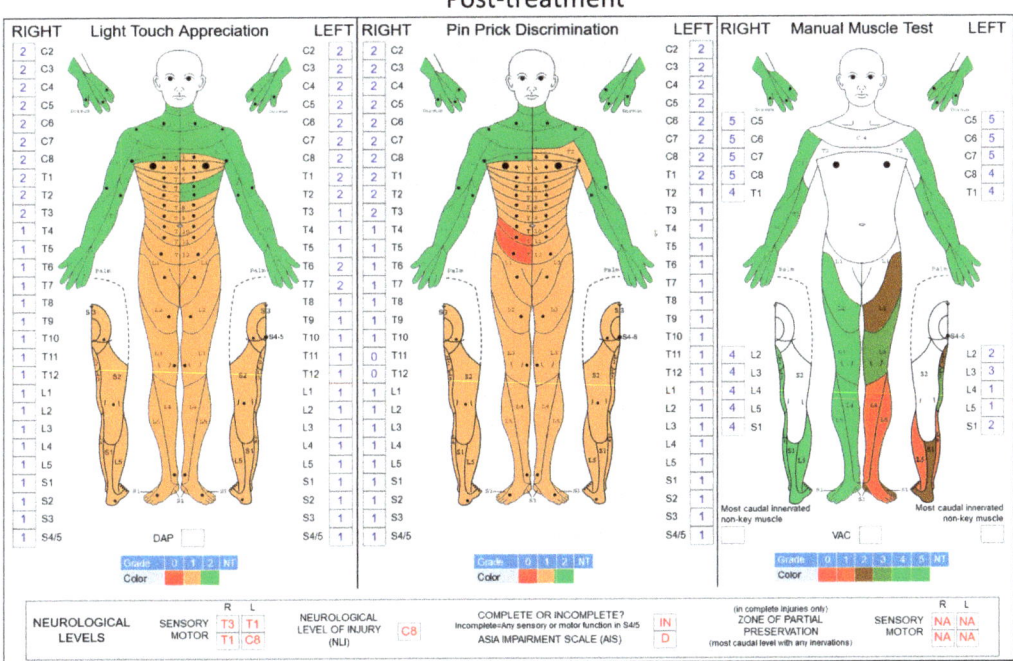

Figure 2. Pre- and post-training assessment of the participant. International Standards for Neurological Classification of Spinal Cord Injuries (ISNCSCI) worksheet scores before and after the treatment. Significant improvements in motor scores (manual muscle test) indicate the renversement of paralysis

of the left lower limb. The total score of the five individual movements (hip flexion, knee extension, ankle dorsiflexion, long toe extension, and ankle plantar flexion) exhibited significant improvements ($p = 0.009$; two-tailed paired t-test) after stimulation treatment compared to the baseline. Significant changes in the light touch appreciation ($p = 0.031$, two-tailed paired t-test) indicate some sensory recovery, while the pin-prick sensations did not change significantly ($p = 0.769$, two-tailed paired t-test) compared to the baseline.

3.2. Restoration of Overground Walking Ability

At the end of the study, we tested the participant's walking ability in a 4-m walking test with a high-speed motion capture system (Vicon Motion Systems Ltd., Oxford, UK) and a wireless EMG system (Trigno Avanti, ADInstruments, Dunedin, New Zealand). Due to long chronic paralysis, the study participant had shortened calf muscles and ankle invertors, which made her unable to place her heels on the ground while standing. To resolve this, we stretched her bilateral dorsiflexors. However, we did not see any significant improvements in the passive ranges of motion of her bilateral ankle eversion and plantarflexion. Hence, our study participant had to utilize ankle–foot orthoses (AFOs) to prevent excessive ankle inversion and plantarflexion during weight-bearing standing and walking. Figure 3 shows the gait pattern and muscle dynamics of the left and right leg during over-ground walking with a walker. Figure 3a shows details of motion and muscle activities, while Figure 3b,c summarizes the overall gait pattern and differences between the left and right legs. Although a clear stepping pattern can be observed, the participant often put her left foot even with the right foot, instead of ahead of the right, for each step (Figure 3a). Gait and muscle dynamics were further analyzed from the motion markers and EMG signals of lower-limb movements. The Stick diagram shows that the left leg had slower steps compared to the right leg, while the right leg had much smoother steps, as observed in the swing phases. This can be further observed in the foot, ankle, and knee position patterns (Figure 3a). Furthermore, the quadriceps and hamstring muscles showed more robust EMG signals on the right leg compared to the left leg. Figure 3b shows the normalized gait cycle of our study participant, illustrating symmetric phase relationships of temporal events and periods.

The gait cycle of the right leg had 80% stance phase (19% initial double support, 31% single support, 30% final double support) and the rest 20% swing phase. Figure 3c summarizes the overall steps analysis. The average stride lengths were 0.339 ± 0.106 and 0.389 ± 0.072 m for the left and right leg ($p = 0.318$, unpaired t-test). Average stride periods were 4.045 ± 0.723 and 4.213 ± 0.370 s for the left and right leg ($p = 0.622$, unpaired t-test). Similarly, average steps per minute (15.273 ± 2.967 and 14.322 ± 1.118 for the left and right legs) were not significantly different ($p = 0.479$, unpaired t-test). The over-ground walking speed of the study participant was 0.107 m/s.

3.3. Improvement of Forward Biking Ability with tES

For active cycling, a motorized bike with the option of both passive and active operation (MOTOmed viva2, RECK-Technik GmbH and Co. KG, Germany) was set at 10 cycles/min. The study participant was asked to try to exceed the speed while tES was delivered at 25 Hz. Over the course of the study, our participant showed a significant improvement in forward ($p < 0.001$; R2 value = 0.945) but not reverse biking speed, suggesting improved leg extensors function in the forward biking direction (Figure 3d). Although both forward and reverse biking could activate quadriceps, the sequence and extent of the muscle recruitment sequence might differ between the two types of biking, which might partly explain the differential findings. We also observed little or no difference in walking ability with and without the tES, suggesting a significant reorganization of spinal–supraspinal networks attributable to the repetitive exposure to spinal neuromodulation concomitant with exposure to a task-specific training paradigm as also observed recently with epidural stimulation [27].

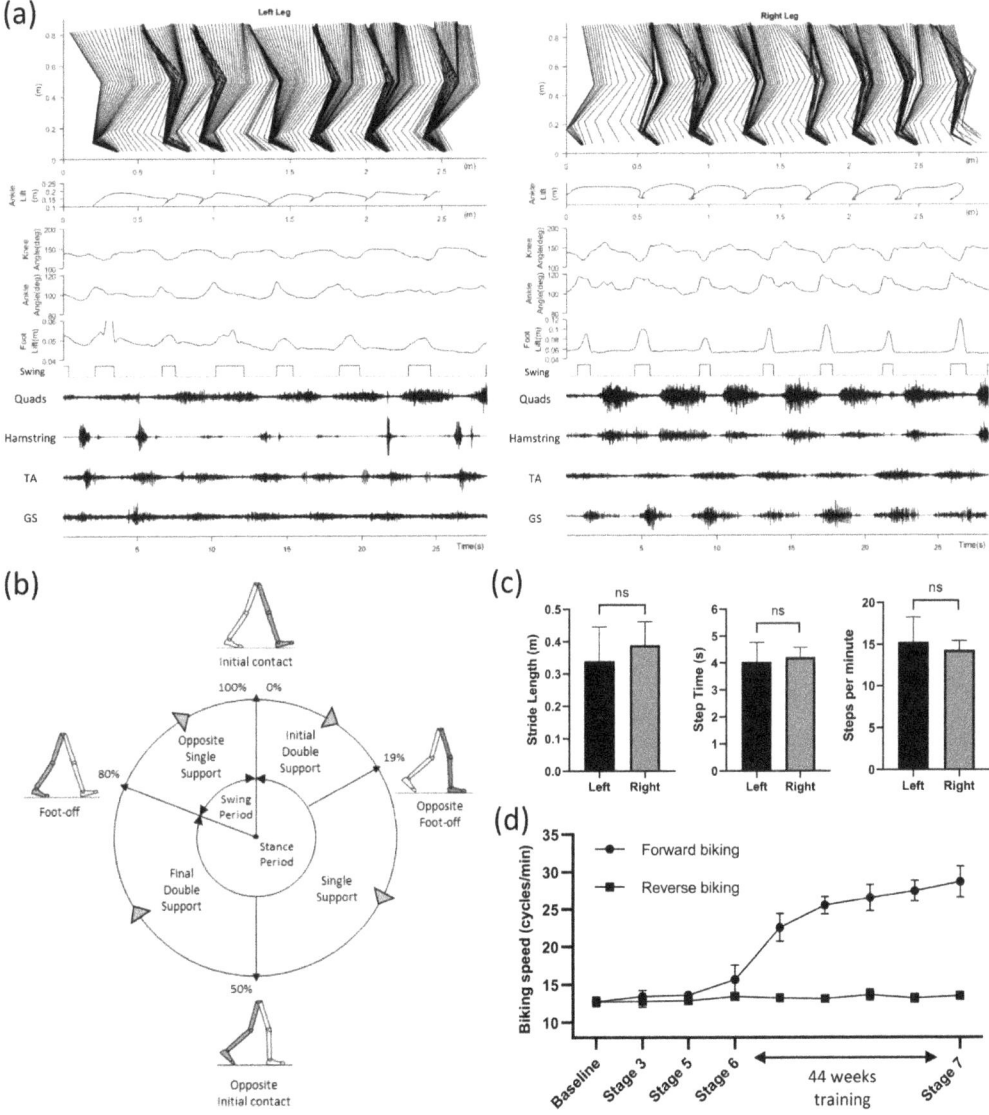

Figure 3. (**a**) Gait pattern and muscle dynamics of the left and right leg during over-ground walking with a walker. Stick diagram decomposition of lower-limb movements (1st row). The position of the ankle shows each stride (2nd row). Knee and ankle angles (3rd to 4th row). Foot lifting off the ground (5th row) is used to determine the stance and swing phase (6th row). Synchronized EMG signals showing activations of the Quadriceps, Hamstring, Tibialis Anterior (TA), and Gastrocnemius (GS) (7th to 10th row). (**b**) Normalized gait cycle of the right leg with 80% stance phase (19% initial double support, 31% single support, 30% final double support) and the rest 20% swing phase. (**c**) Average stride length, step period, and steps per minute (mean ± SD) for both legs. No significant difference was found between the left and right leg for all parameters ($p = 0.318$; $p = 0.622$; and $p = 0.479$; t-tests). (**d**) Average biking speed in forward and backward directions throughout different stages of the study. Significant improvement ($p < 0.001$; R2 value = 0.945; non-linear regression) in forward biking speed is observed during the 44-week discontinuous training period (STAGE 6).

3.4. Secondary Functional Improvements

The results reported by the participant in this study include descriptions of each of the functions noted above, plus noting improvements in sleeping patterns, with less insomnia and more deep sleep; the ability to perform exercises for longer periods and sitting posture also were improved. Throughout the research trial period, the study participant experienced a continuous improvement in the strength of the lower back and core muscles, which allowed her to sit up straighter and perform a variety of daily tasks. While engaging in standing exercises, the study participant gradually reduced her reliance on her hands for support, thus increasing the duration of standing solely on her feet. These enhancements have positive impacts on various aspects of her daily life. The increased lower body strength has helped the study participant to relieve some of the burden of the upper body and improved overall body balance. The participant noted, "Now I sit in a more upright posture and can work longer with less exhaustion". These findings may result in a reduced cost of healthcare throughout life.

4. Discussion

Although researchers all over the world have searched for a cure for spinal cord injury, as yet, there is no known therapy to regenerate a damaged spinal cord [28]. Neuroregeneration, along with anti-inflammatory and preventive therapies, do not yet translate to humans with SCI [29]. In contrast, neurostimulation therapies can often be used for functional restoration and to minimize secondary conditions such as pain, respiratory, and cardiovascular functions, as well as improve gait performance [15,30,31].

Transcutaneous electrical stimulation (tES), a non-invasive method in which stimulating electrodes are placed on the skin to pass an electric current through the tissue underneath, has shown neuromodulatory effects on spinal cord neurocircuits [32]. We have recently shown that by combining locomotor training with tES at the lower thoracic (T11) and upper lumber (L1) spinal levels, an individual with over two decades of chronic paralysis suffering from Brown Séquard Syndrome from a motor-vehicle accident-induced cervical cord injury (C7), regained significant voluntary control on her pelvic limb [25]. In brief, after passing the clinical screening (Figure 1b, STAGE 1), 6 weeks of baseline test with tES were conducted to determine the best stimulation parameters for training (STAGE 2), followed by 16 weeks of training with tES to improve the lower extremity motor functions (STAGE 3). After training, the lower extremity motor score (LEMS) of the pelagic left leg, based on International Standards for Neurological Classification of SCI (ISNCSCI), increased significantly from 0 to 10 ($p < 0.001$; one-way repeated measures ANOVA; post hoc Tukey's multiple comparison test) over the course of 16 weeks of tES and locomotor training. Further, after 6 weeks without stimulation or training (STAGE 4), the improved motor function did not change significantly (ISNCSCI score dropped from 10 to 8), thus sustaining an improved level of functional spinal–supraspinal connectivity. Hence, we further extended the study to examine if we can nurture additional neuronal plasticity and reinforce further motor learning. In particular, we further fine-tuned the stimulation parameters based on the lower extremity muscles' responses to different functional tasks, including weight shifting during standing, reaching with the legs, squats, and reclined sit-ups (Figure 1b, STAGE 5). We found that in extensors-related activities such as standing, the participant responded well with 20 Hz stimulation; while attempting volitional effort during gait training, 25 Hz stimulation frequency was more beneficial along with the other fixed stimulation parameters (101 μsec biphasic pulses with 90 mA stimulation intensity). Stimulation details are shown in Figure 1a.

In a previous study, it was shown that multisite transcutaneous electrical stimulation along with locomotor training improves locomotor function in individuals with incomplete SCI [33]. However, no non-invasive treatment has yet shown restoration of over-ground ambulatory function in a wheelchair-bound individual with SCI. In the present study, the training protocol comprised 44 weeks of variable locomotor training (due to occasional restrictions for the COVID-19 pandemic) along with or without tES (STAGE 6). In the final assessments (STAGE 7), we found that even after this on-and-off training, our participant regained significant voluntary control over her lower extremities, and she could, for the first time, ambulate over-ground with the help of a walker (Pacer Gait Trainer, Rifton, USA) without any stimulation (Supplementary Video S1). Notably, the current study adopted the exercise progression principle in resistance training to improve muscle strength, corticospinal plasticity, and motor skill learning [34,35]. To the best of our knowledge, this is the first demonstration of walking restoration using a non-invasive treatment for an individual with severe chronic SCI.

The quantitative results demonstrating recovery of unassisted mobility over a period of 66 weeks in an individual who has been severely paralyzed and wheelchair-dependent for more than two decades using non-invasive spinal stimulation concomitant with task-specific training is of high significance. This demonstrates that the neuromuscular system is capable of adapting well beyond 6–12 months post-injury, a persistent long-term dogma that is rarely the case. Neuromodulation techniques have been used to successfully treat a variety of neurological conditions, such as spinal cord injury, stroke, multiple sclerosis, and children with cerebral palsy [16,22,36,37]. There is accumulating evidence that neuromodulation electrical modulation improves neuroregeneration and neural repair by affecting nervous system signals, which may help to enhance motor function and motor learning following neurological injury [38,39]. This can be accomplished by specifically controlling, suppressing, or increasing the activity of neurons and neural networks [40].

The success in the sensorimotor recovery of our participant sheds light on the future of non-invasive treatment for SCI paralysis. It also leaves an open question of whether non-invasive spinal cord neuromodulation can work similarly to or, in some individuals, even better than invasive epidural stimulation to restore lost functions, including voluntary movements, standing, over-ground walking, and sensation. If confirmed in future studies, tES could benefit a large population worldwide, to regain a significant level of function even after prolonged periods of paralysis.

We recognize the limitation necessary for interpreting the present data simply because it is a single case study. However, it should be pointed out that the strength of the present data, as in other case studies, by definition, has no valid control. These data do not address the issue of whether these observations imply that they represent some given population of specific subjects. The results are novel and demonstrate a level of plasticity in response to a novel combination of interventions, i.e., a neuromodulation procedure previously demonstrated consistently to transform the level of excitability and functionality of neural networks when combined with a specific series of activity-dependent interventions. The observations present functional levels that have not been previously reported using any intervention in a subject that has been paralyzed for a prolonged period. The present dogma is that such results are impossible, and the medical community routinely responds to patients accordingly. Thus, these results demonstrate what is possible with the new interventional strategy. It is also important because this result was obtained without being dependent on an extensive technological capability and, thus, has the potential of having a high impact in environments with limited medical technologies.

Despite the promising results, the current study had several limitations. Our findings may not be generalized to individuals with different levels or severity of SCI. Future trials with a larger sample size are warranted to validate the positive results in the present study. Furthermore, it remains unclear whether the stimulation location may have differential effects on the treatment outcomes. Future studies should determine the optimal electrode placement locations. Given that the mechanisms underlying the recovery remain unclear, future animal and human mechanistic studies should use advanced imaging technologies to explore the functional mechanisms of such recovery, which will help determine the optimal stimulation parameters for the best treatment outcomes in individuals with SCI.

5. Conclusions

This study shows for the first time how non-invasive spinal cord neuromodulation permanently restores volition control and over-ground ambulatory function in an individual with chronic paralysis. However, future studies are warranted to validate the results in more participants and to better understand the underlying mechanisms. Further explorations of the optimal stimulation parameters and their efficiency in more severely injured individuals are also needed.

Supplementary Materials: The following supporting information can be downloaded at https://www.mdpi.com/article/10.3390/jcm12237362/s1, Video S1: Study participant walks using a walking frame with AFOs (Ankle–Foot Orthoses) after completion of the study. No stimulation therapy was provided during or immediately before walking.

Author Contributions: Conceptualization, M.A., V.R.E. and Y.-P.Z.; methodology, M.A., A.Y.L.W., H.Z. and Y.-P.Z.; formal analysis, M.A., Y.T.L. and M.A.R.; investigation, M.A., Y.T.L., M.A.R., A.Y.L.W. and H.Z.; resources, M.A.; data curation, M.A. and Y.T.L.; writing—original draft preparation, M.A.; writing—review and editing, M.A., Y.T.L., M.A.R. and A.Y.L.W.; visualization, M.A. and V.R.E.; supervision, M.A. and Y.-P.Z.; project administration, M.A.; funding acquisition, M.A. and Y.-P.Z. All authors have read and agreed to the published version of the manuscript.

Funding: The study was supported by the Hong Kong Polytechnic University (UAKB) and the Telefield Charitable Fund (83D1).

Institutional Review Board Statement: The study was conducted in accordance with the Declaration of Helsinki and approved by the Hong Kong Polytechnic University Human Subjects Ethics Sub-committee (HSEARS20190201002, 1 March 2019). The study was registered on ClinicalTrials.gov (Identifier: NCT04171375, 20 November 2019).

Informed Consent Statement: Written informed consent was obtained from the subject involved in the study. Informed consent has been obtained from the study participant to publish this paper.

Data Availability Statement: The data generated from this work can be obtained from the corresponding author upon request.

Acknowledgments: The authors would like to sincerely thank the study participant for her enthusiasm and hard work during the long training sessions. The authors also thank L. N. Wong, N. S. Thoru, V. Nazari, and R. U. Ahmed for their help in training the participant.

Conflicts of Interest: M.A. holds shareholder interest in RehabExo Pty Ltd. and certain inventorship rights on intellectual property owned by RehabExo Pty Ltd. and its subsidiaries. None of the other authors have any conflicts of interest, financial or otherwise, to disclose. The funders had no role in the design of the study, in the collection, analyses, or interpretation of data, in the writing of the manuscript, or in the decision to publish the results.

References

1. Alam, M.; Zheng, Y.P. Motor neuroprosthesis for injured spinal cord: Who is an ideal candidate? *Neural Regen. Res.* **2017**, *12*, 1809–1810. [CrossRef]
2. Cripps, R.A.; Lee, B.B.; Wing, P.; Weerts, E.; Mackay, J.; Brown, D. A global map for traumatic spinal cord injury epidemiology: Towards a living data repository for injury prevention. *Spinal Cord* **2011**, *49*, 493–501. [CrossRef] [PubMed]
3. Hall, A.G.; Karabukayeva, A.; Rainey, C.; Kelly, R.J.; Patterson, J.; Wade, J.; Feldman, S.S. Perspectives on life following a traumatic spinal cord injury. *Disabil. Health J.* **2021**, *14*, 101067. [CrossRef] [PubMed]
4. Anjum, A.; Yazid, M.D.; Fauzi Daud, M.; Idris, J.; Ng, A.M.H.; Selvi Naicker, A.; Ismail, O.H.R.; Athi Kumar, R.K.; Lokanathan, Y. Spinal Cord Injury: Pathophysiology, Multimolecular Interactions, and Underlying Recovery Mechanisms. *Int. J. Mol. Sci.* **2020**, *21*, 7533. [CrossRef] [PubMed]
5. Alam, M.; He, J. Lower-Limb Neuroprostheses: Restoring Walking after Spinal Cord Injury. In *Emerging Theory and Practice in Neuroprosthetics*; Naik, G.R., Guo, Y., Eds.; IGI Global: Hershey, PA, USA, 2014; pp. 153–180.
6. Sezer, N.; Akkuş, S.; Uğurlu, F.G. Chronic complications of spinal cord injury. *World J. Orthop.* **2015**, *6*, 24–33. [CrossRef] [PubMed]
7. Koukoulithras, I.; Alkhazi, A.; Gkampenis, A.; Stamouli, A.; Plexousakis, M.; Drousia, G.; Xanthi, E.; Roussos, C.; Kolokotsios, S. A Systematic Review of the Interventions for Management of Pain in Patients after Spinal Cord Injury. *Cureus* **2023**, *15*, e42657. [CrossRef] [PubMed]

8. Parker, M.A.; Ichikawa, J.K.; Bombardier, C.H.; Hammond, F.M. Association Between Anxiety Symptoms, Depression Symptoms, and Life Satisfaction among Individuals 1 Year after Spinal Cord Injury: Findings from the SCIRehab Project. *Arch. Rehabil. Res. Clin. Transl.* **2022**, *4*, 100211. [CrossRef] [PubMed]
9. Craig, A.; Tran, Y.; Middleton, J. Psychological morbidity and spinal cord injury: A systematic review. *Spinal Cord* **2009**, *47*, 108–114. [CrossRef]
10. Kennedy, P.; Lude, P.; Taylor, N. Quality of life, social participation, appraisals and coping post spinal cord injury: A review of four community samples. *Spinal Cord* **2006**, *44*, 95–105. [CrossRef]
11. Tsai, I.; Graves, D.E.; Chan, W.; Darkoh, C.; Lee, M.-S.; Pompeii, L.A. Environmental barriers and social participation in individuals with spinal cord injury. *Rehabil. Psychol.* **2017**, *62*, 36–44. [CrossRef]
12. Angeli, C.A.; Boakye, M.; Morton, R.A.; Vogt, J.; Benton, K.; Chen, Y.; Ferreira, C.K.; Harkema, S.J. Recovery of over-Ground Walking after Chronic Motor Complete Spinal Cord Injury. *N. Engl. J. Med.* **2018**, *379*, 1244–1250. [CrossRef]
13. Wagner, F.B.; Mignardot, J.-B.; Le Goff-Mignardot, C.G.; Demesmaeker, R.; Komi, S.; Capogrosso, M.; Rowald, A.; Seáñez, I.; Caban, M.; Pirondini, E.; et al. Targeted neurotechnology restores walking in humans with spinal cord injury. *Nature* **2018**, *563*, 65–71. [CrossRef]
14. Patel, S.K.; Gozal, Y.M.; Saleh, M.S.; Gibson, J.L.; Karsy, M.; Mandybur, G.T. Spinal cord stimulation failure: Evaluation of factors underlying hardware explantation. *J. Neurosurg. Spine* **2019**, *32*, 133–138. [CrossRef]
15. Caylor, J.; Reddy, R.; Yin, S.; Cui, C.; Huang, M.; Huang, C.; Ramesh, R.; Baker, D.G.; Simmons, A.; Souza, D.; et al. Spinal cord stimulation in chronic pain: Evidence and theory for mechanisms of action. *Bioelectron. Med.* **2019**, *5*, 12. [CrossRef] [PubMed]
16. Hofstoetter, U.S.; Freundl, B.; Lackner, P.; Binder, H. Transcutaneous Spinal Cord Stimulation Enhances Walking Performance and Reduces Spasticity in Individuals with Multiple Sclerosis. *Brain Sci.* **2021**, *11*, 472. [CrossRef] [PubMed]
17. Kumru, H.; García-Alén, L.; Ros-Alsina, A.; Albu, S.; Valles, M.; Vidal, J. Transcutaneous Spinal Cord Stimulation Improves Respiratory Muscle Strength and Function in Subjects with Cervical Spinal Cord Injury: Original Research. *Biomedicines* **2023**, *11*, 2121. [CrossRef] [PubMed]
18. Salavatian, S.; Kuwabara, Y.; Wong, B.; Fritz, J.R.; Howard-Quijano, K.; Foreman, R.D.; Armour, J.A.; Ardell, J.L.; Mahajan, A. Spinal neuromodulation mitigates myocardial ischemia-induced sympathoexcitation by suppressing the intermediolateral nucleus hyperactivity and spinal neural synchrony. *Front. Neurosci.* **2023**, *17*, 1180294. [CrossRef]
19. Steadman, C.J.; Grill, W.M. Spinal cord stimulation for the restoration of bladder function after spinal cord injury. *Healthc. Technol. Lett.* **2020**, *7*, 87–92. [CrossRef]
20. DiMarco, A.F.; Geertman, R.T.; Tabbaa, K.; Nemunaitis, G.A.; Kowalski, K.E. Effects of Lower Thoracic Spinal Cord Stimulation on Bowel Management in Individuals with Spinal Cord Injury. *Arch. Phys. Med. Rehabil.* **2021**, *102*, 1155–1164. [CrossRef]
21. Qian, Q.; Ling, Y.T.; Zhong, H.; Zheng, Y.-P.; Alam, M. Restoration of arm and hand functions via noninvasive cervical cord neuromodulation after traumatic brain injury: A case study. *Brain Inj.* **2020**, *34*, 1771–1780. [CrossRef]
22. Rahman, M.A.; Tharu, N.S.; Gustin, S.M.; Zheng, Y.-P.; Alam, M. Trans-spinal electrical stimulation therapy for functional rehabilitation after spinal cord injury. *J. Clin. Med.* **2022**, *11*, 1550. [CrossRef] [PubMed]
23. Tharu, N.S.; Alam, M.; Ling, Y.T.; Wong, A.Y.; Zheng, Y.-P. Combined Transcutaneous Electrical Spinal Cord Stimulation and Task-Specific Rehabilitation Improves Trunk and Sitting Functions in People with Chronic Tetraplegia. *Biomedicines* **2023**, *11*, 34. [CrossRef] [PubMed]
24. Martin, R. Utility and Feasibility of Transcutaneous Spinal Cord Stimulation for Patients with Incomplete SCI in Therapeutic Settings: A Review of Topic. *Front. Rehabil. Sci.* **2021**, *2*, 724003. [CrossRef] [PubMed]
25. Alam, M.; Ling, Y.T.; Wong, A.Y.; Zhong, H.; Edgerton, V.R.; Zheng, Y.P. Reversing 21 years of chronic paralysis via non-invasive spinal cord neuromodulation: A case study. *Ann. Clin. Transl. Neurol.* **2020**, *7*, 829–838. [CrossRef]
26. Kraemer, W.J.; Ratamess, N.A. Fundamentals of resistance training: Progression and exercise prescription. *Med. Sci. Sports Exerc.* **2004**, *36*, 674–688. [CrossRef]
27. Peña Pino, I.; Hoover, C.; Venkatesh, S.; Ahmadi, A.; Sturtevant, D.; Patrick, N.; Freeman, D.; Parr, A.; Samadani, U.; Balser, D.; et al. Long-Term Spinal Cord Stimulation after Chronic Complete Spinal Cord Injury Enables Volitional Movement in the Absence of Stimulation. *Front. Syst. Neurosci.* **2020**, *14*, 35. [CrossRef]
28. Pêgo, A.P.; Kubinova, S.; Cizkova, D.; Vanicky, I.; Mar, F.M.; Sousa, M.M.; Sykova, E. Regenerative medicine for the treatment of spinal cord injury: More than just promises? *J. Cell. Mol. Med.* **2012**, *16*, 2564–2582. [CrossRef]
29. Turczyn, P.; Wojdasiewicz, P.; Poniatowski, Ł.A.; Purrahman, D.; Maślińska, M.; Żurek, G.; Romanowska-Próchnicka, K.; Żuk, B.; Kwiatkowska, B.; Piechowski-Jóźwiak, B.; et al. Omega-3 fatty acids in the treatment of spinal cord injury: Untapped potential for therapeutic intervention? *Mol. Biol. Rep.* **2022**, *49*, 10797–10809. [CrossRef]
30. Tefertiller, C.; Rozwod, M.; VandeGriend, E.; Bartelt, P.; Sevigny, M.; Smith, A.C. Transcutaneous Electrical Spinal Cord Stimulation to Promote Recovery in Chronic Spinal Cord Injury. *Front. Rehabil. Sci.* **2022**, *2*, 740307. [CrossRef]
31. Aout, T.; Begon, M.; Jegou, B.; Peyrot, N.; Caderby, T. Effects of Functional Electrical Stimulation on Gait Characteristics in Healthy Individuals: A Systematic Review. *Sensors* **2023**, *23*, 8684. [CrossRef]
32. Gerasimenko, Y.P.; Lu, D.C.; Modaber, M.; Zdunowski, S.; Gad, P.; Sayenko, D.G.; Morikawa, E.; Haakana, P.; Ferguson, A.R.; Roy, R.R.; et al. Noninvasive Reactivation of Motor Descending Control after Paralysis. *J. Neurotrauma* **2015**, *32*, 1968–1980. [CrossRef]

33. Samejima, S.; Caskey, C.D.; Inanici, F.; Shrivastav, S.R.; Brighton, L.N.; Pradarelli, J.; Martinez, V.; Steele, K.M.; Saigal, R.; Moritz, C.T. Multisite Transcutaneous Spinal Stimulation for Walking and Autonomic Recovery in Motor-Incomplete Tetraplegia: A Single-Subject Design. *Phys. Ther.* **2022**, *102*, pzab228. [CrossRef] [PubMed]
34. Dost, G.; Dulgeroglu, D.; Yildirim, A.; Ozgirgin, N. The effects of upper extremity progressive resistance and endurance exercises in patients with spinal cord injury. *J. Back Musculoskelet. Rehabilit.* **2014**, *27*, 419–426. [CrossRef] [PubMed]
35. Christiansen, L.; Larsen, M.N.; Madsen, M.J.; Grey, M.J.; Nielsen, J.B.; Lundbye-Jensen, J. Long-term motor skill training with individually adjusted progressive difficulty enhances learning and promotes corticospinal plasticity. *Sci. Rep.* **2020**, *10*, 15588. [CrossRef]
36. Singh, G.; Lucas, K.; Keller, A.; Martin, R.; Behrman, A.; Vissarionov, S.; Gerasimenko, Y.P. Transcutaneous Spinal Stimulation From Adults to Children: A Review. *Top. Spinal Cord Inj. Rehabil.* **2022**, *29*, 16–32. [CrossRef]
37. Powell, M.P.; Verma, N.; Sorensen, E.; Carranza, E.; Boos, A.; Fields, D.P.; Roy, S.; Ensel, S.; Barra, B.; Balzer, J.; et al. Epidural stimulation of the cervical spinal cord for post-stroke upper-limb paresis. *Nat. Med.* **2023**, *29*, 689–699. [CrossRef]
38. Tian, T.; Zhang, S.; Yang, M. Recent progress and challenges in the treatment of spinal cord injury. *Protein Cell* **2023**, *14*, 635–652. [CrossRef] [PubMed]
39. Hu, M.; Hong, L.; Liu, C.; Hong, S.; He, S.; Zhou, M.; Huang, G.; Chen, Q. Electrical stimulation enhances neuronal cell activity mediated by Schwann cell derived exosomes. *Sci. Rep.* **2019**, *9*, 4206. [CrossRef]
40. Flores, Á.; López-Santos, D.; García-Alías, G. When Spinal Neuromodulation Meets Sensorimotor Rehabilitation: Lessons Learned From Animal Models to Regain Manual Dexterity after a Spinal Cord Injury. *Front. Rehabil. Sci.* **2021**, *2*, 755963. [CrossRef]

Disclaimer/Publisher's Note: The statements, opinions and data contained in all publications are solely those of the individual author(s) and contributor(s) and not of MDPI and/or the editor(s). MDPI and/or the editor(s) disclaim responsibility for any injury to people or property resulting from any ideas, methods, instructions or products referred to in the content.

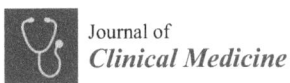

Systematic Review

The Impact of Machine Learning and Robot-Assisted Gait Training on Spinal Cord Injury: A Systematic Review and Meta-Analysis

Dewa Putu Wisnu Wardhana [1,*], Sri Maliawan [1], Tjokorda Gde Bagus Mahadewa [1], Rohadi Muhammad Rosyidi [2] and Sinta Wiranata [3]

1. Neurosurgery Division, Department of Surgery, Faculty of Medicine, Universitas Udayana, Prof. Dr. IGNG Ngoerah General Hospital, Denpasar 80113, Indonesia
2. Department of Neurosurgery, Medical Faculty, Mataram University, West Nusa Tenggara General Hospital, Mataram 84371, Indonesia
3. Faculty of Medicine, Universitas Udayana, Denpasar 80232, Indonesia
* Correspondence: wisnu_wardhana@unud.ac.id; Tel.: +62-8174732149

Abstract: Introduction: Spinal cord injury (SCI) is a significant and transforming event, with an estimated annual incidence of 40 cases per million individuals in North America. Considering the significance of accurate diagnosis and effective therapy in managing SCI, Machine Learning (ML) and Robot-Assisted Gait Training (RAGT) technologies hold promise for enhancing optimal practices and elevating the quality of care. This study aims to determine the impact of the ML and RAGT techniques employed on the outcome results of SCI. Methods: We reviewed four databases, including PubMed, Scopus, ScienceDirect, and the Cochrane Central Register of Controlled Trials (CENTRAL), until 20 August 2023. The keywords used in this study encompassed the following: a comprehensive search was executed on research exclusively published in the English language: machine learning, robotics, and spinal cord injury. Results: A comprehensive search was conducted across four databases, identifying 2367 articles following rigorous data filtering. The results of the odd ratio (OR) and confidence interval (CI) of 95% for the ASIA Impairment Scale, or AIS grade A, were 0.093 (0.011–0.754, $p = 0.026$), for AIS grade B, 0.875 (0.395–1.939, $p = 0.743$), for AIS grade C, 3.626 (1.556–8.449, $p = 0.003$), and for AIS grade D, 8.496 (1.394–51.768, $p = 0.020$). The robotic group exhibited a notable reduction in AS (95% CI = −0.239 to −0.045, $p = 0.004$) and MAS (95% CI = −3.657 to −1.066, $p \leq 0.001$) measures. This study also investigated spasticity and walking ability, which are significant. Conclusions: The ML approach exhibited enhanced precision in forecasting AIS result scores. Implementing RAGT has been shown to impact spasticity reduction and improve walking ability.

Keywords: spinal cord injury; machine learning; robot-assisted gait training

1. Introduction

Spinal cord injury (SCI) is a significant and transforming event, with an estimated annual incidence of 40 cases per million individuals in North America [1]. Following the occurrence of an injury, there are physiological repercussions that impact several body systems and are frequently accompanied by a substantial risk of mortality. Previous studies have reported inconsistent findings about the rates of in-hospital mortality, which have been shown to range from 3% to 13%. Similarly, the 1 year mortality rates after SCI have been estimated to range from 5% to 10% [2–5]. Numerous research studies have previously elucidated predictive features and algorithms for evaluating the probability of death after SCI. However, there is currently a shortage of prognostic instruments tailored specifically to the SCI patient cohort that may be conveniently employed in a clinical environment [2,5–8]. Apart from its utility in informing clinical decision-making and facilitating patient and family talks, a predictive tool may also serve as a valuable instrument in clinical research by accounting for the possible influence of distinct patient and injury variables on the mortality risk of study participants.

Considering the significance of accurate diagnosis and effective therapy in managing SCI, Machine Learning (ML) and Robot-Assisted Gait Training (RAGT) technologies hold promise for enhancing optimal practices and elevating the quality of care. The numerical value is provided by the user [9,10]. ML is often regarded as the most promising field within the domain of artificial intelligence (AI). It encompasses using algorithms to automatically generate predictions or outputs by analyzing the attributes of given inputs [11]. ML possesses inherent advantages in processing large datasets compared to traditional statistical approaches. They exhibit greater precision and reproducibility than conventional models and even skilled operators. ML can potentially uncover nuanced information that may not be perceptible to the human eye in specific image-related activities [11,12]. The user's text is too short to be rewritten academically. In the current era characterized by large-scale datasets, ML techniques can significantly enhance diagnostic accuracy and prognosis [13].

Clinicians consistently face challenges in rehabilitating patients to improve pain management, reduce stiffness, and increase walking capacity. The application of RAGT in rehabilitation has experienced increased prevalence due to its ability to transcend the constraints imposed by the extent of an individual's muscle paralysis. The provision of recurrent and functional task training by RAGT has been found to elicit increased activity in the sensorimotor cortex (specifically, S1 and S2) and the cerebellar areas [14,15]. The convergence of advancements in fundamental neuroscience and technology innovation has presented neurosurgery with distinctive prospects for utilizing ML and RAGT in research and clinical settings to enhance patient care [16].

Moreover, using customized or precision medicine in the context of patients with SCI seems beneficial in customizing expectations and treatment strategies, considering the intrinsic diversity observed within this group in terms of outcomes, functional prognosis, and the rehabilitation process [17–19]. This study comprehensively aims to examine the impact of ML on predicting AIS score outcomes and RAGT on rehabilitation outcomes. The focus was on research endeavors to enhance therapeutic advancements and develop predictive models.

2. Material and Methods

2.1. Search Strategy

The PRISMA [20] systematically reviewed four databases, including PubMed, Scopus, ScienceDirect, and the Cochrane Central Register of Controlled Trials (CENTRAL), until 20 August 2023. The MeSH phrases and keywords used in this study encompassed the following: a comprehensive search was executed on research exclusively published in the English language: machine learning, robotics, and spinal cord injury. The reference lists of the published works were examined to identify potential areas for further investigation. In instances where duplicate studies were identified, preference has been given to studies with larger sample sizes. Each study produced the subsequent findings: (1) the initial name and year of publication; (2) the nation and total sample; (3) type of study design; (4) level of injury; (5) ASIA Impairment Scale (AIS) grade; (6) intervention; and (7) outcome.

2.2. Data Selection

Three reviewers (D.P.W.W., S.M., and T.G.B.M.) independently performed the selection. The conflict among the first three reviewers was settled by the establishment of a consensus by the fourth and fifth reviewers. Exclusion of studies occurred in cases where essential outcome measures were absent or not assessed. The included papers should be: (1) a paper that investigated ML and RAGT; (2) research given information on ML and RAGT as well as outcome status; (3) studies that provide the computation data for the calculation of the total sample, mean, and standard deviation (SD); and (4) a full-text article. The protocol for this review was registered in PROSPERO, with the registration number CRD42023464103. The publication was subsequently developed according to PRISMA principles.

2.3. Data Extraction

The relevant data were extracted using a pre-established Google Sheets Excel Online form by two reviewers (D.P.W.W. and S.W.) who worked independently. Any discrepancies were identified and resolved through consensus with a senior reviewer (S.M.). When data was absent or doubts arose, we initiated electronic correspondence with the authors via email to acquire the necessary data.

2.4. Risk of Bias

Two authors (D.P.W.W. and S.M.) independently evaluated the bias quality of the chosen randomized controlled trials (RCTs) using the Cochrane risk of bias assessment methodology [20]. Two authors have used the Newcastle Ottawa Scale (NOS) [21] to evaluate the chosen articles' methodological quality independently. We divided the articles' overall quality into moderate (4–6) and high (7–9). Any potential conflicts were effectively resolved by open dialogue and the attainment of mutual agreement facilitated by the involvement of the third author (S.W.).

2.5. Statistical Analysis

RCTs and non-RCTs were categorized into separate groups and subjected to individual studies afterward. The treatment impact was analyzed using Comprehensive Meta-Analysis (CMA) version 3 through statistical analysis. The mean differences (MD), odds ratio (OR), and 95% CI were computed for outcome measures. We use a random effect model for the analysis. The application of a random effect model offers distinct advantages over a fixed effect model due to its ability to effectively capture the entirety of the population under study.

3. Results
3.1. Search Results and Study Characteristics

A comprehensive search was conducted across four databases, identifying 2367 articles following rigorous data filtering. A cumulative sum of 127 papers was deemed ineligible for inclusion in the study due to their failure to match the predetermined criteria for research inclusion in Figure 1. Ultimately, a total of 19 publications were selected for further research. The combined sample size of the papers included in this study was 1508 patients. The sample comprised 16 publications utilizing ML techniques and three articles using RAGT techniques. The articles were sourced from various nations, including the USA, Canada, Japan, Italy, Spain, Republic of Korea, and Switzerland.

The analysis incorporated both RCT and non-RCT study designs. The outcomes examined in the RAGT group encompassed measures such as the Ashworth Scale (AS), Modified Ashworth Scale (MAS), Visual Analog Scale (VAS), Lower Extremity Motor Score (LEMS), 6 Minute Walk Test (6MWT), 10 Meter Walk Test (10MWT), and Timed Up and Go Test (TUG). In the context of the ML group, an examination was conducted on the AIS grade result. The highest marks obtained from the collection of 13 articles are AIS C and D. The OR (95% CI) analysis was employed for the ML group. In contrast, the mean differences (MD) were utilized for the RAGT group. The features of the studies are presented in Tables 1 and 2.

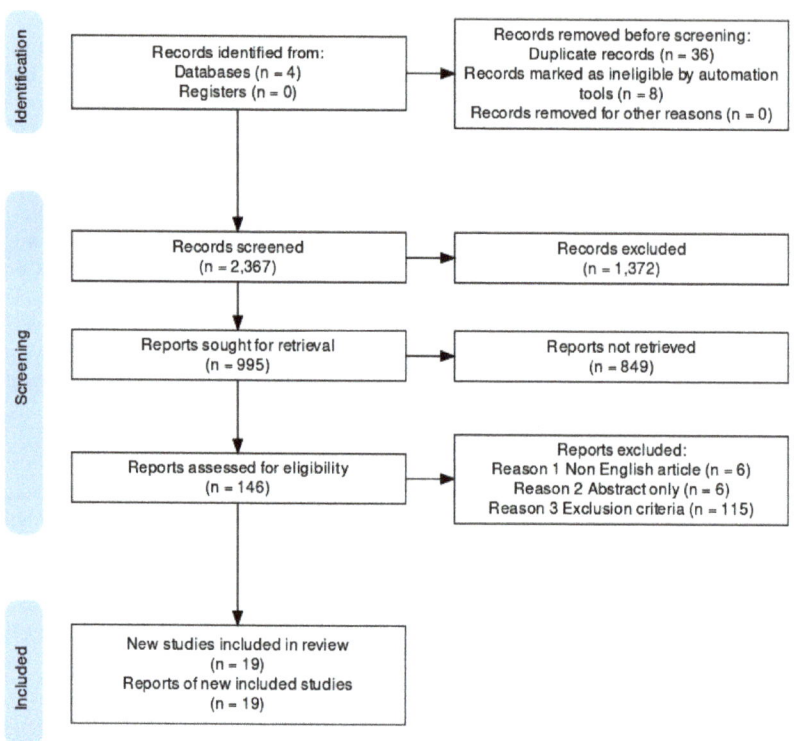

Figure 1. The flowchart depicts the process of selecting studies.

Table 1. RAGT concise overview of the chosen papers' key characteristics and bias risk.

Author, Year	Country	Total Sample (TS)	Study Design	Intervention	Outcome	Level of Injury	NOS
Hornby 2005 [22]	USA	30	RCT	The utilization of robotic assistance in BWSTT and therapist-assisted BWSTT. The intervention involved engaging in overground ambulation via a mobile suspension device for three 30 min weekly sessions over 8 weeks.	LEMS, 6MWT	AIS B, C, and D. The level of damage is located above the tenth thoracic vertebra (T10).	-
Wirz 2005 [23]	USA	20	Single group	The Lokomat (DGO) intervention consisted of an 8 week duration, with participants attending three to five sessions per week, each lasting 45 min.	AS, LEMS, 6MWT, 10MWT, and TUG	AIS C and D. The level of injury is at L1 or above.	7

Table 1. Cont.

Author, Year	Country	Total Sample (TS)	Study Design	Intervention	Outcome	Level of Injury	NOS
Field 2011 [24]	USA	64	RCT	The participants engaged in a training regimen for 12 weeks, with a frequency of 5 days per week. The training program encompassed four distinct modalities, namely treadmill-based training with manual help (TM), treadmill-based training with stimulation (TS), overground training with motivation (OG), and treadmill-based training with robotic assistance (LR).	LEMS	AIS C and D. The level of damage is located at or above the tenth thoracic vertebra (T10).	-
Alcobendas 2012 [25]	Spain	75	RCT	The study consisted of a total of 40 sessions conducted over 8 weeks. Each session lasted for approximately 1 h and involved a Lokomat group intervention. Specifically, participants spent 30 min utilizing the Lokomat device within each session, followed by an additional 30 min of normal physical treatment. The overground group implemented a standardized biological treatment protocol for one hour.	VAS, LEMS, 6MWT, and 10MWT	AIS C and D. The range of injuries observed in the individual spans from the second cervical vertebra (C2) to the twelfth thoracic vertebra (T12).	-
Aach 2014 [26]	Germany	8	Pre-post experimental design	HAL had been used for 90 days, with a frequency of five weekly sessions.	LEMS, 6MWT, 10MWT, and TUG	ASIA A. Degree of damage: T8 to L2	7
del-Ama 2014 [27]	Switzerland	3	Pilot study	The Kinesis system was implemented during the first week, whereas no intervention was delivered the following week.	AS, VAS, 6MWT, and 10MWT	AIS A and D. Injuries impact the spinal levels encompassing L1 and L2.	8
Labruyère 2014 [28]	Switzerland	9	RCT	The first group underwent 16 sessions of RAGT using the Lokomat device, followed by an additional 16 strength training sessions. Group 2 received the intervention in reverse order.	VAS, LEMS, and 10MWT	AIS C and D. The extent of the injury ranges from the fourth cervical vertebra (C4) to the eleventh thoracic vertebra (T11).	-
Niu 2014 [29]	USA	40	RCT	The experimental group underwent twelve 1 h Lokomat training sessions over one month, whereas the control group did not receive any interventions.	TUG	AIS B, C, and D. The level of damage is located above the tenth thoracic vertebra (T10).	-

Table 1. Cont.

Author, Year	Country	Total Sample (TS)	Study Design	Intervention	Outcome	Level of Injury	NOS
Shin 2014 [30]	South Korea	53	RCT	In four weeks, the RAGT group received three 40 min sessions per week of RAGT in addition to regular physiotherapy. The conventional group received physiotherapy twice daily, five days per week.	LEMS	AIS D. The level of injury is classified as upper motor neuron (UMN) involvement.	-
Varoqui 2014 [31]	USA	30	RCT	The Lokomat group participated in three weekly sessions for four weeks, each lasting one hour. The control group, on the other hand, did not receive any intervention.	6MWT, 10MWT, TUG	AIS C and D. The level of damage is located above the tenth thoracic vertebra (T10).	-
Duffell 2015 [32]	USA	56	RCT	The study involved allocating participants with an incomplete SCI into three groups: a control group receiving no intervention, a group receiving Lokomat intervention, and a group receiving tizanidine intervention.	TUG	AIS C and D The level of damage is located above the tenth thoracic vertebra (T10).	-
Lam 2015 [33]	Canada	15	RCT	The Lokomat-assisted BWSTT intervention was conducted for 45 min, three times a week, for three months.	6MWT, 10MWT	AIS C and D. Exclusion criteria encompassed individuals with lower motoneuron damage or lesion levels than T11.	-
Stampacchia 2016 [34]	Italy	21	Single group	The robotic exoskeleton (Ekso GT) exercise lasted approximately 40 min.	MAS, VAS	AIS A, B, and D. The observed lesions were located at the low cervical level (C7), dorsal level, and high lumbar level (L1–L2).	7
Mazzoleni 2017 [35]	Italy	7	Single group	The study consisted of 20 sessions, with a frequency of three sessions per week. The first set of sessions utilized a FES cycling system called Pegaso. It was followed by another group of 20 sessions, again with a frequency of three sessions per week, where participants used an overground robotic exoskeleton called the Ekso GT.	MAS, VAS, 6MWT, 10MWT, and TUG	AIS A. Injury severity: T4–T12	7

Table 1. Cont.

Author, Year	Country	Total Sample (TS)	Study Design	Intervention	Outcome	Level of Injury	NOS
Watanabe 2019 [36]	Japan	2	Case report	HAL has been used 3–4 times weekly for eight sessions. It is performed with regular physical therapy, each lasting approximately 20–30 min.	MAS, LEMS	AIS C and D Injury severity: T8–T10, L1	7
Wirz 2017 [37]	USA	21	RCT	The intervention group received a training duration of 50 min per session, while the control group had a training duration of 25 min per session using the Lokomat device. Both groups underwent training sessions 3–5 days per week for a total period of 8 weeks.	10MWT	AIS B and C. C4 to T12 are affected.	-

AS: Ashworth Scale; MAS: Modified Ashworth Scale; VAS: Visual Analog Scale; 6MWT: 6 Minute Walk Test; 10MWT: 10 Meter Walking Test; LEMS: Lower Extremity Motor Score; TUG: Timed Up And Go Test; BWSTT: Body Weight-Supported Treadmill Training; HAL: Hybrid Assistive Limb; FES: Functional Electrical Stimulation; AIS: ASIA Impairment Scale; SCI: Spinal Cord Injury; NOS: Newcastle Ottawa Scale.

3.2. Bias Assessment

All studies considered in the analysis demonstrate a minimal likelihood of selection bias. The existence of a wide range of rehabilitation procedures in numerous research studies has led to a significant occurrence of performance and detection bias. All research investigations demonstrate a low-risk level of attrition and reporting bias. Several studies exhibit a lack of clarity concerning potential biases, including issues related to loss of follow-up in Figure 2, Tables 1 and 2.

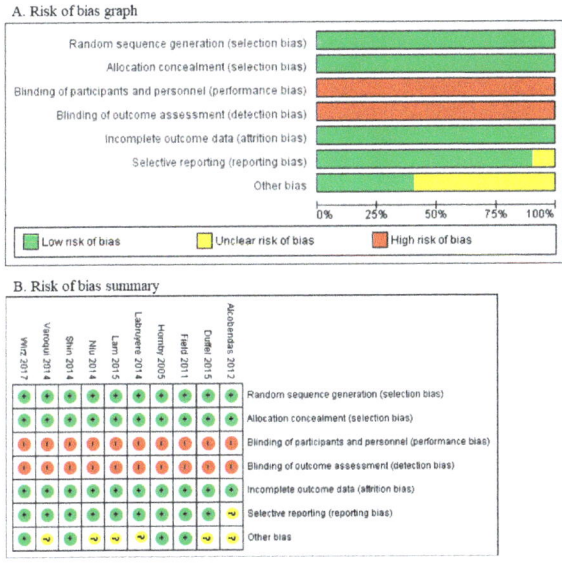

Figure 2. The risk of bias include the study are Alcobendas et al., 2012 [25]; Duffel et al., 2015 [32]; Field et al., 2011 [24]; Hornby et al., 2005 [22]; Labruyère et al., 2014 [28]; Lam et al., 2015 [33]; Niu et al., 2014 [29]; Shin et al., 2014 [30]; Varoqui et al., 2014 [31]; Wirz et al., 2017 [37].

3.3. Analysis of the ML Group

The analysis of all AIS grades A, B, C, and D included three RCT articles that fulfilled the inclusion criteria. We gathered data on the ability of ML to forecast outcomes based on the AIS score upon the patient's initial hospital admission. We categorized these results into two groups: unimproved and improved in the AIS score. According to the findings of a meta-analysis, predicting using ML in SCI patients with AIS grade A does not improve their condition after re-evaluation following therapy. It may happen due to the presence of a complete injury. The results of the OR CI 95% for AIS grade A were 0.093 (0.011–0.754, $p = 0.026$).

Meanwhile, in AIS B, several patients demonstrated progress in the forest plot, but this outcome is because there is no significant difference of 0.875 (0.395–1.939, $p = 0.743$). Considerable improvement in AIS grade C was 3.626 (1.556–8.449, $p = 0.003$), and AIS grade D was 8.496 (1.394–51.768, $p = 0.020$). The final result is shown in Figures 3–6.

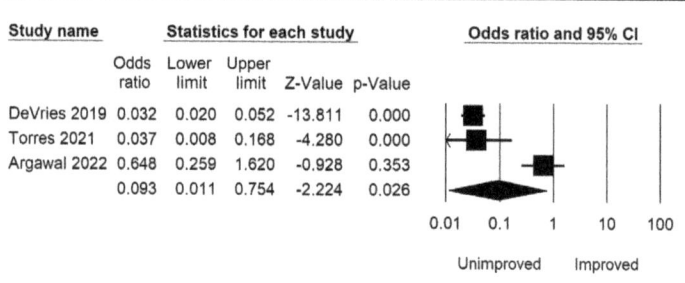

Figure 3. Forest plot of AIS grade A using OR ratio analysis between unimproved and improved prediction groups. The square box represents the point estimate for the respective study, while the horizontal line is the 95% CI. The diamonds represent pooled results. DeVries et al., 2009 [38]; Torres et al., 2021 [39]; Agarwal et al., 2022 [40].

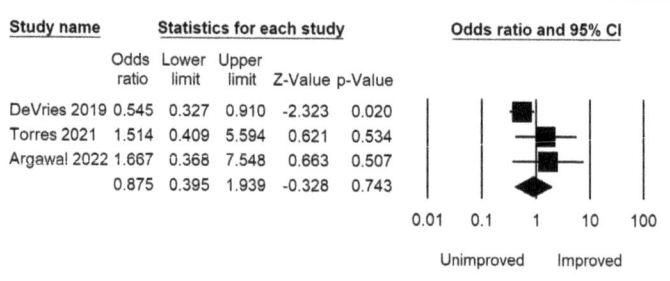

Figure 4. Forest plot of AIS grade B using OR ratio analysis between unimproved and improved prediction groups. The square box represents the point estimate for the respective study, while the horizontal line is the 95% CI. The diamonds represent pooled results. DeVries et al., 2009 [38]; Torres et al., 2021 [39]; Agarwal et al., 2022 [40].

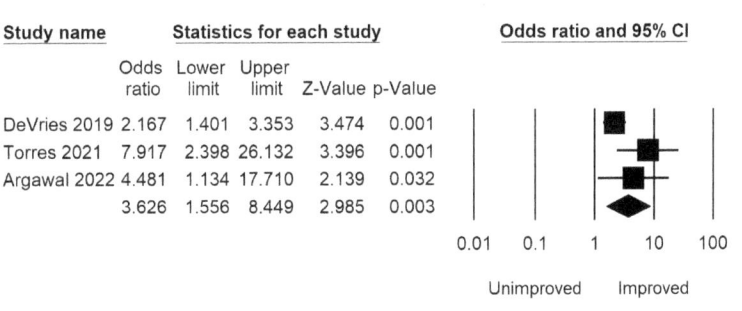

Figure 5. Forest plot of AIS grade C using OR ratio analysis between unimproved and improved prediction groups. The square box represents the point estimate for the respective study, while the horizontal line is the 95% CI. The diamonds represent pooled results. DeVries et al., 2009 [38]; Torres et al., 2021 [39]; Agarwal et al., 2022 [40].

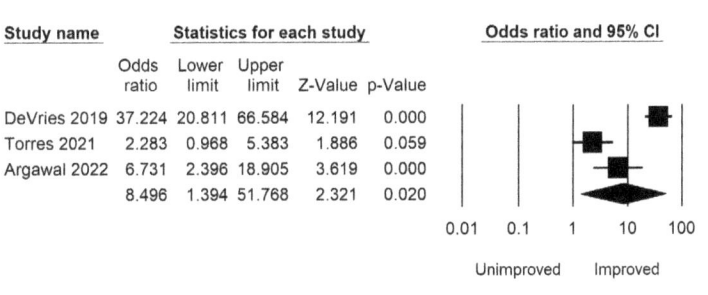

Figure 6. Forest plot of AIS grade D using OR ratio analysis between unimproved and improved prediction groups. The square box represents the point estimate for the respective study, while the horizontal line is the 95% CI. The diamonds represent pooled results. DeVries et al., 2009 [38]; Torres et al., 2021 [39]; Agarwal et al., 2022 [40].

3.4. Analysis of the RAGT Group

Four RCTs [23,28,30,32] were conducted to evaluate the effects of interventions on spasticity. In the conducted investigations, all participants' spasticity levels were categorized as mild, as indicated by a MAS score ranging from 0 to 2. Furthermore, it was noted that there were no significant alterations in spasticity levels following the implementation of RAGT. The robotic group exhibited a notable reduction in AS (95% CI = −0.239 to −0.045, $p = 0.004$) and MAS (95% CI = −3.657 to −1.066, $p \leq 0.001$) measures. The pooled MD using MAS and AS was −2.149 and −0.142, respectively (Figures 7 and 8).

We also analyzed the pain parameter using the VAS variable. The findings from the analysis of the primary outcomes of pain following RAGT are depicted in Figure 9, consisting of two RCTs [28,32] and three non-RCTs [22,29,37]. Despite the observed trend indicating a potential reduction in pain in the robotic group, there was no statistically significant difference between the robotic and control groups. This lack of significance was consistent in the analysis ($p = 0.243$). The pooled MD was −1.418. The studies included in the research reported various pain levels, varying from mild to moderate.

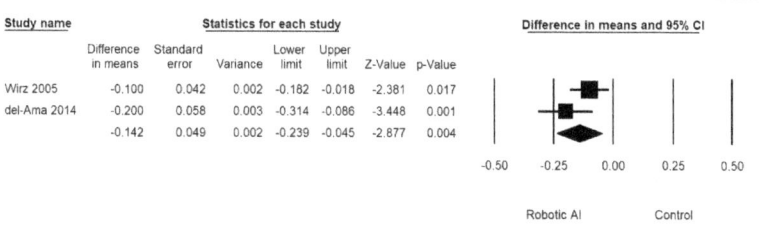

Figure 7. Forest plot of AS using standardized mean difference analysis between robotic and control groups. The square box represents the mean differences for the respective study, while the horizontal line is the 95% CI. The diamonds represent pooled results. Wirz et al., 2005 [23]; del-Ama et al., 2014 [27].

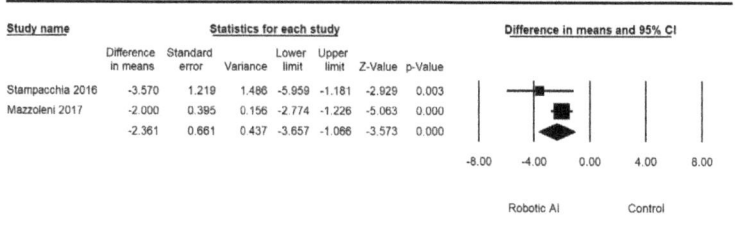

Figure 8. Forest plot of MAS using standardized mean difference analysis between robotic and control groups. The square box represents the mean differences for the respective study, while the horizontal line is the 95% CI. The diamonds represent pooled results. Stampacchia et al., 2016 [34]; Mazzoleni et al., 2017 [35].

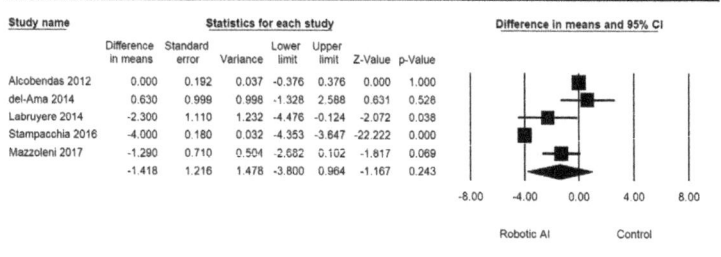

Figure 9. Forest plot of VAS using standardized mean difference analysis between robotic and control groups. The square box represents the mean differences for the respective study, while the horizontal line is the 95% CI. The diamonds represent pooled results. Alcobendas et al., 2012 [25]; del-Ama et al., 2014 [27]; Labruyère et al., 2014 [28]; Stampacchia et al., 2016 [34]; Mazzoleni et al., 2017 [35].

Table 2. ML concise overview of the chosen papers' key characteristics and bias risk.

Author, Year	Country	Total Sample (TS)	Study Design	Intervention	Outcome	AIS Grade	NOS
DeVries 2019 [38]	Canada	862	Retrospective	The comparison of unsupervised MLA and LR, utilizing comprehensive neurological data for total admission, did not reveal any clinically significant disparities in functional prediction compared to previous models.	The F1-score has been demonstrated to possess greater reliability in evaluating algorithms than the area under the operating curve.	AIS A, B, C, and D	8
Torres 2021 [39]	USA	118	Retrospective	A similar network has been developed among patients to predict neurological recovery following spinal cord damage, focusing on MAP recorded before surgery.	The findings from the network analysis indicate that deviations from the optimal MAP range, either in the form of hypotension or hypertension, during surgical procedures are correlated with a reduced probability of achieving neurological recovery.	AIS A, B, C, D, and E	8
Agarwal 2022 [40]	USA	74	Retrospective	This study uses a deep-tree-based machine learning approach to evaluate the impact of intraoperative MAP and vasopressor administration on enhancing neurological outcomes in individuals with acute spinal cord injury.	An association between a MAP ranging from 80 to 96 mmHg and enhanced neurological function has been observed. Conversely, 93 min or more spent outside the MAP range of 76 to 104 mmHg had been associated with a worse outcome.	AIS A, B, C, D, and E	7

MLA: Machine Learning Algorithms; LR: Logistic Regression; MAP: Mean Arterial Pressure; NOS: Newcastle Ottawa Scale.

This study investigated walking ability by combining the LEMS, 6MWT, 10MWT, and TUG group analyses. In the LEMS analysis, we found five RCTs [22,24,25,28,29] and three non-RCTs [23,26,37] with statistically significant beneficial effects in favor of the robotic group (95% [CI] = 0.515 to 2.995, $p \leq 0.05$). The mean difference is 1.755, as depicted in Figure 10. The 6MWT is a commonly used assessment tool in four RCTs [22,25,30,32], and four non-RCTs [23,26,27,34] were conducted to evaluate the 6MWT. Irrespective of the type of study design, there was a significant increase in walking distance in the group that received robotic assistance. The CI is 95% (21.665–69.884, $p \leq 0.001$), with MD 45.774, as shown in Figure 11. The 10MWT comprises five RCTs [25,28,30,32,36] and five non-RCTs [23,26,27,34,37]. The 10MWT demonstrated a substantial improvement in the robotic group, as indicated by CI 95% 0.015–0.117, $p = 0.012$, with MD 0.066, as shown in Figure 12. The TUG study comprised a total of three RCTs [28,30,31]. The findings indicated a noteworthy enhancement in favor of the robotic group, with a CI of 95% −21.742 to 5.225,

$p = 0.230$. The MD obtained by pooling the data using a random effects model was -8.258, as shown in Figure 13.

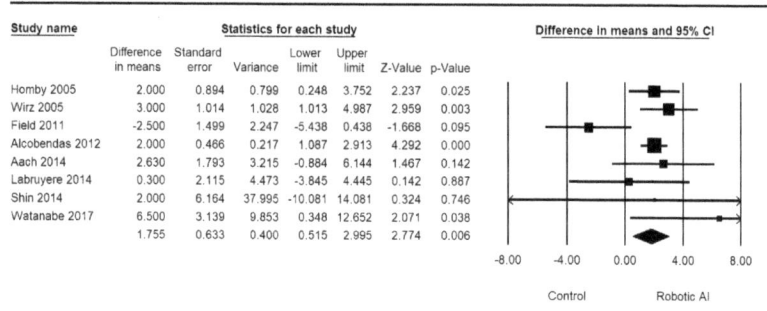

Figure 10. Forest plot of LEMS using standardized mean difference analysis between robotic and control groups. The square box represents the mean differences for the respective study, while the horizontal line is the 95% CI. The diamonds represent pooled results. Hornby et al., 2005 [22]; Wirz et al., 2005 [23]; Field et al., 2011 [24]; Alcobendas et al., 2012 [25]; Aach et al., 2014 [26]; Labruyère et al., 2014 [28]; Shin et al., 2014 [30]; Watanabe et al., 2019 [36].

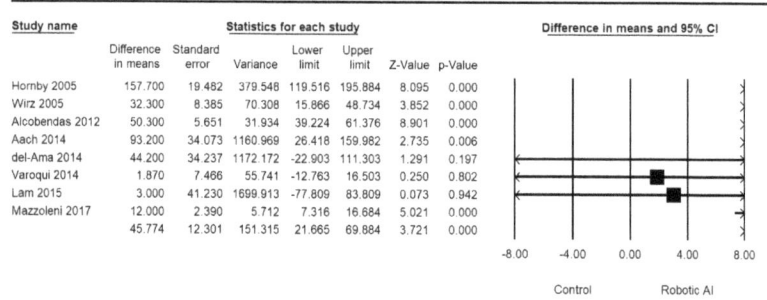

Figure 11. Forest plot of 6MWT using standardized mean difference analysis between robotic and control groups. The square box represents the mean differences for the respective study, while the horizontal line is the 95% CI. The diamonds represent pooled results. Hornby et al., 2005 [22]; Wirz et al., 2005 [23]; Alcobendas et al., 2012 [25]; Aach et al., 2014 [26]; del-Ama et al., 2014 [27]; Varoqui et al., 2014 [31]; Lam et al., 2015 [33]; Mazzoleni et al., 2017 [35].

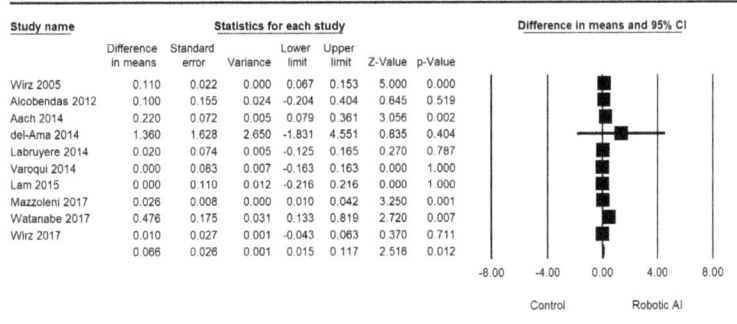

Figure 12. Forest plot of 10MWT using standardized mean difference analysis between robotic and control groups. The square box represents the mean differences for the respective study, while the horizontal line is the 95% CI. The diamonds represent pooled results. Wirz et al., 2005 [23]; Alcobendas et al., 2012 [25]; Aach et al., 2014 [26]; del-Ama et al., 2014 [27]; Labruyère et al., 2014 [28]; Varoqui et al., 2014 [31]; Lam et al., 2015 [33]; Mazzoleni et al., 2017 [35]; Watanabe et al., 2019 [36]; Wirz et al., 2017 [37].

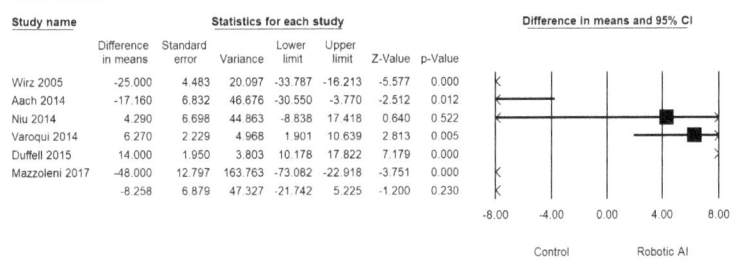

Figure 13. Forest plot of TUG using standardized mean difference analysis between robotic and control groups. The square box represents the mean differences for the respective study, while the horizontal line is the 95% CI. The diamonds represent pooled results. Wirz et al., 2005 [23]; Aach et al., 2014 [26]; Niu et al., 2014 [29]; Varoqui et al., 2014 [31]; Duffel et al., 2015 [32]; Mazzoleni et al., 2017 [35].

4. Discussion

The findings demonstrated encouraging outcomes in forecasting the improvement of AIS. Clinicians have used the AIS to categorize SCI and assess the extent of recovery. It may involve documenting enhancements, such as an improvement in AIS grade or deteriorations [41]. Within the confines of a conventional clinical environment, the primary determinants recognized for the prognostication of SCI recovery encompass patient age, patient gender, duration of hospitalization, manner of hospital release, SCI classification, procedural timing, nature of procedure, and presence of comorbidities. The prognosis of SCI is typically assessed using bedside evaluation and MRI or through classic clinical analysis, such as the calculation of odds ratios [42]. Hence, it is possible to identify the factors that can predict the recovery of SCI by incorporating the initial AIS scores into ML algorithms. This framework leverages big data and precision medicine, serving as a valuable tool for clinicians to enhance the overall prognosis of SCI patients. The current ML study [43] demonstrates a higher test accuracy of 73.6% than the MRI accuracy of 71.4%. A few studies [43–47] collectively utilize a patient sample size that is one to two times larger and incorporates a comprehensive evaluation of feature importance. Furthermore, even considering all AIS grades and employing a far less complex model that can be readily implemented, the outcomes are generally similar or superior.

The reduction of spasticity can be attributed to various theoretical frameworks. The RAGT technique elicits rhythmic movements in the lower limbs and offers sensory input. Prior research has indicated that rhythmic passive exercise has the potential to cause the reorganization of spinal circuitry and reduce stiffness in individuals with SCI [12]. The potential impact of repetitive elements within a therapy program on the enhancement of spasticity and locomotor function through the stimulation of spinal locomotor centers has been suggested [48]. Repetitive functional task training, sometimes called RAGT, represents a form of intervention that involves repeating available tasks. The mechanisms above could explain the observed reduction in spasticity resulting from RAGT [48]. As previously mentioned, despite decreasing spasticity, RAGT improves the detection of rhythmic muscle activations.

Furthermore, it is worth considering the significance of weight bearing as a contributing component. RAGT offers assistance that enables individuals to apply load to their lower extremities while engaging in training activities. The application of weight bearing on the lower limbs and the subsequent increase in muscle activation can positively impact the recovery of lower extremity motor function in individuals with LEMS. Furthermore, the findings of this meta-analysis indicate that the 6MWT can enhance endurance levels without imposing the strain associated with deliberate muscular contractions [34]. As evidenced by the findings of the LEMS improvement results, enhanced lower extremity strength probably contributes to an augmentation in walking speed, as observed in the 10MWT variable [49].

5. Limitations

One constraint of the analysis is the methodology employed for data collection in non-RCTs, particularly in the context of informing predictive modeling. It is generally acknowledged that prospective approaches are more suitable for developing accurate predictive models. The existing body of literature on this subject is minimal and exhibits variability in both topic and research design, hindering the possibility of conducting a meta-analysis or facilitating direct comparisons. Undoubtedly, the degree of injury has been demonstrated as a fundamental determinant in predicting the long-term functional result. Ultimately, models must undergo external validation and be meticulously implemented before their utilization and dependence in clinical settings. Regrettably, the identified articles lacked specific descriptions of the symptoms exhibited by patients. Furthermore, most of the research evaluated treatment efficacy solely during a predetermined timeframe, impeding our ability to examine this aspect comprehensively. The limitations of our study include the potential for future research to explore and offer additional insights into the symptoms and follow-up duration.

6. Conclusions

The ML approach exhibited enhanced precision in forecasting AIS result scores. The implementation of RAGT has been shown to positively impact the reduction of spasticity and the improvement of walking ability. The implementation of RAGT has been proven to be beneficial in the normalization of muscle tone and enhancement of lower extremity function. The presence of variability among individuals with SCI presents a distinct and advantageous prospect for AI to facilitate desired results and evaluate risk within this specific group of patients.

Author Contributions: Participated in formulation and development of the study's conceptualization and design, D.P.W.W., S.M. and S.W.; actively involved in the process of performing searches within databases and then extracting material that was deemed relevant and of interest, T.G.B.M. and R.M.R.; participated in the process of analyzing and interpreting data, D.P.W.W. and S.W.; manuscript—draft, S.M., S.W. and T.G.B.M. The article has been critically reviewed by R.M.R. and D.P.W.W. All authors have read and agreed to the published version of the manuscript.

Funding: This research received no external funding.

Institutional Review Board Statement: Not applicable.

Informed Consent Statement: Not applicable.

Data Availability Statement: This study did not include generating or analyzing new data. Sharing data is neither relevant nor appropriate to this article's subject matter.

Conflicts of Interest: The authors declare no conflict of interest.

References

1. Lee, B.B.; Cripps, R.A.; Fitzharris, M.; Wing, P.C. The Global Map for Traumatic Spinal Cord Injury Epidemiology: Update 2011, Global Incidence Rate. *Spinal Cord* **2014**, *52*, 110–116. [CrossRef] [PubMed]
2. Fallah, N.; Noonan, V.K.; Waheed, Z.; Rivers, C.S.; Plashkes, T.; Bedi, M.; Etminan, M.; Thorogood, N.P.; Ailon, T.; Chan, E.; et al. Development of a Machine Learning Algorithm for Predicting In-Hospital and 1-Year Mortality after Traumatic Spinal Cord Injury. *Spine J.* **2022**, *22*, 329–336. [CrossRef]
3. Varma, A.; Hill, E.G.; Nicholas, J.; Selassie, A. Predictors of Early Mortality after Traumatic Spinal Cord Injury: A Population-Based Study. *Spine* **2010**, *35*, 778–783. [CrossRef] [PubMed]
4. Chamberlain, J.D.; Meier, S.; Mader, L.; von Groote, P.M.; Brinkhof, M.W.G. Mortality and Longevity after a Spinal Cord Injury: Systematic Review and Meta-Analysis. *Neuroepidemiology* **2015**, *44*, 182–198. [CrossRef]
5. Cao, Y.; Krause, J.S.; DiPiro, N. Risk Factors for Mortality after Spinal Cord Injury in the USA. *Spinal Cord* **2013**, *51*, 413–418. [CrossRef]
6. Shibahashi, K.; Nishida, M.; Okura, Y.; Hamabe, Y. Epidemiological State, Predictors of Early Mortality, and Predictive Models for Traumatic Spinal Cord Injury: A Multicenter Nationwide Cohort Study. *Spine* **2019**, *44*, 479–487. [CrossRef]
7. Azarhomayoun, A.; Aghasi, M.; Mousavi, N.; Shokraneh, F.; Vaccaro, A.R.; Haj Mirzaian, A.; Derakhshan, P.; Rahimi-Movaghar, V. Mortality Rate and Predicting Factors of Traumatic Thoracolumbar Spinal Cord Injury; A Systematic Review and Meta-Analysis. *Bull. Emerg. Trauma* **2018**, *6*, 181–194. [CrossRef] [PubMed]
8. Bank, M.; Gibbs, K.; Sison, C.; Kutub, N.; Papatheodorou, A.; Lee, S.; Stein, A.; Bloom, O. Age and Other Risk Factors Influencing Long-Term Mortality in Patients With Traumatic Cervical Spine Fracture. *Geriatr. Orthop. Surg. Rehabil.* **2018**, *9*, 2151459318770882. [CrossRef]
9. Raju, B.; Jumah, F.; Ashraf, O.; Narayan, V.; Gupta, G.; Sun, H.; Hilden, P.; Nanda, A. Big Data, Machine Learning, and Artificial Intelligence: A Field Guide for Neurosurgeons. *J. Neurosurg.* **2020**, *135*, 373–383. [CrossRef] [PubMed]
10. Mesbah, S.; Ball, T.; Angeli, C.; Rejc, E.; Dietz, N.; Ugiliweneza, B.; Harkema, S.; Boakye, M. Predictors of Volitional Motor Recovery with Epidural Stimulation in Individuals with Chronic Spinal Cord Injury. *Brain A J. Neurol.* **2021**, *144*, 420–433. [CrossRef]
11. Jordan, M.I.; Mitchell, T.M. Machine Learning: Trends, Perspectives, and Prospects. *Science* **2015**, *349*, 255–260. [CrossRef]
12. Chang, M.; Canseco, J.A.; Nicholson, K.J.; Patel, N.; Vaccaro, A.R. The Role of Machine Learning in Spine Surgery: The Future Is Now. *Front. Surg.* **2020**, *7*, 54. [CrossRef]
13. Galbusera, F.; Casaroli, G.; Bassani, T. Artificial Intelligence and Machine Learning in Spine Research. *JOR Spine* **2019**, *2*, e1044. [CrossRef]
14. Sliwinski, C.; Nees, T.A.; Puttagunta, R.; Weidner, N.; Blesch, A. Sensorimotor Activity Partially Ameliorates Pain and Reduces Nociceptive Fiber Density in the Chronically Injured Spinal Cord. *J. Neurotrauma* **2018**, *35*, 2222–2238. [CrossRef]
15. Winchester, P.; McColl, R.; Querry, R.; Foreman, N.; Mosby, J.; Tansey, K.; Williamson, J. Changes in Supraspinal Activation Patterns Following Robotic Locomotor Therapy in Motor-Incomplete Spinal Cord Injury. *Neurorehabil. Neural Repair* **2005**, *19*, 313–324. [CrossRef]
16. Obermeyer, Z.; Emanuel, E.J. Predicting the Future—Big Data, Machine Learning, and Clinical Medicine. *N. Engl. J. Med.* **2016**, *375*, 1216–1219. [CrossRef] [PubMed]
17. Khan, O.; Badhiwala, J.H.; Grasso, G.; Fehlings, M.G. Use of Machine Learning and Artificial Intelligence to Drive Personalized Medicine Approaches for Spine Care. *World Neurosurg.* **2020**, *140*, 512–518. [CrossRef] [PubMed]
18. Dietz, N.; Wagers, S.; Harkema, S.J.; D'Amico, J.M. Intrathecal and Oral Baclofen Use in Adults With Spinal Cord Injury: A Systematic Review of Efficacy in Spasticity Reduction, Functional Changes, Dosing, and Adverse Events. *Arch. Phys. Med. Rehabil.* **2023**, *104*, 119–131. [CrossRef]

19. Ter Wengel, P.V.; Post, M.W.M.; Martin, E.; Stolwijk-Swuste, J.; Hosman, A.J.F.; Sadiqi, S.; Vandertop, W.P.; Öner, F.C. Neurological Recovery after Traumatic Spinal Cord Injury: What Is Meaningful? A Patients' and Physicians' Perspective. *Spinal Cord* **2020**, *58*, 865–872. [CrossRef] [PubMed]
20. Higgins, J.P.T.; Altman, D.G. Assessing Risk of Bias in Included Studies. In *Cochrane Handbook for Systematic Reviews of Interventions*; Wiley: Hoboken, NJ, USA, 2008; pp. 187–241. ISBN 9780470712184.
21. Stang, A. Critical Evaluation of the Newcastle-Ottawa Scale for the Assessment of the Quality of Nonrandomized Studies in Meta-Analyses. *Eur. J. Epidemiol.* **2010**, *25*, 603–605. [CrossRef] [PubMed]
22. Hornby, T.G.; Campbell, D.D.; Zemon, D.H.; Kahn, J.H. Clinical and Quantitative Evaluation of Robotic-Assisted Treadmill Walking to Retrain Ambulation after Spinal Cord Injury. *Top. Spinal Cord Inj. Rehabil.* **2005**, *11*, 1–17. [CrossRef]
23. Wirz, M.; Zemon, D.H.; Rupp, R.; Scheel, A.; Colombo, G.; Dietz, V.; Hornby, T.G. Effectiveness of Automated Locomotor Training in Patients with Chronic Incomplete Spinal Cord Injury: A Multicenter Trial. *Arch. Phys. Med. Rehabil.* **2005**, *86*, 672–680. [CrossRef] [PubMed]
24. Field-Fote, E.C.; Roach, K.E. Influence of a Locomotor Training Approach on Walking Speed and Distance in People with Chronic Spinal Cord Injury: A Randomized Clinical Trial. *Phys. Ther.* **2011**, *91*, 48–60. [CrossRef] [PubMed]
25. Alcobendas-Maestro, M.; Esclarín-Ruz, A.; Casado-López, R.M.; Muñoz-González, A.; Pérez-Mateos, G.; González-Valdizán, E.; Martín, J.L.R. Lokomat Robotic-Assisted Versus Overground Training Within 3 to 6 Months of Incomplete Spinal Cord Lesion: Randomized Controlled Trial. *Neurorehabilit. Neural Repair* **2012**, *26*, 1058–1063. [CrossRef]
26. Aach, M.; Cruciger, O.; Sczesny-Kaiser, M.; Höffken, O.; Meindl, R.C.; Tegenthoff, M.; Schwenkreis, P.; Sankai, Y.; Schildhauer, T.A. Voluntary Driven Exoskeleton as a New Tool for Rehabilitation in Chronic Spinal Cord Injury: A Pilot Study. *Spine J. Off. J. North Am. Spine Soc.* **2014**, *14*, 2847–2853. [CrossRef]
27. Del-Ama, A.J.; Gil-Agudo, Á.; Pons, J.L.; Moreno, J.C. Hybrid Gait Training with an Overground Robot for People with Incomplete Spinal Cord Injury: A Pilot Study. *Front. Hum. Neurosci.* **2014**, *8*, 298. [CrossRef] [PubMed]
28. Labruyère, R.; Van Hedel, H.J.A. Strength Training versus Robot-Assisted Gait Training after Incomplete Spinal Cord Injury: A Randomized Pilot Study in Patients Depending on Walking Assistance. *J. NeuroEngineering Rehabil.* **2014**, *11*, 4. [CrossRef]
29. Niu, X.; Varoqui, D.; Kindig, M.; Mirbagheri, M.M. Prediction of Gait Recovery in Spinal Cord Injured Individuals Trained with Robotic Gait Orthosis. *J. Neuroeng. Rehabil.* **2014**, *11*, 42. [CrossRef]
30. Shin, J.C.; Kim, J.Y.; Park, H.K.; Kim, N.Y. Effect of Robotic-Assisted Gait Training in Patients with Incomplete Spinal Cord Injury. *Ann. Rehabil. Med.* **2014**, *38*, 719–725. [CrossRef]
31. Varoqui, D.; Niu, X.; Mirbagheri, M.M. Ankle Voluntary Movement Enhancement Following Robotic-Assisted Locomotor Training in Spinal Cord Injury. *J. Neuroeng. Rehabil.* **2014**, *11*, 46. [CrossRef]
32. Duffell, L.D.; Brown, G.L.; Mirbagheri, M.M. Interventions to Reduce Spasticity and Improve Function in People With Chronic Incomplete Spinal Cord Injury: Distinctions Revealed by Different Analytical Methods. *Neurorehabilit. Neural Repair* **2015**, *29*, 566–576. [CrossRef]
33. Lam, T.; Pauhl, K.; Ferguson, A.; Malik, R.N.; Krassioukov, A.; Eng, J.J. Training with Robot-Applied Resistance in People with Motor-Incomplete Spinal Cord Injury: Pilot Study. *J. Rehabil. Res. Dev.* **2015**, *52*, 113–129. [CrossRef]
34. Stampacchia, G.; Rustici, A.; Bigazzi, S.; Gerini, A.; Tombini, T.; Mazzoleni, S. Walking with a Powered Robotic Exoskeleton: Subjective Experience, Spasticity and Pain in Spinal Cord Injured Persons. *NeuroRehabilitation* **2016**, *39*, 277–283. [CrossRef] [PubMed]
35. Mazzoleni, S.; Battini, E.; Rustici, A.; Stampacchia, G. An Integrated Gait Rehabilitation Training Based on Functional Electrical Stimulation Cycling and Overground Robotic Exoskeleton in Complete Spinal Cord Injury Patients: Preliminary Results. In Proceedings of the 2017 International Conference on Rehabilitation Robotics (ICORR), London, UK, 17–20 July 2017; IEEE: Piscataway, NJ, USA; pp. 289–293. [CrossRef]
36. Watanabe, H.; Marushima, A.; Kawamoto, H.; Kadone, H.; Ueno, T.; Shimizu, Y.; Endo, A.; Hada, Y.; Saotome, K.; Abe, T.; et al. Intensive Gait Treatment Using a Robot Suit Hybrid Assistive Limb in Acute Spinal Cord Infarction: Report of Two Cases. *J. Spinal Cord Med.* **2019**, *42*, 395–401. [CrossRef]
37. Wirz, M.; MacH, O.; Maier, D.; Benito-Penalva, J.; Taylor, J.; Esclarin, A.; DIetz, V. Effectiveness of Automated Locomotor Training in Patients with Acute Incomplete Spinal Cord Injury: A Randomized, Controlled, Multicenter Trial. *J. Neurotrauma* **2017**, *34*, 1891–1896. [CrossRef] [PubMed]
38. DeVries, Z.; Hoda, M.; Rivers, C.S.; Maher, A.; Wai, E.; Moravek, D.; Stratton, A.; Kingwell, S.; Fallah, N.; Paquet, J.; et al. Development of an Unsupervised Machine Learning Algorithm for the Prognostication of Walking Ability in Spinal Cord Injury Patients. *Spine J.* **2020**, *20*, 213–224. [CrossRef] [PubMed]
39. Torres-Espín, A.; Haefeli, J.; Ehsanian, R.; Torres, D.; Almeida, C.A.; Huie, J.R.; Chou, A.; Morozov, D.; Sanderson, N.; Dirlikov, B.; et al. Topological Network Analysis of Patient Similarity for Precision Management of Acute Blood Pressure in Spinal Cord Injury. *eLife* **2021**, *10*, e68015. [CrossRef]
40. Agarwal, N.; Aabedi, A.A.; Torres-Espin, A.; Chou, A.; Wozny, T.A.; Mummaneni, P.V.; Burke, J.F.; Ferguson, A.R.; Kyritsis, N.; Dhall, S.S.; et al. Decision Tree–Based Machine Learning Analysis of Intraoperative Vasopressor Use to Optimize Neurological Improvement in Acute Spinal Cord Injury. *Neurosurg. Focus* **2022**, *52*, E9. [CrossRef]
41. Chay, W.; Kirshblum, S. Predicting Outcomes After Spinal Cord Injury. *Phys. Med. Rehabil. Clin.* **2020**, *31*, 331–343. [CrossRef]

42. Burns, A.S.; Marino, R.J.; Flanders, A.E.; Flett, H. Clinical Diagnosis and Prognosis Following Spinal Cord Injury. In *Handbook of Clinical Neurology*; Elsevier: Amsterdam, The Netherlands, 2012; Volume 109, pp. 47–62. [CrossRef]
43. Okimatsu, S.; Maki, S.; Furuya, T.; Fujiyoshi, T.; Kitamura, M.; Inada, T.; Aramomi, M.; Yamauchi, T.; Miyamoto, T.; Inoue, T.; et al. Determining the Short-Term Neurological Prognosis for Acute Cervical Spinal Cord Injury Using Machine Learning. *J. Clin. Neurosci.* **2022**, *96*, 74–79. [CrossRef] [PubMed]
44. Inoue, T.; Ichikawa, D.; Ueno, T.; Cheong, M.; Inoue, T.; Whetstone, W.D.; Endo, T.; Nizuma, K.; Tominaga, T. XGBoost, a Machine Learning Method, Predicts Neurological Recovery in Patients with Cervical Spinal Cord Injury. *Neurotrauma Rep.* **2020**, *1*, 8–16. [CrossRef] [PubMed]
45. Chou, A.; Torres-Espin, A.; Kyritsis, N.; Huie, J.R.; Khatry, S.; Funk, J.; Hay, J.; Lofgreen, A.; Shah, R.; McCann, C.; et al. Expert-Augmented Automated Machine Learning Optimizes Hemodynamic Predictors of Spinal Cord Injury Outcome. *PLoS ONE* **2022**, *17*, e0265254. [CrossRef] [PubMed]
46. Fan, G.; Liu, H.; Yang, S.; Luo, L.; Wang, L.; Pang, M.; Liu, B.; Zhang, L.; Han, L.; Rong, L. Discharge Prediction of Critical Patients with Spinal Cord Injury: A Machine Learning Study with 1485 Cases 2021. *medRxiv* 2021. [CrossRef]
47. Buri, M.; Tanadini, L.G.; Hothorn, T.; Curt, A. Unbiased Recursive Partitioning Enables Robust and Reliable Outcome Prediction in Acute Spinal Cord Injury. *J. Neurotrauma* **2022**, *39*, 266–276. [CrossRef] [PubMed]
48. Dietz, V.; Sinkjaer, T. Spasticity. In *Handbook of Clinical Neurology*; Elsevier: Amsterdam, The Netherlands, 2012; Volume 109, pp. 197–211. [CrossRef]
49. Barbeau, H.; Danakas, M.; Arsenault, B. The Effects of Locomotor Training in Spinal Cord Injured Subjects: A Preliminary Study. *Restor. Neurol. Neurosci.* **1993**, *5*, 81–84. [CrossRef] [PubMed]

Disclaimer/Publisher's Note: The statements, opinions and data contained in all publications are solely those of the individual author(s) and contributor(s) and not of MDPI and/or the editor(s). MDPI and/or the editor(s) disclaim responsibility for any injury to people or property resulting from any ideas, methods, instructions or products referred to in the content.

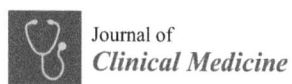

Article

Impact of Robotic-Assisted Gait Therapy on Depression and Anxiety Symptoms in Patients with Subacute Spinal Cord Injuries (SCIs)—A Prospective Clinical Study

Alicja Widuch-Spodyniuk [1], Beata Tarnacka [2,*], Bogumił Korczyński [1] and Justyna Wiśniowska [3]

[1] Research Institute for Innovative Methods of Rehabilitation of Patients with Spinal Cord Injury in Kamien Pomorski, Health Resort Kamien Pomorski, 72-400 Kamień Pomorski, Poland; alicjamariawiduch@gmail.com (A.W.-S.)
[2] Department of Rehabilitation, Medical University of Warsaw, 02-091 Warsaw, Poland
[3] Department of Rehabilitation, Eleonora Reicher National Institute of Geriatrics, Rheumatology and Rehabilitation, 02-637 Warsaw, Poland; justyna.wisniowska@spartanska.pl
* Correspondence: btarnacka@wum.edu.pl

Abstract: Background: Mood disorders, especially depression, and emotional difficulties such as anxiety are very common problems among patients with spinal cord injuries (SCIs). The lack of physical training may deteriorate their mental state, which, in turn, has a significant impact on their improvement in functioning. The aim of the present study was to examine the influence of innovative rehabilitation approaches involving robotic-assisted gait therapy (RAGT) on the depression and anxiety symptoms in patients with SCI. Methods: A total of 110 participants with subacute SCIs were enrolled in this single-center, single-blinded, single-arm, prospective study; patients were divided into experimental (robotic-assisted gait therapy (RAGT)) and control (conventional gait therapy with dynamic parapodium (DPT)) groups. They received five training sessions per week over 7 weeks. At the beginning and end of therapy, the severity of depression was assessed via the Depression Assessment Questionnaire (KPD), and that of anxiety symptoms was assessed via the State–Trait Anxiety Inventory (STAI X-1). Results: SCI patients in both groups experienced significantly lower levels of anxiety- and depression-related symptoms after completing the seven-week rehabilitation program (KPD: $Z = 6.35$, $p < 0.001$, $r = 0.43$; STAI X-1: $Z = -6.20$, $p < 0.001$, $r = 0.42$). In the RAGT group, post-rehabilitation measurements also indicated an improvement in psychological functioning (i.e., decreases in depression and anxiety and an increase in self-regulation (SR)). Significant results were noted for each variable (STAI X-1: $Z = -4.93$; KPD: $Z = -5.26$; SR: $Z = -3.21$). In the control group, there were also decreases in the effects on depression and state anxiety and an increase in self-regulation ability (STAI X-1: $Z = -4.01$; KPD: $Z = -3.65$; SR: $Z = -2.83$). The rehabilitation modality did not appear to have a statistically significant relationship with the magnitude of improvement in the Depression Assessment Questionnaire (KPD) (including self-regulation) and State–Trait Anxiety Inventory (STAI) scores. However, there were some significant differences when comparing the groups by the extent and depth of the injury and type of paralysis. Moreover, the study did not find any significant relationships between improvements in physical aspects and changes in psychological factors. Conclusions: Subjects in the robotic-assisted gait therapy (RAGD) and dynamic parapodium training (DPT) groups experienced decreases in anxiety and depression after a 7-week rehabilitation program. However, the rehabilitation modality (DPT vs. RAGT) did not differentiate between the patients with spinal cord injuries in terms of the magnitude of this change. Our results suggest that individuals with severe neurological conditions and complete spinal cord injuries (AIS A, according to the Abbreviated Injury Scale classification) may experience greater benefits in terms of changes in the psychological parameters after rehabilitation with RAGT.

Keywords: spinal cord injury; robotic rehabilitation; coordinative rehabilitation; depression; mood; anxiety

Citation: Widuch-Spodyniuk, A.; Tarnacka, B.; Korczyński, B.; Wiśniowska, J. Impact of Robotic-Assisted Gait Therapy on Depression and Anxiety Symptoms in Patients with Subacute Spinal Cord Injuries (SCIs)—A Prospective Clinical Study. *J. Clin. Med.* **2023**, *12*, 7153. https://doi.org/10.3390/jcm12227153

Academic Editors: Mohit Arora and Ashley Craig

Received: 30 August 2023
Revised: 10 November 2023
Accepted: 10 November 2023
Published: 17 November 2023

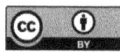

Copyright: © 2023 by the authors. Licensee MDPI, Basel, Switzerland. This article is an open access article distributed under the terms and conditions of the Creative Commons Attribution (CC BY) license (https://creativecommons.org/licenses/by/4.0/).

1. Introduction

There are approximately 10.5 new traumatic spinal cord injury (SCI) diagnoses per 100,000 people worldwide each year [1]. Based on epidemiological data for Poland, the majority of people in this population are males (the sex ratio is 2.5 females to 6 males), the average age is >40 years and the most common cause of injury is traffic accidents [2,3]. Spinal cord injuries directly lead to losses of or limitations to the motor and sensory functions at the level of injury and below. Secondary symptoms are usually sphincter dysfunction, chronic neuropathic pain, autonomic dysreflexia, respiratory failure, sexual dysfunction, digestive disorders and respiratory failure [4]. Direct and secondary somatic symptoms after SCI, as well as the loss of independence and the need to reorganize functioning in family, social and professional life, can affect the deterioration in the psychological well-being, including quality of life, body image (attitudes toward the body at the level of thoughts, emotions and behavior), self-confidence, belief in their own abilities and perception of their social attractiveness [5–9]. The most-frequently described psychiatric symptoms are anxiety, lowered mood and clinical depression. The second most described mental problems are anxiety disorders, including generalized anxiety disorder (GAD) and post-traumatic stress disorder (PTSD). It is estimated to affect approximately 15–32% of people with SCIs, depending on the measure used [10]. The risk rate for depression among SCI patients undergoing inpatient treatment ranges between 20 and 43%, and the average of the results obtained from different studies is 30% [11]; therefore, the prevalence of anxiety and depression among people with spinal cord injuries is higher than in the general population [11].

Rehabilitation, other regular exercise and physical activity significantly reduced stress and depression-related symptoms, and improved quality of life and social interactions [12,13]. They may also have preventive effects on the quality-of-life declines after a spinal injury, reducing pain and increasing sense of control, fitness and performance [12,13]. The endocannabinoid system (i.e., its components, pathways and ligands) may have preventive and therapeutic effects on neurological impairment and neurodegenerative diseases, as well as on mood and affect [14,15]. 2-Arachidonoylglycerol (2-AG) signaling to this system has an important role in adaptation to stress, anxiety, and depressive behavior (Sibers, Balchin, Badse). 2-AG is a full agonist of cannabinoid receptors (CB1 and CB2) and acts as a retrograde eCB signaling molecule [14,16]. Isometric exercise, prolonged and regular physical activity have been shown to increase the serum levels of the Endocannabinoids (eCBs) anandamide (AEA) and (2-AG) [14–18].

Due to the breadth and diversity of health problems after SCI, early, intensive and, above all, multispecialty assistance is essential. An early coordinated rehabilitation program makes it possible to anticipate its implications in terms of somatic and psychological health in the form of reduced anxiety and depression [19–21].

One of the most important and desirable goals of rehabilitation after SCI (regardless of the level, depth of the injury, time since the injury, and age of the patient) is to achieve the ability to maintain an upright position and regain the gait function [22,23]. Patients after SCI use orthoses or wheelchairs in order to transfer from one place to another. Standing and walking bring a lot of benefits to SCI patients, such as prevention of pressure sores, cardiovascular events, decreasing bone osteoporosis and improving the function of the digestive system. The upright position not only has an effect on secondary physical symptoms, but it is also related to improved quality of life, self-confidence and a sense of independence [24,25]. Conventional SCI rehabilitation (in terms of uprighting and gait re-education) involves dynamic parapodium therapy (DPT) [26]. Parapodium is a device that supports gait therapy and allows the patient to achieve an upright position or gait training. The patient's movement consists of a pendulum motion (from side to side), which deviates significantly from the correct gait pattern [27]. The robotic-assisted gait therapy (RAGT) is mostly used for lower-extremity and body-weight-supported treadmill training. It offers a number of advantages, including the ability to start therapy early after an injury, and it is therapeutic for people with significant lower limb paralysis. In addition, it allows for the adjustment of parameters such as the speed, weight-bearing relief (intensity) and length of the training session to suit the patient's current capabilities, and it allows for the accurate monitoring of the patient's progress. Robotic-assisted gait training uses stationary devices, such as the Lokomat device and exoskeletons. The U.S. Food and Drug Administration defines a powered exoskeleton as follows: it "(...) is a prescription device that is composed of an external, powered, motorized orthosis that is placed over a person's paralyzed or weakened lower extremity limb(s) for medical purposes" [28]. There are two groups of exoskeletons: assistive exoskeletons and rehabilitation exoskeletons. A rehabilitation exoskeleton is a device that provides support for the patient's total body weight [29]. It is an equally promising, safe and well-tolerated method of therapy for patients with neurological disorders, including post-spinal-cord-injury (SCI) patients [30–33]. Modern multifaceted rehabilitation using RAGT not only has a beneficial effect on improving the sensorimotor, kinematic and autonomic functions, but it also allows for a greater sense of control over one's own body and independence, thereby contributing to an improvement in psychological functioning and the subjective assessment of one's quality of life [5,34–41].

During this therapy, metabolic energy expenditure and fatiguability in paraplegic persons is much more pronounced in comparison with RAGT. The walking speed of an SCI patient with such orthosis is significantly less than that of normal walking, or RAGT therapy. Robotic therapy allows for a much greater number of steps. In most gait orthosis, the high value of the force is transmitted to the upper limb joints, which can increase shoulder pain incidence. Although dynamic parapodium training DPT is widely used, there is only one study that has compared rehabilitation with DPT versus rehabilitation with RAGT. The results of the study showed that both DPT and RAGT rehabilitation can improve the gait function (WISCI II) and muscle strength (MS). However, patients with RAGT therapy achieved significantly higher scores for the above parameters [26]. Rehabilitation robots are increasingly being used to rehabilitate people with spinal cord injuries. Conventional SCI rehabilitation (in terms of uprighting and gait re-education) uses training with a dynamic parapodium [26]. The dynamic parapodium is a device that allows the patient to achieve an upright position while still allowing them to move. However, the dynamic parapodium has its limitations. The patient's movement consists of a pendulum motion (from side to side), which deviates significantly from the correct gait pattern [27].

There are few studies describing rehabilitation using RAGT that include mental status. There have been no previous studies in the literature comparing the effects of RAGT vs. DPT therapy on psychological aspects. Moreover, most of previous studies focused on quality of life rather than emotional difficulties or affective disorders, or they include people with other neurological disorders, such as multiple sclerosis or stroke [42–48]. The results of these trials are often inconclusive. Some studies suggest an association between RAGT and a reduction in depressive symptoms and increase in quality of life, while others have found no such association. Others emphasize its relevance to and equivalence with biological and social factors [33,49–52]. Relatively few studies have been conducted on the efficacy of rehabilitation with RAGT on groups of patients with spinal cord injuries; however, the analyses conducted so far are promising, especially for patients with significant hemiparesis [22,31,35,47,53–59]. The researchers emphasize that RAGT should not replace conventional rehabilitation but complement it [49,50,60–62]. The rehabilitation procedures have also not been delineated in terms of the duration, frequency and intensity of training, among others [63].

In addition, we set out to see if patients with paraplegia present different levels of anxiety and depression than patients with tetraplegia in patients from the experimental and control groups. Simultaneously, the type of rehabilitation is significant in terms of changes in the symptoms of depression and state anxiety in patients with different degrees of injury on the Abbreviated Injury Scale (AIS) (AIS A vs. AIS B, C, D). Patients with spinal cord injury differ significantly in their neurological status, which has a major impact on their potential abilities and functional status [64–66]. In this study, we decided to divided patients into separate groups according to the AIS classification (AIS A with complete injury and AIS B, C, D with incomplete injury) and the type of paralysis (tetraplegia and paraplegia).

All study patients received psychological support, including cognitive behavioral therapy (CBT). CBT therapy has been scientifically proven to be effective in changing maladaptive thinking and behavioral patterns that contribute to people's psychological problems [67].

In this study, we assumed the following hypotheses:

1. Both the rehabilitation group with DPT (S0) and the rehabilitation group with RAGT (S1) will show significant improvements in the severity of symptoms related to depression and state anxiety;
2. Patients in the experimental group (S1) will achieve greater improvements in the psychological indicators (severity of depression-related symptoms and state anxiety) compared to those in the control group (S0);
3. The improvement in the psychological parameters (i.e., the decrease in symptoms related to depression and state anxiety) will have a significant relationship with the improvement in the gait function and functional independence after SCI.

Based on the available research, we hypothesized that SCI patients would experience less anxiety and lower levels of depression-related symptoms after both forms of therapy, but that they would do so to a greater extent after RAGT [5,12,13,19,20,41,62,68]. The main objective of our study was to analyze the association of RAGT rehabilitation with symptoms related to depression and anxiety, as well as with clinical status. In addition, we assessed whether the level and extent of the injury and the type of paralysis affect the magnitude of changes in the symptom levels of depression and anxiety (the condition after the 7-week rehabilitation program), and whether the changes in these parameters are related to improvements in the medical parameters (i.e., functional independence and mobility and the extent of the recovery of the gait function).

2. Materials and Methods

2.1. Study Protocol

This study was a single-blinded, prospective, clinical study. The study was conducted according to the Declaration of Helsinki committee and obtained approval from the Ethical Board of the District Medical Chamber in Szczecin, Poland (Nr OIL-Sz/MF/KB/452/05/07/2018; Nr OIL-SZ/MF/KB/450/UKP/10/2018). Before being accepted into the study, all participants underwent medical examinations conducted by physicians specialized in neurological physical rehabilitation and medicine, physiotherapists and a psychologist.

Medical inclusion criteria included the following: time since injury ranging from 3 months to 2 years; the general condition of the patient defined as conscious, able to cooperate with the physiotherapist and adapted to the upright position; complete and incomplete SCIs (cervical, thoracic or lumbar) with preserved flexion and extension functions at the elbow and wrist; surgical stabilization of the spine in the phase of completed bone fusion; no contraindications to rehabilitation arising from, among other things, venous thrombosis, pulmonary embolism, orthostatic hypotension, epilepsy or infection; body weight not exceeding 120 kg; height between 150 and 190 cm. Exclusion criteria included the following: high and complete tetraplegia and very low lumbar spine injury; lack of completion of bone fusion after established spinal stabilization; lack of completed bone fusion after spine surgery; respiratory insufficiency, circulatory insufficiency III and New York Heart Association (NYHA) class IV; osteoporosis; lower-limb shortening of more than 2 cm; the presence of decubitus ulcers, deep abrasions or skin lesions that could be exacerbated by the robotic system; intensive spasticity (4 points on the Ashworth scale) and muscle contractures that make it impossible to conduct robotic rehabilitation; past or present neurological disorders (i.e., traumatic spinal stroke, multiple sclerosis, childhood cerebral palsy); symptoms of recurrent autonomic dysreflexia. In the psychological studies, additional exclusion criteria were the finding of a reduced general level of intellectual functioning preventing the completion of the questionnaire tests and an age below 16 years (there is no normalization of the psychological tools used for this age group).

All patients underwent two physiotherapeutic, medical and psychological assessments each by professionals unfamiliar with the purpose of the study at the beginning and end of the 7-week treatment program. Research tools with proven validity and reliability were used to verify the hypotheses. The research procedure followed scheme No. 1 each time. Medical, physical and neurological examination included medical history and questionnaire tests using the Spinal Cord Independence Measure, version III (SCIM-III), and the Walking Index for Spinal Cord Injury, version II (WISCI-II). The test procedure was carried out using The American Spinal Cord Injury Association (ASIA) Impairment Scale (AIS). The psychological examination included a structured interview and the administration of surveys using questionnaires (including the Depression Assessment Questionnaire (KPD) and State–Trait Anxiety Inventory (STAI X-1)). To standardize the research procedure, the psychologist read the questionnaire questions and marked the answers. This was necessary due to the motor difficulties of some patients (i.e., problems marking answers or turning pages).

2.2. Physiotherapy and Psychological Intervention

The rehabilitation program consisted of two phases lasting three weeks each, with a one-week break in between. Rehabilitation interventions took place six days a week. Psychological activities were held once a week and included individual sessions (targeting the patients' needs and difficulties based on their resources) and group therapy.

Patients were enrolled in two groups by coin toss: a control group (S0) subjected to conventional gait therapy with DPT, and an experimental group subjected to rehabilitation using RAGT. The mentioned therapies lasted 30 min each. Patients enrolled in the experimental group (S1) received RAGT sessions using the EKSO-GT exoskeleton (model EKSO 1 by Ekso Bionics, San Rafael, CA, USA; year of manufacture: 2014) or Lokomat Pro (model LO218 by Hocoma AG, Volketswil, Switzerland; year of manufacture: 2014) in addition to the general standard physiotherapy training program based on proprioceptive neuromuscular facilitation. All participants from the Lokomat group with incomplete SCIs started with 60% body weight support and an initial treadmill speed of 1.5 km/h. Patients with complete SCIs started with 90–100% body weight support. In patients with the EKSO-GT, a minimum of 100 steps was required per session for DPT 20. All patients in both the S0 and S1 groups received psychological support; meetings were held three times during the cycle of the seven-week rehabilitation program, and 50-min individual sessions based on cognitive–behavioral-therapy (CBT) techniques were held at least once a week (at least eight times during the course of the camp). In general, CBT therapy is aimed at changing maladaptive patterns of thinking and behavior [67]. The program and purpose of the meetings were tailored to each patient's needs and problems and were closely coordinated with the patient. In addition to individual meetings, weekly 90-min group therapy meetings were conducted based on the CBT method rational behavior therapy using motivational interviewing and mindfulness-based cognitive therapy. The group therapy was aimed at the general difficulties faced by people after SCI, as well as at exchanging information, supporting other patients and receiving feedback from them.

2.3. Participants

Patients self-reported from all over the country to participate in the study. They agreed to participate and signed an informed consent form before the study. Based on the criteria, three patients did not qualify for the psychological testing. One of the subjects had moderate intellectual disabilities and two of them were under the age of 16 years (scheme No. 1).

A simple randomization method was used to assign patients to comparison groups. The random assignment to groups was performed by a medical staff member, unaware of the study's purpose (a blinded investigator). The medical team, paramedical team and psychologist were unaware of the purpose of the study when performing the treatment and therapeutic measures (single blinding).

A total of 110 patients completed the study; 79 of them were assigned to the S1 group participating in rehabilitation with RAGT, including 62 men and 17 women, and 31 were assigned to the S0 group, including 27 men and 4 women. The disproportion in the number of control group patients was caused by patients resigning when they were not assigned to RAGD rehabilitation group (see Table 1). Also, the situation caused by the COVID-19 pandemic caused 11 patients in the S0 group to not complete the rehabilitation cycle.

Table 1. Characteristics of the study group.

Group	S0 (N = 31; 28.2%)	S1 (N = 79; 71.8%)	p-Value
Sex			
Women	4 (12.9%)	17 (21.5%)	0.301
Men	27 (87.1%)	62 (78.5%)	
Education			
Enrolled in education	2 (6.5%)	4 (5.1%)	
Elementary	0 (0.0%)	2 (2.5%)	
Vocational	6 (19.4%)	7 (8.9%)	0.554 *
Secondary	6 (19.4%)	19 (24.1%)	
Higher	17 (54.8%)	47 (59.5%)	
Accommodation			
Countryside	8 (25.8%)	22 (28.6%)	
Small town	7 (22.6%)	20 (26.0%)	0.912
Medium-size town	6 (19.4%)	11 (14.3%)	
Big city	10 (32.3%)	24 (31.2%)	
Marital status			
Lack of partner	5 (16.1%)	22 (27.8%)	
Informal relationship	5 (16.1%)	15 (19%)	0.338
Formal relationship	21 (67.7%)	42 (53.2%)	
Cause of injury			
Vehicle accident	12 (38.7%)	24 (30.8%)	
Fall < 1 m	2 (6.5%)	5 (6.4%)	
Fall > 1 m	8 (25.8%)	29 (37.2%)	
Dive	2 (6.5%)	2 (2.6%)	0.089 *
Violence-related trauma	0 (0.0%)	1 (1.3%)	
Body crushing	4 (12.9%)	1 (1.3%)	
Others	3 (9.7%)	16 (20.5%)	
Level of neurological impairment			
Cervical	8 (25.8%)	16 (20.3%)	0.811
Thoracic	15 (48.4%)	42 (53.2%)	
Lumbar	8 (25.8%)	21 (26.6%)	
Extent of spinal injury according to The Abbreviated Injury Scale (AIS)			
AIS A	14 (45.2%)	30 (38.0%)	0.489
AIS B/C/D	17 (54.8%)	49 (62.2%)	0.666
Type of paralysis			
Paraplegia	25 (80.6%)	64 (81.0%)	0.965
Tetraplegia	6 (19.4%)	15 (19.0%)	
Age			
Median (IQR)	37.0 (22)	36 (23)	0.666
Time from accident (months)			
Median (IQR)	13 (13)	12 (11)	0.433

*—Fisher's exact test.

Comparisons of the S0 and S1 groups with sociodemographic and other characteristic variables showed that there were no differences between the groups at the initial level. In both groups, the majority were men and people with higher education, in formal relationships. The largest group was made up of respondents living in large cities. The most common cause of injury was a fall from a height of more than 1 m. The main level of the neurological damage was Th. The median ages were 37 (S0) and 36 (S1) years, and the median times since the accident, respectively, were 13 and 12 months.

The study flowchart is shown in Figure 1.

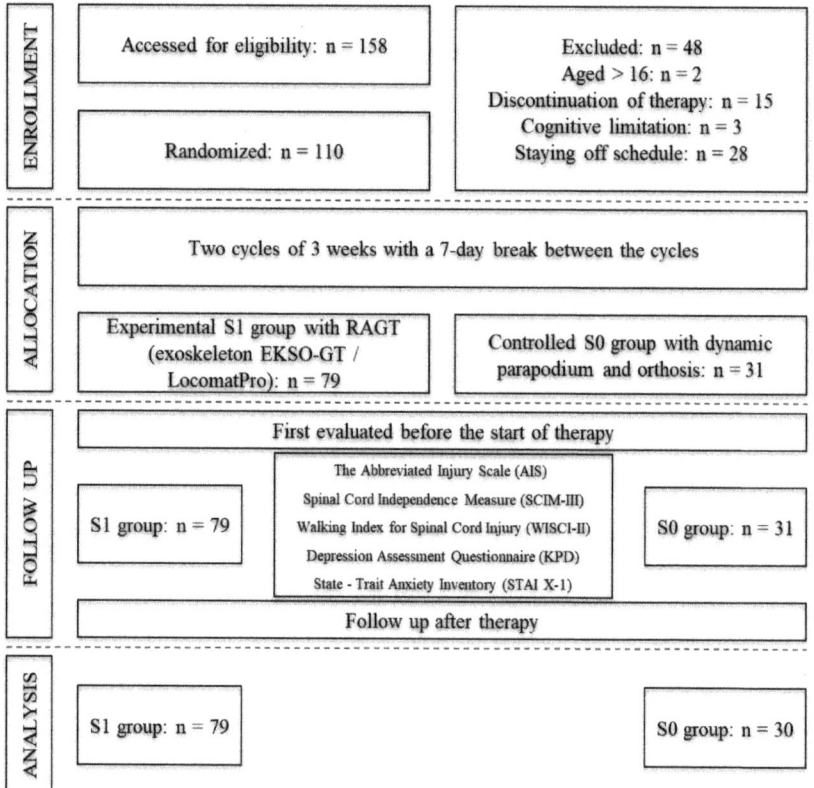

Figure 1. Flowchart of details of patients' recruitment.

2.3.1. Primary Outcome Measures

In this analysis, the primary outcome measures were the overall depression severity scores and the anxiety severity status measure, while the second-order indicators were the individual depression symptom severity scores, the scores for the level of functional independence and mobility after SCI and the gait function measure.

To estimate the severity of the depression symptoms, the Depression Assessment Questionnaire (KPD) by E. Łojek, J. Stańczak, A. Wójcik was used. The KPD measures the severity of depression and its individual symptoms and includes an additional scale to assess the subjects' self-regulatory abilities. Its theoretical basis is based on data on the symptoms and mechanisms of depression in accordance with international diagnostic criteria. The overall score (WO) of the KPD indicates the general severity of the depression. Possible scores range from 60 (no depression) to 240 (severe depression). A WO of 130 points is the cutoff between a normal score and a score suggesting depressive disorders [69].

To measure anxiety as a state, the STAI X-1 by C.D. Spielberger, R.L. Gorsuch and R.E. Lushene was used. State anxiety is understood as tension related to a current situation. Possible scores range from 20 (low anxiety) to 80 (high anxiety) [70].

2.3.2. Secondary Outcome Measures

Additional scales of the KPD were used to measure the severity of individual depressive symptoms. The KPD consists of five scales: DPUE—Cognitive deficits and energy loss (refers to symptoms associated with decreased learning performance and impaired attention and memory performance, as well as deterioration in psychomotor functions and loss of energy; the range of scores is from 19 to 76 points); MSPA—Thinking about death, pessimism and alienation (refers to the measurement of the severity of the loss of meaning in life, social withdrawal and emotions with negative signs; the lowest possible raw score is 15 and the highest is 60, indicating the very high severity of the described symptoms); PWNL—Guilt and anxiety tension (measures the severity of fear, anxiety and related emotional tension and the tendency to blame oneself for various situations, behaviors and thoughts, and it also allows for an estimation of one's level of self-esteem and sense of social attractiveness; the score range is from 16 to 64); OPSZ—Psychosomatic symptoms and decline in interest (refers to the subjective assessment of one's somatic and mental health, and it also allows for a determination of the decrease in previous interests (anhedonia); the range of raw scores is from 10 to 40); SR—Self-regulation (an additional scale used to measure a subject's emotional and cognitive resources protecting them from depression; the minimum number of points possible is 15 and the maximum is 60). The sum of the scores of the first four scales affects the overall score of the severity of the symptoms associated with depression (WO) [69].

In order to diagnose and assess the neurological and functional statuses, tests were conducted using the following measures: The AIS, which was used to assess the motor and sensory functions; we divided patients according to the AIS to A, B, C, D or E subgroups, where AIS A refers to complete SCI and AIS B, C and D refer to incomplete SCI [71]. The Walking Index for Spinal Cord Injury (WISCI-II), which was used to measure the improvement in the gait function of our patients after SCI. It is the most sensitive measure in terms of changes in the gait ability compared to other leading measurement scales [72]. The index provides an assessment of the level of the gait function. A level of 0 indicates the inability to stand and participate in walking, and a level of 21 indicates the ability to walk without the use of aids, orthoses or assistance from others [73]. The Spinal Cord Independence Measure, version III (SCIM-III), was used for functional assessment because it is a reliable and accurate scale for assessing skills in the daily functioning of patients with spinal cord injuries, with proven adequacy in group studies [74], and it is the only comprehensive scale for assessing the ability of patients to perform basic daily activities. Version III contains 19 tasks divided into three areas: self-care; breathing and sphincter control; mobility. The total score ranges from 0 (indicating total dependence) to 100 (indicating total independence) [75].

2.4. Statistical Analyses

In this study, continuous data are presented as mean values and standard deviations (SDs) and categorical data are presented as percentages. Distributions were checked, and descriptive statistics of the quantitative variables were calculated. The normality of the distributions was tested with the Shapiro–Wilk test, but the skewness and kurtosis values were also considered. Due to the violation of the assumptions of normal distribution and numerous outlier observations exceeding the third standard deviation, analyses were based on non-parametric tests. Comparisons of the nominal and ordinal variables for the group characteristics were based on chi-square tests of independence along with Fisher's exact test. In addition, correlation analyses with Spearman's rho coefficient were performed to assess the relationships between the variables. In order to determine the effect size used to measure the impact of the strength of the relationship between the independent variables studied and dependent variables, we adopted cutoff values at significance levels of $p < 0.001$, $p < 0.01$ and $p < 0.05$. The effect size results were determined and interpreted as correlation values: 0.00–0.19: "very weak"; 0.20–0.39: "weak"; 0.40–0.59: "moderate"; 0.60–0.79: "strong"; 0.80–1.0: "very strong" [76].

Quantitative analysis of group characteristics and normality of distribution tests were performed on a group of 110 individuals. However, further comparative analyses were performed on a group of 109 people due to missing data for one person at the second measurement in the S0 group n = 30 (see Figure 1).

Differences in the state anxiety and depression indicators between the pre-rehabilitation and post-rehabilitation measurements were tested using the Mann–Whitney U test. Similarly, this analysis was performed with the division into control and experimental groups (S0 n = 30 vs. S1 n = 79) using Wilcoxon rank-sum and signed-rank tests for this purpose. Differences in functional indices (WISCI-II and SCIM-III) were also tested separately in groups S0 and S1 and between the study groups (S0 and S1) using the Wilcoxon rank tests and Mann–Whitney U test. Next, we tested whether there were relationships between the changes that occurred between the measures of the functional indicators (WISCI-II, SCIM-III) and changes in mental health (STAI X-1, KPD). Spearman's rho correlation analyses were performed for this purpose. Measures of anxiety and depression before and after rehabilitation were also compared, as well as changes in the anxiety and depression divided into the S0 and S1 groups and according to the AIS classification of spinal cord injury, so that four groups were compared: S0 AIS A (n = 13); S0 AIS B, C, D (n = 17); S1 AIS A (n = 30); S1 AIS B, C, D (n = 49). This analysis was then performed between subjects with two types of paralysis: paraplegia (n = 89) and tetraplegia (n = 20). These analyses were performed using a series of Wilcoxon signed-rank tests and Mann–Whitney U tests.

The present study did not perform a comparative analysis between the degree of paralysis (paraplegia vs. tetraplegia) and AIS scale scores (AIS A vs. AIS B, C, D) based on the division into study groups (S0 vs. S1) in terms of changes in the psychological parameter scores. This was due to the different sizes of the groups (S0 vs. S1; Table 1). The distribution by AIS vs. the range of paralysis was as follows: paraplegia: group S0, n = 25; group S1, n = 64; tetraplegia: group S0, n = 6; group S1, n = 15.

In summary, a total of 158 subjects qualified for our prospective, single-blind clinical trial based on specific inclusion and exclusion criteria. However, 48 people dropped out during the study (see Figure 1). A total od 110 subjects completed the study (see Table 1). However, 109 individuals were included in the analyses due to missing data. The analyses were performed using the IBM SPSS Statistics package, version 25.

The subjects underwent medical, physiotherapeutic and psychological examinations twice (at the beginning and at the end of the rehabilitation program). Statistical analysis was performed using non-parametric tests. A probability level of $p > 0.05$ was assumed.

3. Results

As mentioned above, 158 people qualified for the study and 110 completed it. However, 109 people were included in the statistical analyses because one person in the control group missed the second measurement (Figure 1).

In the present research, all the patients had neurological impairments after SCIs. In the S0 and S1 groups, totals of 25% and 20.3% of patients had neurological impairments at the cervical level, respectively, 48.4 and 53.2% had neurological impairments at the thoracic level, respectively, and 25.8 and 26.6% had neurological impairments at the lumbar level, respectively.

3.1. Severity of State Anxiety and Depression after 7-Week Rehabilitation Program

The results provided in Table 2 (the severity of the state anxiety ($Z = -6.20$, $p < 0.001$) and general depression ($Z = 6.35$, $p < 0.001$) symptoms and all the depression factors (DPUE, MSPA, PWLN, OPSZ)) were significantly decreased after the 7-week rehabilitation program, compared with the first measurement, regardless of the type of rehabilitation. The ability to self-regulate also increased significantly. The moderate effect size of rehabilitation was obtained in both the severity of depression ($r = 0.42$) and state anxiety ($r = 0.43$). Similarly, a moderate effect size in the PWLN depression factor and a weak effect size of rehabilitation in DPUE, MSPA, OPSZ and SR were obtained.

Table 2. Changes in state anxiety and depression across the study sample.

Variables	The Whole Group		
	Baseline, Median (IQR)	Final Median (IQR)	Size Effect
the State–Trait Anxiety Inventory Subscale (STAI x-1)	35.00 (13.00)	31.00 (8.50)	0.42 ***
Depression Assessment Questionnaire (KPD)	89.00 (34.00)	80.50 (29.50)	0.43 ***
Cognitive deficits and energy loss and alienation (DPUE)	29.00 (10.00)	26.50 (7.50)	0.35 ***
Thinking about death, pessi mism (MSPA)	19.00 (8.00)	17.00 (5.50)	0.35 ***
Guilt and anxiety tension (PWLN)	27.00 (8.00)	24.50 (10.00)	0.43 ***
Psychosomatic symptoms and decline in interest (OPSZ)	16.00 (7.00)	13.00 (6.50)	0.32 ***
Self-regulation (SR)	46.00 (8.00)	49.00 (10.00)	0.29 ***

Abbreviations: IQR: interquartile range; size effect: r. *** $p < 0.001$.

3.1.1. Differences in State Anxiety, Depression and Functionality in Comparison to the Type of Rehabilitation

The results in Table 3 show significant increases in all the general depression symptoms and depression and state anxiety factors after 7 weeks of rehabilitation in both the experimental and control groups. In the RAGT group, the effect size of rehabilitation was moderate for anxiety and all the KPD subscales, except PWLN and SR. For PWLN and SR, a weak effect size of the RAGT rehabilitation was obtained.

Table 3. Changes in state anxiety and depression and changes in functioning rates by type of rehabilitation.

Variables	S0 (n = 30)			S1 (n = 79)			S0 (n = 30)	S1 (n = 79)	Size Effect
	Baseline, Median (IQR)	Final Median (IQR)	Size Effect	Baseline, Median (IQR)	Final Median (IQR)	Size Effect	Change Median (IQR)	Change Median (IQR)	
STAI X-1	35.50 (10.00)	31.00 (8.50)	0.52 ***	32.00 (13.00)	26.00 (5.00)	0.39 ***	5.00 (5.50)	4.00 (9.00)	0.05
KPD	90.50 (34.00)	80.50 (29.50)	0.47 ***	85.00 (30.00)	78.00 (26.00)	0.42 ***	5.50 (12.00)	6.00 (11.00)	0.04
DPUE	29.00 (10.00)	26.50 (7.50)	0.42 **	27.00 (10.00)	26.00 (8.00)	0.32 ***	2.50 (5.00)	2.00 (5.00)	0.09
MSPA	19.50 (8.00)	17.00 (5.50)	0.38 **	19.00 (5.00)	17.00 (4.00)	0.34 ***	2.00 (3.75)	1.00 (2.00)	0.07
PWLN	27.50 (9.00)	24.50 (10.00)	0.40 **	25.00 (9.00)	21.00 (8.00)	0.45 ***	11.00 (8.25)	10.00 (5.00)	0.14
OPSZ	16.00 (8.00)	13.00 (6.50)	0.40 **	15.00 (6.00)	14.00 (5.00)	0.28 ***	1.50 (4.00)	1.00 (4.00)	0.12
SR	46.00 (9.00)	49.00 (10.00)	0.37 **	46.00 (7.00)	47.00 (8.00)	0.26 **	3.00 (4.25)	2.00 (4.00)	0.11
WISCI	0.00 (4.00)	0.50 (5.75)	0.26 *	2.00 (11.00)	6.00 (15.00)	0.41 ***	0.00 (0.00)	0.00 (3.00)	0.24 *
SCIM	63.50 (27.25)	66.50 (22.25)	0.50 ***	64.00 (20.00)	70.00 (24.00)	0.56 ***	4.00 (8.25)	5.00 (7.00)	0.07

Abbreviations: S0: control group; S1: experimental group; IQR: interquartile range. The change for SR was based on the P2–P1 difference, and the changes for the other variables were based on the P1–P2 difference. Size effect: r. *** $p < 0.001$; ** $p < 0.01$; * $p < 0.05$.

Table 3 also shows the differences in the results in the functional scales tested between the WISCI-II and SCIM-III separately in the S0 and S1 subgroups. There was an improvement in the clinical-functioning tests in the S0 group in the second measurement compared with the first. In the S1 group, there was also a significant improvement in the patients' clinical functioning after RAGT rehabilitation, but with greater effects on the WISCI-II scale ($Z = -5.17$; $p < 0.001$) and SCIM-III scale ($Z = 6.99$; $p < 0.001$). The effect sizes of RAGT rehabilitation on the WISCI-II ($r = 0.41$) and SCIM-III ($r = 0.56$) scales were moderate. Intergroup comparisons (S0 vs. S1) in terms of functional impairment showed a greater improvement in the S1 group, but only for the WISCI-II scale. The effect size of RAGT rehabilitation was weak. There were no statistically significant differences for the SCIM-III between the S0 and S1 groups ($Z = -0.69$; $p = 0.487$).

3.1.2. Functional and Mental Status Correlation

Table 4 shows the relationships between the changes that occurred between the measurements in the functional indicators (WISCI-II, SCIM-III) and changes in mental health (STAI X-1, KPD). There was no significant relationship between the somatic and mental functioning changes.

Table 4. Correlations of functional changes (SCIM and WISCI) with changes in mental health (STAI X-1 and KPD).

Change	S0 (n = 30)				S1 (n = 79)			
	Change, STAI X-1		Change, KPD		Change, STAI		Change, KPD	
	r_s	p	r_s	p	r_s	p	r_s	p
SCIM	−0.29	0.152	−0.16	0.422	0.17	0.233	0.08	0.573
WISCI	0.03	0.902	0.04	0.841	−0.02	0.870	−0.15	0.281

3.2. Severity of State Anxiety and Depression according to Neurological Impairment (AIS)

The anxiety and depression comparisons before and after rehabilitation in all the patients and subgroups according to the AIS classification are provided in Table 5. The results indicate significant increases in self-regulation and decreases in anxiety and depression in both the experimental and control groups.

Table 5. Changes in state anxiety and depression according to rehabilitation type and spinal cord injury classification.

S0	ASIA-A (n = 13)			ASIA-B, C, D (n = 17)			ASIA-A	ASIA-B, C, D	
	Baseline, Median (IQR)	Final Median (IQR)	Size Effect	Baseline, Median (IQR)	Final Median (IQR)	Size Effect	Change, Median (IQR)	Change, Median (IQR)	Size Effect
STAI X-1	32.00 (7.50)	27.00 (7.50)	0.60 **	38.00 (8.50)	33.00 (11.50)	0.48 **	5.00 (6.50)	5.00 (6.50)	0.07
KPD	78.00 (24.00)	78.00 (24.00)	0.28	97.00 (38.50)	84.00 (40.00)	0.59 ***	4.00 (10.00)	10.00 (16.50)	0.34
DPUE	27.00 (11.00)	24.00 (9.00)	0.37	35.00 (13.50)	28.00 (13.50)	0.47 **	2.00 (3.50)	4.00 (7.50)	0.25
MSPA	16.00 (5.50)	17.00 (3.50)	0.07	21.00 (13.00)	18.00 (10.50)	0.56 **	0.00 (3.50)	2.00 (4.00)	0.45 *
PWLN	23.00 (6.5)	24.00 (8.50)	0.37	28.00 (6.50)	25.00 (11.50)	0.44 *	11.00 (7.00)	15.00 (9.50)	0.16
OPSZ	16.00 (5.00)	13.00 (5.00)	0.34	19.00 (8.50)	12.00 (9.00)	0.43 *	1.00 (5.00)	2.00 (4.50)	0.05
SR	47.00 (5.50)	49.00 (9.00)	0.34	45.00 (11.50)	48.00 (12.50)	0.38 *	2.00 (4.50)	3.00 (7.50)	0.14
S1	ASIA-A (n = 30)			ASIA-B, C, D (n = 49)			ASIA-A	ASIA-B, C, D	
	Baseline, Median (IQR)	Final Median (IQR)	Size Effect	Baseline, Median (IQR)	Final Median (IQR)	Size Effect	Change, Median (IQR)	Change, Median (IQR)	Size Effect
STAI X-1	31.50 (11.50)	26.00 (2.75)	0.41 **	33.00 (12.00)	26.00 (6.00)	0.38 ***	4.00 (8.25)	3.00 (8.50)	<0.01
KPD	80.50 (33.75)	75.50 (23.50)	0.44 **	86.00 (27.00)	79.00 (31.00)	0.40 ***	6.00 (12.25)	6.00 (10.00)	<0.01
DPUE	26.50 (10.25)	26.00 (5.75)	0.30 **	28.00 (10.50)	26.00 (10.50)	0.33 **	2.00 (5.50)	2.00 (4.00)	0.04
MSPA	17.00 (5.00)	16.00 (4.00)	0.39 **	19.00 (5.50)	18.00 (4.50)	0.32 **	1.00 (2.00)	1.00 (2.00)	<0.01
PWLN	24.50 (7.50)	19.00 (7.50)	0.44 **	26.00 (10.00)	22.00 (10.00)	0.44 ***	9.50 (6.00)	11.00 (4.50)	0.11
OPSZ	14.00 (7.50)	14.00 (5.25)	0.30 **	15.00 (5.50)	14.00 (5.50)	0.27 **	1.00 (4.00)	1.00 (4.00)	0.02
SR	47.00 (6.00)	47.50 (9.00)	0.26 *	44.00 (8.00)	46.00 (9.50)	0.25 *	1.50 (4.25)	2.00 (4.50)	0.04

Abbreviations: S0: control group; S1: experimental group; IQR: interquartile range. The change for SR was based on the P2–P1 difference, and the changes for the other variables were based on the P1–P2 difference. Size effect: r. *** $p < 0.001$; ** $p < 0.01$; * $p < 0.05$.

In the S0 and AIS A group of patients, there was a significant decrease in the state anxiety after rehabilitation with a strong effect size (Z = −3.07; $p = 0.002$; r = 0.60). However, there were no significant differences between the measurements of general depressive symptoms (Z = −1.45; $p = 0.147$). Among patients in the S0 and AIS B, C, D group, the effects sizes of DPT for the general depression score and MSPA subscale were strong. The impacts of DPT on other depression factors (DPUE, PWLN, OPSZ and SR) were moderate. In the S1 and AIS A and S1 and AIS B, C, D groups, significant decreases were also observed for each depression and state anxiety measurement. In the S1 with AIS A group, the effect size was weak for self-regulation (r = 0.26). The effect size of RAGT rehabilitation was of moderate strength for the other KPD subscales (DPUE, MSPA, PWLN, OPSZ) and STAI X-1. The S1 and AIS B, C, D group also showed statistically significant decreases in depression and anxiety symptoms between the two measures, and an increase in SR.

In addition, Table 5 presents a comparison of the AIS (AIS A vs. AIS B, C, D) groups and depression and anxiety indicators separately in the S0 and S1 groups. It turns out, in the S0 group, a greater reduction in MSPA in AIS B, C, D than in AIS A was observed ($Z = -2.46$; $p = 0.014$). The effect size of the DPT was moderate ($r = 0.45$). There were no significant differences between the two groups in the other KPD subscales (DPUE, PWLN, OPSZ, SR). In contrast, the comparison between the RAGT groups (AIS A vs. AIS B, C, D) showed that the severity of changes in anxiety and depression was quite similar. The groups did not differ in self-regulation.

3.3. Severity of State Anxiety and Depression according to the Type of Paralysis

The differences between the subjects with two types of paralyses (tetraplegia vs. paraplegia) for the anxiety and depression indicators are presented in Table 6.

Table 6. Changes in state anxiety and depression depending on the type of paralysis.

Variables	Paraplegia (n = 89)			Tetraplegia (n = 20)			Paraplegia (n = 89)	Tetraplegia (n = 20)	Size Effect
	Baseline, Median (IQR)	Final Median (IQR)	Size Effect	Baseline, Median (IQR)	Final Median (IQR)	Size Effect	Change Median (IQR)	Change Median (IQR)	
STAI X-1	33.00 (13.00)	26.00 (7.00)	0.40 ***	35.00 (13.00)	28.00 (6.75)	0.49 **	4.00 (7.00)	3.50 (8.75)	<0.01
KPD	86.00 (29.00)	79.00 (25.50)	0.42 ***	92.50 (36.25)	81.50 (31.00)	0.49 **	6.00 (13.00)	7.00 (8.50)	<0.01
DPUE	28.00 (9.50)	26.00 (7.00)	0.36 ***	26.00 (13.00)	25.00 (13.50)	0.28	2.00 (4.50)	1.50 (5.50)	0.06
MSPA	19.00 (5.50)	17.00 (4.00)	0.35 ***	18.50 (6.75)	18.00 (4.00)	0.32 *	1.00 (2.00)	0.50 (3.50)	0.06
PWLN	26.00 (8.50)	22.00 (8.50)	0.43 ***	25.50 (12.00)	23.00 (10.75)	0.47 **	10.00 (6.00)	10.50 (7.00)	0.03
OPSZ	15.00 (6.50)	13.00 (5.00)	0.30 ***	16.50 (7.75)	14.00 (5.50)	0.41 **	1.00 (4.00)	2.00 (3.75)	0.11
SR	46.00 (9.00)	47.00 (10.00)	0.22 **	46.00 (7.50)	49.00 (8.75)	0.55 ***	1.00 (4.00)	3.00 (5.50)	0.20 *

Abbreviations: IQR: interquartile range. The change for SR was based on the P2–P1 difference, and the changes in the other variables were based on the P1–P2 difference. Size effect: r. *** $p < 0.001$; ** $p < 0.01$; * $p < 0.05$.

The results indicated a significant decrease in the levels of state anxiety ($Z = -5.40$; $p < 0.001$; $r = 0.40$) and depression ($Z = -5.59$; $p < 0.001$; $r = 0.42$), including an increase in self-regulation ($Z = -2.95$, $p = 0.003$, $r = 0.22$), among people with paraplegia. The effect size on SR was weak, while the effects on the other subscales of the KPD and STAI X-1 were moderate.

In the patients with tetraplegia, there were significant decreases in the state anxiety, general depression indicators and MSPA, PWLN, OPSZ and SR subscales. Only on the MSPA subscale were there were no significant differences between the two measurements. An increase in self-regulation after the rehabilitation program was obtained ($Z = -3.48$; $p < 0.001$). Among those with tetraplegia, there was also a decrease in the severity of symptoms related to depression and state anxiety, and an increase in the self-regulatory capacity. The effect size was strong for SR but moderate for the other KPD and STAI subscales. The patients with tetraplegia also showed decreases in anxiety ($Z = -3.08$; $p = 0.002$) and the total scores for depression ($Z = -3.07$; $p = 0.002$), as well as in other subscales, except for the DPUE index. In this group of patients, there was also an increase in self-regulation ($Z = -3.48$; $p < 0.001$) after rehabilitation. The effect was strong for SR but moderate for other significant differences (i.e., general KPD scores, MSPA, PWLN and OPSZ subscales and STAI X-1).

The differences in the anxiety and depression between the groups with different types of paralyses are provided in Table 6. The results indicate that subjects with paraplegia were characterized by a smaller increase in self-regulation compared to subjects with tetraplegia. The significant differences between the groups were obtained with low size effects. No differences between the groups were observed for the other KPD subscales (DPUE, MSPA, PWLN, OPSZ) or state anxiety.

The present study did not perform a comparative analysis between the degree of paralysis (paraplegia vs. tetraplegia) and AIS scale scores (AIS A vs. AIS B, C, D) based on the division into study groups (S0 vs. S1) in terms of changes in the psychological parameter scores. This was due to the different sizes of the groups (S0 vs. S1; Table 2). The distribution by AIS vs. the range of paralysis was as follows: paraplegia: group S0, n = 25; group S1, n = 64; tetraplegia: group S0, n = 6; group S1, n = 15.

In summary, after the seven-week rehabilitation program, all patients studied achieved significant improvements in anxiety state (STAI—X1) and depression (i.e., in terms of total scores and all symptoms of depression), as well as an increase in Self-regulation (see Table 2).

Analysis of changes in psychological factors (STAI X-1, KPD) and functional status (SCIM III) and improvement in gait function (WISCI—II) after a seven-week rehabilitation program showed improvement in all parameters studied in both study groups (S0 and S1), as seen in Table 3.

Intergroup comparisons (S1 vs. S0) for functional improvement (SCIM, WISCI) showed significantly greater improvement in gait function (WISCI-II) in the S1 group compared to the S0 group. No significant between-group differences were found for SCIM-III, as seen in Table 3.

Correlation analysis showed no significant relationship between functional changes (SCIM-III and WISCI-II) and changes in psychological parameters (STAI X-1, KPD), as seen in Table 4.

Comparison of measures of psychological factors before and after rehabilitation (STAI X1, KPD) divided into four groups (i.e., S0 AIS A; S0 AIS B,C,D; S1 AIS A; S1 AIS B,C,D) showed a significant decrease in anxiety and depression, as well as an increase in Self-regulation in the groups studied, except for the S0 AIS A group, where only a significant decrease in state anxiety (STAI X-1) was observed (no differences were observed between the measures of depression, including self-regulation, in this group), as seen in Table 5.

Group comparisons according to neurological impairment (AIS A vs. AIS B, C, D) separately for each research group (S0 and S1) showed no significant differences for any of the variables tested, except for a greater change in the MSPA (Thinking about death, pessimism and alienation, KPD subscale) in the S0 group, as seen in Table 5.

An analogous analysis of the differences in psychological factors by type of paralysis (tetraplegia and paraplegia) showed that in people with tetraplegia, there was a significant decrease in anxiety and depression and all their symptoms except DPUE (Cognitive deficits and Energy loss, KPD subscale), and an increase in Self-regulation. However, in people with paraplegia, there was a significant change in every parameter tested. Intergroup comparisons did not show significant differences for state anxiety (STAI-X1) and general depression scores and its individual KPD symptoms. However, it was observed that people with tetraplegia had a significantly higher increase in Self-regulation ability compared to people with paraplegia. (See Table 6).

4. Discussion

4.1. The Impact of a 7-Week Rehabilitation Program on Functionality and Severity of Depression and State Anxiety

Our study showed significant decreases in the state anxiety and symptoms of depression and increases in self-regulation in the patients in both groups (S0 and S1) after a 7-week rehabilitation program. However, no significant difference was observed between the groups according to the type of rehabilitation (RAGT vs. DPT). Although no differences were found between the types of rehabilitation (RAGT vs. DPT) in reducing the severity of the state anxiety and symptoms of depression, it can be speculated from the results that robotic rehabilitation may be particularly important for patients with complete spinal cord injuries (AIS A). After robotic rehabilitation, a decrease in the severity of the state anxiety and a decrease in the level of perceived symptoms of depression were observed in both patients with complete SCIs and those with incomplete SCIs. In addition, we also noted no significant statistical association between the functional independence and psychological factors. A statistically significant difference was observed only for the WISCI-II scale. Patients in the rehabilitation group with RAGT achieved a greater improvement in gait function. We analyzed the association of the medical parameters with the psychological variables. We found that the improvements in the gait function (WISCI II) and functional independence (SCIM-III) were unrelated to improvements in the depression (KPD), state anxiety as a condition (STAI X-1) and self-regulation (KPD) scores.

Both, RAGT and DPT rehabilitations reduced state anxiety and depression symptoms. The mechanism for reducing depression and anxiety symptoms could be related to general fitness and performance improvement after rehabilitation. SCI patients recovered independence in everyday activities, which improved their moods and reduced their anxiety severity. In addition, rehabilitation and other regular exercise and physical activity are significantly associated with lower levels of stress and depressive symptoms, increased social participation and improvement in quality of life. They may also have a preventive effect on the decline in quality of life after spinal cord injury, primarily by reducing the patient's pain levels, increasing their feelings of control and mastery and improving their fitness and performance In addition, as mentioned in the introduction, rehabilitation and other regular physical activity are significantly associated with improvement of emotional and affective states, improvement of quality of life (primarily by reducing pain levels, increasing sense of control and mastery, improving fitness and efficiency and increasing participation in social life) [12,13]. It can also be assumed that improvement of anxiety and symptoms of depression is a natural process of recovery and adaptation to disability [77]. In addition, the time since injury and adaptation to new living conditions through the introduction of practical training, such as the independent use of handicapped accessible cars, improving wheelchair mobility, etc., may have a positive impact on the emotional and affective state of spinal cord injury patients.

It can also be assumed that the improvement in the psychological parameters of both study groups may have been influenced by their therapeutic interactions with CBT. This hypothesis appears to be supported by the results of studies and meta-analyses that show improvements in, among others, anxiety and depression in people with spinal cord injuries following CBT [78–80].

The present study did not show an association between improvements in the gait function and functional independence after SCI and symptoms of anxiety and depression. These aspects are not correlated, which may be partly explained by the patients' subjective assessments of their health. The perceptions of health and objective physical-condition functional assessments were not the same among the SCI participants.

In opposite to our findings, the results of a review and meta-analysis by den Brave, M., et al. (2023) indicated improvement in depression-related outcomes after RAGT training [68]. Our results are also different from those obtained by Shahin et al. (2017), who noted a statistically significant difference between subjects rehabilitated with RAGT and those rehabilitated using conventional methods with DPT. This discrepancy may be due to the use of a different measurement tool and the size of the study group [81]. The referenced study was conducted on a group of forty people (N = 40) and depression was measured using the Beck Depression Inventory. However, other meta-analyses and retrospective studies indicate that there is insufficient evidence of an association between robotic rehabilitation and reductions in depression or improvements in quality of life [47]. Nevertheless, our results are largely consistent with other studies indicating that all rehabilitation interactions have beneficial effects on psychological well-being, emotional state and mood, and on lowering depressive symptoms. Many researchers emphasize that the most optimal results in re-educating gait and improving the overall functioning of patients with SCIs are obtained with conventional rehabilitation and the coordinated interaction of multiple specialist combinations [65,81]. This is due, among other things, to the peculiarities of neurological disorders, the physical effects of which are multi-systemic, translating into psycho-sociological aspects.

4.2. State Anxiety/Depression Status and Neurological Impairment, Depth of Injury and Type of Paralysis

Patients who participated in rehabilitation with the dynamic parapodium (S0) showed statistically significant reductions only in the level of state anxiety, while no improvements in the symptoms of depression were observed in patients with complete SCIs (AIS A). As we emphasized above, patients rehabilitated with RAGT with complete SCIs (AIS A) and incomplete impairment (AIS B, C, D) experienced reductions in both state anxiety and symptoms of depression, in contrast to patients with complete impairment (AIS A), who reported only reductions in state anxiety.

In the present study, there was also a significantly greater decrease in symptoms related to thinking about death and feeling alienated (moderate effect) in the control group among patients with incomplete spinal cord injuries compared with those with complete injuries (AIS A) according to the AIS A classification. Perhaps this can be explained by their improved neurological condition, which is important for greater mobility and independence. This allows patients to participate more in social life and feel higher levels of hope and satisfaction with life, and to make plans for the future.

Additionally, we observed no significant differences between the groups by type of paralysis (paraplegia vs. tetraplegia) in the reductions in state anxiety and symptoms of depression. The only difference was in the increase in self-regulation when comparing improvements by type of paralysis (i.e., paraplegia vs. tetraplegia). The results showed a greater increase in self-regulation in people with tetraplegia. The higher increase in the self-regulation abilities of people with tetraplegia can perhaps be explained by the initial low expectation of being able to change their condition and the low confidence in their ability to achieve their rehabilitation goals. Medical and paramedical staff are geared towards providing positive reinforcement, jointly setting motivating and satisfactory but realistic rehabilitation goals and giving patients the hope of achieving them, which positively influences the patients' growth in self-confidence and self-control and their subjective belief in their own self-efficacy in coping [72]. Hopes for the coordinated rehabilitation program allow us to anticipate its implications in the psychological dimension in the form of reductions in state anxiety and depression (i.e., common symptoms co-occurring with spinal cord injury) [21]. Psychological support and assistance are, according to many studies, as important as rehabilitation in the quest to improve the quality of life of people with spinal cord injuries [82].

4.3. General Discussion

Our study showed that all the study patients experienced fewer anxiety- and depression-related symptoms after the 7-week rehabilitation program. However, we did not observe significant differences between the groups (DPT vs. RAGT). The data obtained allow us to assume that RAGT can be recommended to patients with severe neurological conditions and total spinal cord injuries within the context of their emotional and affective states. Our research also suggests that an individual's perception of their own health and their actual physical health may not be the same. We can also assume that psychological support during rehabilitation is an essential part of the process.

There are several limitations to this study: (1) First of all, a sample size was not estimated before the start of the study. Despite this, a very large group of SCI patients participated in study. (2) Patients were self-recruited, which may have falsified the representativeness of this group among the general population of people with SCIs. (3) There were disproportionate numbers of patients between the experimental and control groups, and between those with complete and incomplete SCIs. This was mainly due to the decision of many patients to withdraw from the rehabilitation program after being informed that they had been assigned to the control group (DPT). Many patients hoped to have the opportunity to participate in robotic therapy. (4) There was a lack of qualitative control for and quantitative measurement of the patient-reported fear of falling that was experienced during exoskeleton rehabilitation. (5) Due to the patients' motor disabilities, the psychologist read the questionnaire questions, which may have disturbed the objectivity of the survey results. (6) The strict inclusion and exclusion criteria may have limited the reliability of generalizing the results to the general population. (7) It is also worth mentioning that non-parametric tests were used in this analysis, although the power of these tests (calculated as 1 minus the probability of making a 2nd degree error: an error of the second type, which involves accepting a null hypothesis that is in fact false. The probability of making an error of the second type is denoted by the symbol β. The values of α (the significance level) and β are related in such a way that a decrease in the probability of α causes an increase in the probability of β) is lower than for parametric tests. However, in some cases, their use is a better or even necessary choice. In the present study, the quantitative variables had a non-normal distribution, and the averages in the study groups were not equal or similar.

Future research should pay attention to the adaptation of the tools that measure mental health status to the special needs and difficulties of SCI patients or consider the validation of the existing instruments in this group of patients. Important research issues related to people with spinal cord injuries that should be considered in future studies are as follows: sexual problems; chronic pain; spastic tension vs. neuroticism and anxiety; the relationship of motivation levels on the outcomes of rehabilitation progress, anxiety and depression among caregivers and families of people with SCI; the social adaptation and socioeconomic functioning of patients post-institutional rehabilitation.

5. Conclusions

In conclusion, both types of rehabilitation (RAGT and DPT) appeared to be associated with reductions in anxiety- and depression-related symptoms. Rehabilitation with RAGT contributes to the strengthening the self-regulation abilities of patients with tetraplegia.

Author Contributions: Conceptualization, A.W.-S. and B.T.; methodology, A.W.-S., B.T. and B.K.; software, A.W.-S.; formal analysis, A.W.-S.; investigation, A.W.-S., B.T. and B.K.; data curation, A.W.-S., B.T. and B.K.; writing, A.W.-S., B.T. and J.W.; draft preparation, A.W.-S., B.T. and J.W.; writing—review and editing, B.T. and J.W.; visualization, A.W.-S.; supervision, B.T. and J.W.; project administration, B.T. and B.K. All authors have read and agreed to the published version of the manuscript.

Funding: This study was supported by a grant from the National Center for Research and Development, Poland (Nr POIR.01.01.01-00-0848/17-00).

Institutional Review Board Statement: The study was conducted in accordance with the Declaration of Helsinki and approved by the Ethics Committee of the District Medical Chamber in Szczecin (Poland) (Nr OIL-Sz/MF/KB/452/05/07/2018; Nr OIL-SZ/MF/KB/450/UKP/10/2018). The study was not preregistered before commencement.

Informed Consent Statement: Informed consent was obtained from all subjects involved in the study.

Data Availability Statement: Data are contained within the article.

Conflicts of Interest: The authors declare no conflict of interest.

References

1. Kumar, R.; Lim, L.; Mekary, R.A.; Rattani, A.; Dewan, M.C.; Sharif, Y.S.; Osorio-Fonseca, E.; Park, K.B. Traumatic Spinal Injury: Global Epidemiology and Worldwide Volume. *World Neurosurg.* **2018**, *113*, e345–e363. [CrossRef]
2. Tederko, P.; Jagodziński, R.; Krasuski, M.; Tarnacka, B. People with Spinal Cord Injury in Poland, Country Report. *Am. J. Phys. Med. Rehabil.* **2017**, *96*, 102–105. [CrossRef] [PubMed]
3. Wysocka, B.; Ślusarz, R.; Haor, B. Epidemiology of spinal cord injury in the own material of the Emergency Room in Włocławek: A retrospective study. *Neurol. Neurol. Nurs.* **2012**, *1*, 109–118.
4. Holanda, L.J.; Silva, P.M.M.; Amorim, T.C.; Lacerda, M.O.; Simão, C.R.; Morya, E. Robotic assisted gait as a tool for rehabilitation of individuals with spinal cord injury: A systematic review. *J. Neuroeng. Rehabil.* **2017**, *14*, 126. [CrossRef] [PubMed]
5. Maggio, M.G.; Naro, A.; De Luca, R.; Latella, D.; Balletta, T.; Caccamo, L.; Pioggia, G.; Bruschetta, D.; Calabrò, R.S. Body Representation in Patients with Severe Spinal Cord Injury: A Pilot Study on the Promising Role of Powered Exoskeleton for Gait Training. *J. Pers. Med.* **2022**, *12*, 619. [CrossRef] [PubMed]
6. Van Diemen, T.; van Leeuwen, C.; van Nes, I.; Geertzen, J.; Post, M. Body Image in Patients with Spinal Cord Injury during Inpatient Rehabilitation. *Arch. Phys. Med. Rehabil.* **2017**, *98*, 1126–1131. [CrossRef] [PubMed]
7. Craig, A.; Tran, Y.; Wijesuriya, N.; Middleton, J. Fatigue and tiredness in people with spinal cord injury. *J. Psychosom. Res.* **2012**, *73*, 205–210. [CrossRef]
8. Kalpakjian, C.Z.; Toussaint, L.T.; Albright, K.J.; Bombardier, C.H.; Krause, J.K.; Tate, D.G. Patient health Questionnaire-9 in spinal cord injury: An examination of factor structure as related to gender. *J. Spinal Cord Med.* **2009**, *32*, 147–156. [CrossRef]

9. Anderson, K.D. Targeting Recovery: Priorities of the Spinal Cord-Injured Population. *J. Neurotrauma* **2004**, *21*, 1371–1383. [CrossRef]
10. Le, J.; Dorstyn, D. Anxiety prevalence following spinal cord injury: A meta-analysis. *Spinal Cord* **2016**, *54*, 570–578. [CrossRef]
11. Craig, A.; Tran, Y.; Middleton, J. Psychological morbidity and spinal cord injury: A systematic review. *Spinal Cord* **2009**, *47*, 108–114. [CrossRef] [PubMed]
12. Hicks, A.L.; Martin, K.A.; Ditor, D.S.; Latimer, A.E.; Craven, C.; Bugaresti, J.; McCartney, N. Long-term exercise training in persons with spinal cord injury: Effects on strength, arm ergometry performance and psychological well-being. *Spinal Cord* **2003**, *41*, 34–43. [CrossRef] [PubMed]
13. Swank, C.; Holden, A.; McDonald, L.; Driver, S.; Callender, L.; Bennett, M.; Sikka, S. Foundational ingredients of robotic gait training for people with incomplete spinal cord injury during inpatient rehabilitation (FIRST): A randomized controlled trial protocol. *PLoS ONE* **2022**, *17*, e0267013. [CrossRef]
14. Charytoniuk, T.; Zywno, H.; Konstantynowicz-Nowicka, K.; Berk, K.; Bzdega, W.; Chabowski, A. Can Physical Activity Support the Endocannabinoid System in the Preventive and Therapeutic Approach to Neurological Disorders? *Int. J. Mol. Sci.* **2020**, *21*, 4221. [CrossRef] [PubMed]
15. Bedse, G.; Hill, M.N.; Patel, S. 2-Arachidonoylglycerol Modulation of Anxiety and Stress Adaptation: From grass roots to novel therapeutics. *Biol. Psychiatry* **2020**, *88*, 520–530. [CrossRef] [PubMed]
16. Katona, I.; Freund, T.F. Multiple Functions of Endocannabinoid Signaling in the Brain. *Annu. Rev. Neurosci.* **2012**, *35*, 529–558. [CrossRef]
17. Siebers, M.; Biedermann, S.V.; Bindila, L.; Lutz, B.; Fuss, J. Exercise-induced euphoria and anxiolysis do not depend on endogenous opioids in humans. *Psychoneuroendocrinology* **2021**, *126*, 105173. [CrossRef]
18. Balchin, R.; Linde, J.; Blackhurst, D.; Rauch, H.L.; Schönbächler, G. Sweating away depression? *The impact of intensive exercise on depression. J. Affect. Disord.* **2016**, *200*, 218–221.
19. Ong, B.; Wilson, J.R.; Henzel, M.K. Management of the Patient with Chronic Spinal Cord Injury. *Med. Clin. N. Am.* **2020**, *104*, 263–278. [CrossRef]
20. Alizo, G.; Sciarretta, J.D.; Gibson, S.; Muertos, K.; Holmes, S.; Denittis, F.; Cheatle, J.; Davis, J.; Pepe, A. Multidisciplinary team approach to traumatic spinal cord injuries: A single institution's quality improvement project. *Eur. J. Trauma Emerg. Surg.* **2018**, *44*, 245–250. [CrossRef]
21. Craig, A.; Perry, K.N.; Guest, R.; Tran, Y.; Dezarnaulds, A.; Hales, A.; Ephraums, C.; Middleton, J. Prospective Study of the Occurrence of Psychological Disorders and Comorbidities After Spinal Cord Injury. *Arch. Phys. Med. Rehabil.* **2015**, *96*, 1426–1434. [CrossRef]
22. Fleerkotte, B.M.; Koopman, B.; Buurke, J.H.; van Asseldonk, E.H.F.; van der Kooij, H.; Rietman, J.S. The effect of impedance-controlled robotic gait training on walking ability and quality in individuals with chronic incomplete spinal cord injury: An explorative study. *J. Neuroeng. Rehabil.* **2014**, *11*, 26. [CrossRef] [PubMed]
23. Ditunno, P.L.; Patrick, M.; Stineman, M.; Ditunno, J.F. Who wants to walk? Preferences for recovery after SCI: A longitudinal and cross-sectional study. *Spinal Cord* **2008**, *46*, 500–506. [CrossRef] [PubMed]
24. Daunoraviciene, K.; Adomaviciene, A.; Svirskis, D.; Griškevičius, J.; Juocevicius, A. Necessity of early-stage verticalization in patients with brain and spinal cord injuries: Preliminary study. *Technol. Health Care* **2018**, *26*, 613–623. [CrossRef]
25. Nordström, B.; Nyberg, L.; Ekenberg, L.; Näslund, A. The psychosocial impact on standing devices. *Disabil. Rehabil. Assist. Technol.* **2014**, *9*, 299–306. [CrossRef] [PubMed]
26. Tarnacka, B.; Korczyński, B.; Frasuńska, J. Impact of Robotic Assisted Gait Training in Subacute Spinal Cord Injury Patients on Outcome Measure. *Diagnostics* **2023**, *13*, 1966. [CrossRef]
27. Roque, A.; Tomczyk, A.; De Maria, E.; Putze, F.; Moucek, R.; Fred, A.; Gamboa, H. *Biomedical Engineering Systems and Technologies: 12th International Joint Conference, BIOSTEC 2019, Prague, Czech Republic, 22–24 February 2019*; Springer Nature: Berlin, Germany, 2019.
28. Available online: https://www.accessdata.fda.gov/scripts/cdrh/cfdocs/cfPCD/classification.cfm?ID=PHL (accessed on 2 June 2023).
29. Duddy, D.; Doherty, R.; Connolly, J.; Loughrey, J.; Condell, J.; Hassan, D.; Faulkner, M. The Cardiorespiratory Demands of Treadmill Walking with and without the Use of Ekso GT™ within Able-Bodied Participants: A Feasibility Study. *Int. J. Environ. Res. Public Health* **2022**, *19*, 6176. [CrossRef]
30. Høyer, E.; Opheim, A.; Jørgensen, V. Implementing the exoskeleton Ekso GT™ for gait rehabilitation in a stroke unit–feasibility, functional benefits and patient experiences. *Disabil. Rehabil. Assist. Technol.* **2020**, *17*, 473–479. [CrossRef] [PubMed]
31. Swank, C.; Sikka, S.; Driver, S.; Bennett, M.; Callender, L. Feasibility of integrating robotic exoskeleton gait training in inpatient rehabilitation. *Disabil. Rehabil. Assist. Technol.* **2019**, *15*, 409–417. [CrossRef]
32. Toderita, A.; Vlase, S. Reliability Study on PUR Injection Machine. *Procedia Manuf.* **2020**, *46*, 885–890. [CrossRef]
33. Federici, S.; Meloni, F.; Bracalenti, M.; De Filippis, M.L. The effectiveness of powered, active lower limb exoskeletons in neurorehabilitation: A systematic review. *NeuroRehabilitation* **2015**, *37*, 321–340. [CrossRef]
34. Mirbagheri, M.M.; Kindig, M.; Niu, X.; Varoqui, D.; Conaway, P. Robotic-locomotor training as a tool to reduce neuromuscular abnormality in spinal cord injury: The application of system identification and advanced longitudinal modeling. In Proceedings of the 2013 IEEE 13th International Conference on Rehabilitation Robotics (ICORR), Seattle, WA, USA, 24–26 June 2013. [CrossRef]

35. Moll, F.; Kessel, A.; Bonetto, A.; Stresow, J.; Herten, M.; Dudda, M.; Adermann, J. Use of Robot-Assisted Gait Training in Pediatric Patients with Cerebral Palsy in an Inpatient Setting—A Randomized Controlled Trial. *Sensors* **2022**, *22*, 9946. [CrossRef] [PubMed]
36. Ustinova, K.; Chernikova, L.; Bilimenko, A.; Telenkov, A.; Epstein, N. Effect of robotic locomotor training in an individual with Parkinson's disease: A case report. *Disabil. Rehabil. Assist. Technol.* **2011**, *6*, 77–85. [CrossRef] [PubMed]
37. Raigoso, D.; Céspedes, N.; Cifuentes, C.A.; del-Ama, A.J.; Múnera, M. A Survey on Socially Assistive Robotics: Clinicians' and Patients' Perception of a Social Robot within Gait Rehabilitation Therapies. *Brain Sci.* **2021**, *11*, 738. [CrossRef]
38. Donati, A.R.C.; Shokur, S.; Morya, E.; Campos, D.S.F.; Moioli, R.C.; Gitti, C.M.; Augusto, P.B.; Tripodi, S.; Pires, C.G.; Pereira, G.A.; et al. Long-term training with a brain-machine Interface-based gait protocol induces partial neurological recovery in paraplegic patients. *Sci. Rep.* **2016**, *6*, 30383. [CrossRef]
39. Hartigan, C.; Kandilakis, C.; Dalley, S.; Clausen, M.; Wilson, E.; Morrison, S.; Etheridge, S.; Farris, R. Mobility Outcomes Following Five Training Sessions with a Powered Exoskeleton. *Top. Spinal Cord Inj. Rehabil.* **2015**, *21*, 93–99. [CrossRef] [PubMed]
40. Juszczak, M.; Gallo, E.; Bushnik, T. Examining the Effects of a Powered Exoskeleton on Quality of Life and Secondary Impairments in People Living With Spinal Cord Injury. *Top. Spinal Cord Inj. Rehabil.* **2018**, *24*, 336–342. [CrossRef] [PubMed]
41. Rodríguez-Fernández, A.; Lobo-Prat, J.; Font-Llagunes, J.M. Systematic review on wearable lower-limb exoskeletons for gait training in neuromuscular impairments. *J. Neuroeng. Rehabil.* **2021**, *18*, 22. [CrossRef]
42. Bragoni, M.; Broccoli, M.; Iosa, M.; Morone, G.; De Angelis, D.; Venturiero, V.; Coiro, P.; Pratesi, L.; Mezzetti, G.; Fusco, A.; et al. Influence of psychologic features on rehabilitation outcomes in patients with subacute stroke trained with robotic-aided walking therapy. *Am. J. Phys. Med. Rehabil.* **2013**, *92*, 16–25. [CrossRef]
43. Kozlowski, A.J.; Fabian, M.; Lad, D.; Delgado, A.D. Feasibility and Safety of a Powered Exoskeleton for Assisted Walking for Persons With Multiple Sclerosis: A Single-Group Preliminary Study. *Arch. Phys. Med. Rehabil.* **2017**, *98*, 1300–1307. [CrossRef]
44. Ozsoy-Unubol, T.; Ata, E.; Cavlak, M.; Demir, S.; Candan, Z.; Yilmaz, F. Effects of Robot-Assisted Gait Training in Patients With Multiple Sclerosis: A Single-Blinded Randomized Controlled Study. *Am. J. Phys. Med. Rehabil.* **2021**, *101*, 768–774. [CrossRef] [PubMed]
45. Alashram, A.R.; Annino, G.; Padua, E. Robot-assisted gait training in individuals with spinal cord injury: A systematic review for the clinical effectiveness of Lokomat. *J. Clin. Neurosci.* **2021**, *91*, 260–269. [CrossRef] [PubMed]
46. Straudi, S.; Fanciullacci, C.; Martinuzzi, C.; Pavarelli, C.; Rossi, B.; Chisari, C.; Basaglia, N. The effects of robot-assisted gait training in progressive multiple sclerosis: A randomized controlled trial. *Mult. Scler. J.* **2016**, *22*, 373–384. [CrossRef] [PubMed]
47. Wier, L.M.; Hatcher, M.S.; Triche, E.W.; Lo, A.C. Effect of Robot-Assisted Versus Conventional Body-Weight-Supported Treadmill Training on Quality of Life for People With Multiple Sclerosis. *J. Rehabil. Res. Dev.* **2011**, *48*, 483. [CrossRef] [PubMed]
48. Middleton, J.; Tran, Y.; Craig, A. Relationship between quality of life and self-efficacy in persons with spinal cord injuries. *Arch. Phys. Med. Rehabil.* **2007**, *88*, 1643–1648. [CrossRef] [PubMed]
49. Shin, J.C.; Kim, J.Y.; Park, H.K.; Kim, N.Y. Effect of Robotic-Assisted Gait Training in Patients With Incomplete Spinal Cord Injury. *Ann. Rehabil. Med.* **2014**, *38*, 719–725. [CrossRef] [PubMed]
50. Ma, D.-N.; Zhang, X.-Q.; Ying, J.; Chen, Z.-J.; Li, L.-X. Efficacy and safety of 9 nonoperative regimens for the treatment of spinal cord injury. *Medicine* **2017**, *96*, 8679. [CrossRef]
51. Çinar, Ç.; Yildirim, M.A.; Öneş, K.; Gökşenoğlu, G. Effect of robotic-assisted gait training on functional status, walking and quality of life in complete spinal cord injury. *Int. J. Rehabil. Res.* **2021**, *44*, 262–268. [CrossRef]
52. Mustafaoglu, R.; Erhan, B.; Yeldan, I.; Gunduz, B.; Tarakci, E. Does robot-assisted gait training improve mobility, activities of daily living and quality of life in stroke? A single-blinded, randomized controlled trial. *Acta Neurol. Belg.* **2020**, *120*, 335–344. [CrossRef]
53. Calabrò, R.S.; Billeri, L.; Ciappina, F.; Balletta, T.; Porcari, B.; Cannavò, A.; Pignolo, L.; Manuli, A.; Naro, A. Toward improving functional recovery in spinal cord injury using robotics: A pilot study focusing on ankle rehabilitation. *Expert Rev. Med. Devices* **2022**, *19*, 83–95. [CrossRef]
54. Miller, L.; Zimmermann, A.; Herbert, W. Clinical effectiveness and safety of powered exoskeleton-assisted walking in patients with spinal cord injury: Systematic review with meta-analysis. *Med. Devices Evid. Res.* **2016**, *22*, 455–466. [CrossRef] [PubMed]
55. Nam, K.Y.; Kim, H.J.; Kwon, B.S.; Park, J.-W.; Lee, H.J.; Yoo, A. Robot-assisted gait training (Lokomat) improves walking function and activity in people with spinal cord injury: A systematic review. *J. Neuroeng. Rehabil.* **2017**, *14*, 24. [CrossRef] [PubMed]
56. Schwartz, I.; Meiner, Z. Robotic-Assisted Gait Training in Neurological Patients: Who May Benefit? *Ann. Biomed. Eng.* **2015**, *43*, 1260–1269. [CrossRef] [PubMed]
57. Stampacchia, G.; Olivieri, M.; Rustici, A.; D'Avino, C.; Gerini, A.; Mazzoleni, S. Gait rehabilitation in persons with spinal cord injury using innovative technologies: An observational study. *Spinal Cord* **2020**, *58*, 988–997. [CrossRef]
58. Zhang, L.; Lin, F.; Sun, L.; Chen, C. Comparison of Efficacy of Lokomat and Wearable Exoskeleton-Assisted Gait Training in People With Spinal Cord Injury: A Systematic Review and Network Meta-Analysis. *Front. Neurol.* **2022**, *13*, 772660. [CrossRef]
59. Calabrò, R.S.; Reitano, S.; Leo, A.; De Luca, R.; Melegari, C.; Bramanti, P. Can robot-assisted movement training (Lokomat) improve functional recovery and psychological well-being in chronic stroke? Promising findings from a case study. *Funct. Neurol.* **2014**, *29*, 139–141.
60. Hayes, S.C.; James Wilcox, C.R.; Forbes White, H.S.; Vanicek, N. The effects of robot assisted gait training on temporal-spatial characteristics of people with spinal cord injuries: A systematic review. *J. Spinal Cord Med.* **2018**, *41*, 529–543. [CrossRef]

61. Mıdık, M.; Paker, N.; Buğdaycı, D.; Mıdık, A.C. Effects of robot-assisted gait training on lower extremity strength, functional independence, and walking function in men with incomplete traumatic spinal cord injury. *Turk. J. Phys. Med. Rehabil.* **2020**, *66*, 54–59. [CrossRef]
62. Wan, C.; Huang, S.; Wang, X.; Ge, P.; Wang, Z.; Zhang, Y.; Li, Y.; Su, B. Effects of robot-assisted gait training on cardiopulmonary function and lower extremity strength in individuals with spinal cord injury: A systematic review and meta-analysis. *J. Spinal Cord Med.* **2023**, *27*, 1–9. [CrossRef]
63. Contreras-Vidal, J.L.; A Bhagat, N.; Brantley, J.; Cruz-Garza, J.G.; He, Y.; Manley, Q.; Nakagome, S.; Nathan, K.; Tan, S.H.; Zhu, F.; et al. Powered exoskeletons for bipedal locomotion after spinal cord injury. *J. Neural Eng.* **2016**, *13*, 031001. [CrossRef]
64. Rosado-Rivera, D.; Radulovic, M.; Handrakis, J.P.; Cirnigliaro, C.M.; Jensen, A.M.; Kirshblum, S.; Bauman, W.A.; Wecht, J.M. Comparison of 24-hour cardiovascular and autonomic function in paraplegia, tetraplegia, and control groups: Implications for cardiovascular risk. *J. Spinal Cord Med.* **2011**, *34*, 395–403. [CrossRef] [PubMed]
65. Goulet, J.; Richard-Denis, A.; Thompson, C.; Mac-Thiong, J.-M. Relationships between Specific Functional Abilities and Health-Related Quality of Life in Chronic Traumatic Spinal Cord Injury. *Am. J. Phys. Med. Rehabil.* **2018**, *98*, 14–19. [CrossRef] [PubMed]
66. O'Shea, T.M.; Burda, J.E.; Sofroniew, M.V. Cell biology of spinal cord injury and repair. *J. Clin. Investig.* **2017**, *127*, 3259–3270. [CrossRef]
67. Beck, J.S. *Cognitive Behavior Therapy: Basics and Beyond*, 2nd ed.; Guilford Press: New York, NY, USA, 2011.
68. den Brave, M.; Beaudart, C.; de Noordhout, B.M.; Gillot, V.; Kaux, J.-F. Effect of robot-assisted gait training on quality of life and depression in neurological impairment: A systematic review and meta-analysis. *Clin. Rehabil.* **2023**, *37*, 876–890. [CrossRef]
69. Łojek, E.; Stańczak, J.; Wójcik, A. *The Depression Assessment Questionarie. Manual*; Laboratory of Psychological Testing of the Polish Psychological Association: Warsaw, Poland, 2015.
70. Wrześniewski, K.; Jaworska, A.; Sosnowski, T.; Fecenec, D. *State-Trait Anxiety Inventory. Polish Adaptation of STAI. Manual*, 4th ed.; Laboratory of Psychological Testing of the Polish Psychological Association: Warsaw, Poland, 2011.
71. Bell, W.; Meyer, P.R.; Edelstein, D. American Spinal Injury Association (ASIA). *Paraplegia* **1984**, *22*, 45–54. [CrossRef]
72. Opera, J.; Mehlich, K.; Bielecki, A. Zastosowanie Indeksu Chodu po Urazie Rdzenia Kregowego-WISCI. *Ortop. Traumatol. Rehabil.* **2007**, *9*, 122–127.
73. Lam, T.; Noonan, V.K.; Eng, J.J. A systematic review of functional ambulation outcome measures in spinal cord injury. *Spinal Cord* **2008**, *46*, 246–254. [CrossRef]
74. Itzkovich, M.; Shefler, H.; Front, L.; Gur-Pollack, R.; Elkayam, K.; Bluvshtein, V.; Gelernter, I.; Catz, A. SCIM III (Spinal Cord Independence Measure version III): Reliability of assessment by interview and comparison with assessment by observation. *Spinal Cord* **2018**, *56*, 46–51. [CrossRef]
75. Itzkovich, M.; Gelernter, I.; Biering-Sorensen, F.; Weeks, C.; Laramee, M.T.; Craven, B.C.; Tonack, M.; Hitzig, S.L.; Glaser, E.; Zeilig, G.; et al. The Spinal Cord Independence Measure (SCIM) version III: Reliability and validity in a multi-center international study. *Disabil. Rehabil.* **2007**, *29*, 1926–1933. [CrossRef]
76. King, B.; Rosopa, P. *Statistical Reasoning in the Behavioral Sciences*, 6th ed.; John Wiley and Sons: Hoboken, NJ, USA, 2011; ISBN 978-1-118-53263-8.
77. Wrona-Polanska, H. Psychological aspects of informing patients about illness. In *Psychological Dimensions of Health, Crisis and Disease*, 1st ed.; Kubacka-Jasiecka, D., Ostrowski, T.M., Eds.; Jagiellonian University Publishing House: Cracow, Poland, 2005.
78. Mehta, S.; Orenczuk, S.; Hansen, K.T.; Aubut, J.-A.L.; Hitzig, S.L.; Legassic, M.; Teasell, R.W. An Evidence-Based Review of the Effectiveness of Cognitive Behavioral Therapy for Psychosocial Issues Post Spinal Cord Injury. *Rehabil. Psychol.* **2011**, *56*, 15–25. [CrossRef]
79. Mehta, S.; Hadjistavropoulos, H.; Nugent, M.; Karin, E.; Titov, N.; Dear, B.F. Guided internet-delivered cognitive-behaviour therapy for persons with spinal cord injury: A feasibility trial. *Spinal Cord* **2020**, *58*, 544–552. [CrossRef]
80. Dorstyn, D.; Mathias, J.L.; Denson, L. Efficacy of cognitive behavior therapy for the management of psychological outcomes following spinal cord injury A meta-analysis. *J. Health Psychol.* **2010**, *16*, 374–391. [CrossRef] [PubMed]
81. Dorstyn, D.S.; Mathias, J.L.; Denson, L.A. Psychological intervention during spinal rehabilitation: A preliminary study. *Spinal Cord* **2009**, *48*, 756–761. [CrossRef] [PubMed]
82. Shahin, A.A.; Shawky, S.A.; Rady, H.M.; Effat, D.A.; Abdelrahman, S.K.; Mohamed, E.; Awad, R. Effect of Robotic Assisted Gait Training on functional and psychological improvement in patients with Incomplete Spinal Cord Injury. *J. Nov. Physiother. Phys. Rehabil.* **2017**, *4*, 83–86. [CrossRef]

Disclaimer/Publisher's Note: The statements, opinions and data contained in all publications are solely those of the individual author(s) and contributor(s) and not of MDPI and/or the editor(s). MDPI and/or the editor(s) disclaim responsibility for any injury to people or property resulting from any ideas, methods, instructions or products referred to in the content.

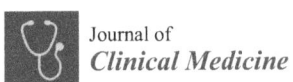

Article

Cortical Mechanisms Underlying Immersive Interactive Virtual Walking Treatment for Amelioration of Neuropathic Pain after Spinal Cord Injury: Findings from a Preliminary Investigation of Thalamic Inhibitory Function

Sylvia M. Gustin [1,2,*], Mark Bolding [3], William Willoughby [3], Monima Anam [4], Corey Shum [5], Deanna Rumble [6], Victor W. Mark [7], Lucie Mitchell [4], Rachel E. Cowan [7], Elizabeth Richardson [8], Scott Richards [7] and Zina Trost [9]

1. NeuroRecovery Research Hub, School of Psychology, University of New South Wales, Sydney 2052, Australia
2. Centre for Pain IMPACT, Neuroscience Research Australia, Sydney 2031, Australia
3. Department of Radiology, University of Alabama at Birmingham, Birmingham, AL 35233, USA
4. Department of Psychiatry and Behavioral Neurobiology, University of Alabama at Birmingham, Birmingham, AL 35233, USA; noriscat.mitchell@gmail.com (L.M.)
5. Immersive Experience Laboratories LLC, Birmingham, AL 35203, USA
6. Department of Psychology and Counseling, University of Central Arkansas, Conway, AR 72035, USA
7. Department of Physical Medicine & Rehabilitation, University of Alabama at Birmingham, Birmingham, AL 35233, USA
8. Department of Behavioral & Social Sciences, University of Montevallo, Montevallo, AL 35115, USA
9. Department of Psychological and Brain Sciences, Texas A&M University, College Station, TX 77843, USA
* Correspondence: s.gustin@unsw.edu.au; Tel.: +61-2-9399-1849

Abstract: Background: Neuropathic pain following spinal cord injury (SCI) affects approximately 60% of individuals with SCI. Effective pharmacological and non-pharmacological treatments remain elusive. We recently demonstrated that our immersive virtual reality walking intervention (VRWalk) may be effective for SCI NP. Additionally, we found that SCI NP may result from a decrease in thalamic γ-aminobutyric-acid (GABA), which disturbs central sensorimotor processing. Objective: While we identified GABAergic changes associated with SCI NP, a critical outstanding question is whether a decrease in SCI NP generated by our VRWalk intervention causes GABA content to rise. Method: A subset of participants ($n = 7$) of our VRWalk trial underwent magnetic resonance spectroscopy pre- and post-VRWalk intervention to determine if the decrease in SCI NP is associated with an increase in thalamic GABA. Results: The findings revealed a significant increase in thalamic GABA content from pre- to post-VRWalk treatment. Conclusion: While the current findings are preliminary and should be interpreted with caution, pre- to post-VRWalk reductions in SCI NP may be mediated by pre- to post-treatment increases in thalamic GABA by targeting and normalizing maladaptive sensorimotor cortex reorganization. Understanding the underlying mechanisms of pain recovery can serve to validate the efficacy of home-based VR walking treatment as a means of managing pain following SCI. Neuromodulatory interventions aimed at increasing thalamic inhibitory function may provide more effective pain relief than currently available treatments.

Keywords: virtual reality; spinal cord injury neuropathic pain; γ-aminobutyric acid; thalamus; MR spectroscopy

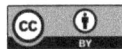

1. Introduction

Approximately 60% of individuals develop neuropathic pain following spinal cord injury (SCI NP). This type of pain is experienced at or below the zone of injury and is described as sharp, burning, and unbearable [1]. It remains persistent and intensifies progressively over time [2,3]. Although pharmacological agents (e.g., serotonin- and noradrenaline-reuptake inhibitors, antiepileptics, and tricyclic antidepressants) are treatment mainstays [4], none of them have consistently proven to be comprehensively effective [5–8]. Furthermore, many pain medications are associated with numerous negative side effects, such as somnolence, sleep disturbances, blurred vision, addiction, abuse, and toxicity [9–11]. Non-pharmacological therapies, such as repetitive transcranial magnetic stimulation, cranial electrotherapy stimulation, transcutaneous electrical nerve stimulation, and psychological interventions, have minimal negative side effects but result in only nominal reductions in pain [12]. As a result, many people with SCI experience ongoing neuropathic pain with no access to effective treatment.

Recently, we demonstrated that an immersive, interactive virtual walking intervention may be an effective treatment for unremitting SCI NP [13]. We pioneered an immersive, interactive virtual reality walking intervention (VRWalk) as a novel extension to visual feedback/illusory walking therapies that have previously been shown to reduce SCI NP [1,14–17]. Through our VRWalk interface, individuals with SCI can, for the first time, freely control their own virtual gait and interact by their own volition with a fully immersive virtual environment. In our study, we compared VRWalk to a passive, non-interactive walking treatment (analogous to previous feedback/illusory walking therapies) in people with SCI NP [13]. Participants in the interactive condition (VRWalk) showed a significant decrease in SCI NP intensity and interference pre- to post-intervention compared with the passive condition [13].

The significant analgesic improvement in participants who experienced VRWalk may be explained by changes occurring in contributing cortical mechanisms. For example, perceiving an environment in an immersive, first-person view activates sensorimotor brain regions more adaptively compared with passive, third-person perspectives [18,19]. This finding is important since SCI NP is associated with structural, functional, and biochemical changes in cortical areas important for sensorimotor processing, such as the thalamus, primary somatosensory cortex (S1), and motor cortex (M1) [20–23]. Animal models have demonstrated the role of thalamic γ-aminobutyric acid (GABA)-ergic processes in inhibiting pain [24–26]. Although data from human studies exhibited a cross-over design, it suggests that a decrease in GABA levels within the thalamic reticular nucleus (TRN) may disturb central sensorimotor processing, which in turn may result in SCI NP [22]. While we have identified thalamic neurochemical changes associated with SCI NP, a critical outstanding question is whether the decrease in SCI NP generated by our novel immersive, interactive VR treatment (VRWalk) is associated with a subsequent rise in GABA levels. To address this question, a subset of participants enrolled in the VRWalk trial [13] underwent magnetic resonance (MR) spectroscopy pre- and post-intervention to determine if the decrease in SCI NP is associated with an increase in thalamic GABA content.

2. Materials and Methods

2.1. Study Design

Single-arm study of neuroimaging data.

2.2. Participants

A pilot subset of seven participants from the interactive condition of the VRWalk trial [13] were randomly selected from the larger cohort and underwent GABA spectroscopy before and after the Interactive Virtual Walking condition at the University of Alabama at Birmingham (UAB) Highlands Hospital. We followed a simple random selection. The research assistant chose a name from the list of interactive VRWalk participants. Pilot funding from the UAB Department of Radiology facilitated imaging of the seven participants. Recruitment procedures, as well as inclusion and exclusion criteria, are fully outlined elsewhere [13]. To summarize, participants from the UAB SCI Model System of Care were included if they had complete paraplegia, as classified by the International Standards for Neurological Classification of Spinal Cord Injury (ISNCSCI). Participants were also included if they endorsed two or more items on the 4-item Spinal Cord Injury Pain Instrument (SCIPI), which has a strong overlap with clinical diagnoses of SCI NP [27].

Items 1–3 of the SCIPI pertain to pain descriptors commonly associated with SCI NP, while Item 4 identifies pain experienced in insensate areas. Eligible participants were between the ages of 18–65, had a diagnosed SCI for at least one year, experienced persistent SCI NP (for 3 months or longer) with a minimum severity of 4/10 on a Numeric Rating Scale (NRS), and had no changes in their pain medication regimen in the past month. Participants were excluded from participating in the VRWalk trial if they had a history of moderate to severe brain injury or severe psychiatric disorder [13] and were further excluded from the present study if they had any contraindication to MRI (e.g., implanted metal clips).

2.3. Regulatory Approvals

The VRWalk study protocol and imaging procedures were approved by the UAB Institutional Review Board (IRB-300001463, 3 May 2019), and all participants provided informed written consent. The VRWalk trial was registered on ClinicalTrials.gov (Identifier: NCT03735017; date of first registration: 8 November 2018). The VRWalk trial was a non-randomized single-arm trial; thus, blinding was not implemented.

2.4. Procedures

Prior to imaging and engaging in the VRWalk intervention, baseline pain intensity interference and disability measures were collected. Participants traveled to UAB to undergo MR spectroscopy prior to starting the VRWalk interactive condition. Following baseline scanning, participants returned to their residences, where they participated in the intervention. Research assistants traveled daily to participants' homes to set up the VR equipment for each session. Participants engaged in two separate 10 min VR gameplay sessions per day, with a minimum of 4 h between sessions, resulting in a total of 20 min of daily VR intervention over a span of 10 days within a two week period. Procedural details regarding delivery schedules have been described previously [13]. Pain intensity, interference, and disability measures were collected again after the last VRWalk session, and participants were brought back to UAB for post-intervention MR spectroscopy scanning.

2.5. Immersive Interactive Virtual Walking Interface

The VR game used in the VRWalk trial, developed by Immersive Experience Labs (IXL), used a cross-platform game engine (Unity Game Engine) and was made available for Windows PC devices. The VR game was hosted on digital distribution software, allowing participants' progression through the VR environment and gameplay to be saved between VR sessions over the entire intervention period. The immersive VR environment consisted of a first-person view from an avatar that could be customized to match participants' own physical characteristics (e.g., skin tone, weight, etc.). A research assistant oversaw each VRWalk session at participants' individual residences, including the research assistant configuring the VR equipment before each session, which is further described elsewhere [13]. The avatar and VR environment were presented to participants via an HTC Vive® Head Mounted Display (HMD) connected to a laptop computer. HTC Vive® includes hand-held controllers with accelerometers that capture actual movement to convert to virtual movement in the 3D VR environment (Figure 1). The HTC Vive® has native a frames per second (fps) rate of 90 fps. The rendering of the environment averaged ~60 fps, which was interpolated with the participant's motion to present 90 fps. In the interactive condition of the VRWalk trial, hand controllers tracked arm movements that were translated into movement of the virtual lower extremities. Progression through the virtual world was incentivized using limited monetary rewards. Details regarding gameplay incentives and how they were awarded have been described previously [13].

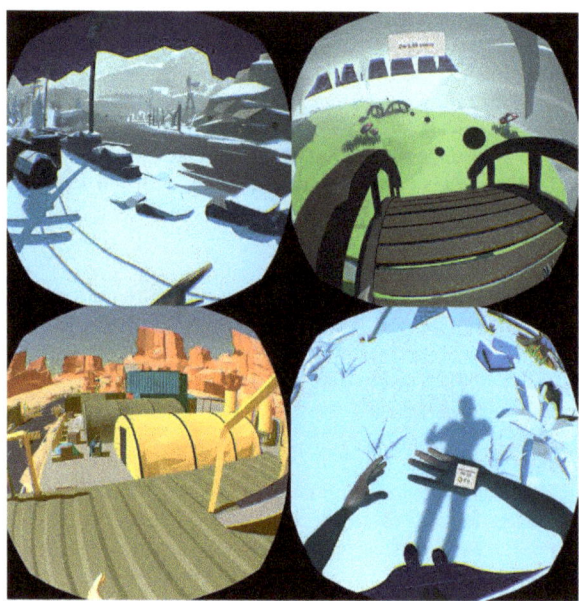

Figure 1. In-game graphics from three open virtual worlds.

2.6. Measures

2.6.1. Chronic Pain Measures

Pain Intensity

Participants' pain intensity was measured via a 0–10 Numeric Rating Scale (NRS), with anchors of 0 = "no pain" and 10 = "worst possible pain" [28,29]. The NRS is a psychometrically sound and frequently used measure that reliably captures changes in pain across time [30–33] and is a recommended measure to use in clinical trials assessing pain as an outcome [34]. In the present study, participants were asked to provide an average NRS rating over the past week before the VRWalk intervention and an average NRS rating one week following the completion of the 10 day intervention. Participants also completed a visual analog scale (VAS [35], 0 = "no pain" and 100 = "worst possible pain") to rate their current level of pain immediately prior to and following the 10 days of intervention. Both NRS and VAS were administered and completed by paper and asked specifically about participants' below-level neuropathic pain.

Pain Disability Index

The Pain Disability Index (PDI) [36] measures the degree of self-reported pain-related disability. Seven items are assessed on a 0–10 NRS in which 0 means no disability, and 10 is maximum disability. The sum of the seven items equals the total score of the PDI, which ranges from 0 to 70, with higher scores reflecting more pain-related disability. The PDI was assessed prior to and following the VRWalk intervention.

Pain Interference

Pain interference describes the extent to which pain restricts or disrupts individuals' physical, mental, and social activities [37]. Pain Interference was assessed using an NRS to measure how much neuropathic pain interfered with day-to-day activities in the last week, ranging from 0 (No Interference) to 10 (Extreme Interference). Pain interference was assessed prior to and after the VRWalk intervention.

Neuropathic Pain Scale

The Neuropathic Pain Scale (NPS) [38] was used to measure the severity of SCI NP symptoms. The NPS encompasses eight items addressing specific NP qualities rated on a 0 to 10 scale (e.g., "not burning" to "the most burning sensation imaginable"). The NPS has good psychometric properties and is recommended for measuring change in SCI-NP in clinical trials [33]. A composite sum of the eight items was used, with higher scores indicating greater severity of SCI-NP. The NPS was collected before and after the VRWalk intervention.

2.7. MR Spectroscopy Measures

GABA-Edited MEscher–GArwood Point RESolved Spectroscopy (MEGA-PRESS) Spectra

Participants laid supine headfirst on the bed of a 3T MRI system (Siemens MAGNETOM Prisma) with their heads immobilized in a 32-channel head coil. A T1-weighted, magnetization-prepared rapid gradient echo (MPRAGE) 3D imaging sequence with 1 mm isotropic voxels was acquired. We used multi-planar reformats (axial, sagittal, coronal) for voxel placement. GABA-edited MEGA-PRESS spectra were acquired from a voxel ($20 \times 20 \times 20$ mm^3) centered in each participant in the right thalamus (Figure 2). While the voxel covered the entire thalamus, the TRN contains nearly all of the GABAergic neurons within the thalamus [39]; thus, any measured GABA content is located in the TRN. The GABA-edited MEGA-PRESS sequence parameters were as follows: repetition time (TR) = 2000 ms, echo time (TE) = 68 ms, 256 averages, and total acquisition time: 20 min. One hundred twenty eight averages were acquired with the MEGA pulse centered at 1.9 ppm (ON) and 128 averages with the pulse centered at 7.5 ppm (OFF). We performed manual shimming, which resulted in line widths of <10 Hz for all spectra. The Siemens Brain Dot Engine auto-align function was used to ensure consistency in the follow-up voxel placement of the same participant and from participant to participant.

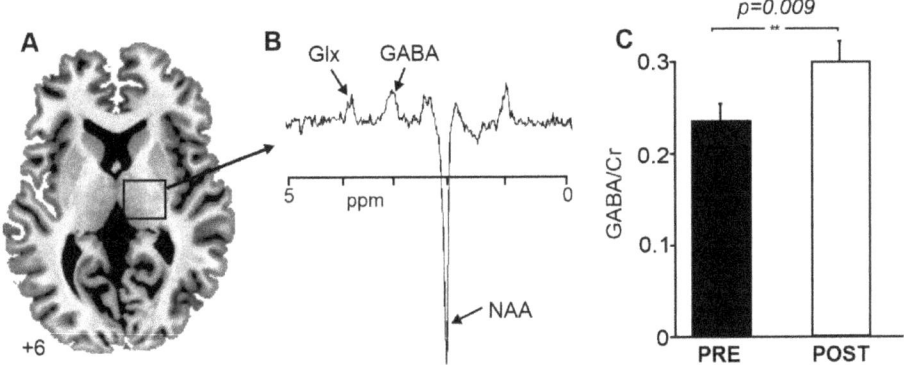

Figure 2. (**A**) Axial slice showing the location from which GABA-edited MEGA-PRESS spectroscopy was performed in the right thalamus of participants. The slice location in the Montreal Neurological Institute space is indicated at the lower left of the image. (**B**) Typical MEGA-PRESS spectrum obtained from the thalamus. (**C**) A plot of the mean (±SD) GABA/creatine ratios in the thalamus of participants prior to and following 10 days of Immersive Interactive Virtual Walking Treatment. Glx: glutamine; GABA: gamma-aminobutyric acid; Cr: Creatine; ppm: parts per million.

2.8. Analysis

2.8.1. GABA-Edited MEGA-PRESS Spectral Analysis

The acquired spectra were analyzed using the Java-based magnetic resonance user interface (jMRUI 6.0, European Union project). We summed the "ON" and "OFF" spectral subsets to produce single "ON" and "OFF" 68 ms sub-spectra for each spectra dataset. These 68 ms sub-spectra were then subtracted, resulting in GABA-edited MEGA-Press difference spectra to measure GABA concentration at 3.01 ppm. The GABA-edited MEGA-PRESS difference spectra were phased with respect to both the zero- and first-order phases. GABA was quantified using AMARES, a nonlinear least-square fitting algorithm operating in the time domain. Peak fitting for GABA was performed after manually defining the center frequency and line width of the GABA peak and modeling the GABA peak as a singlet. We used Lorentzian curves to obtain the peak amplitude for this resonance.

The "OFF" spectral subsets were summed, producing a single "OFF" 68 ms sub-spectra for each spectra dataset to measure creatine concentration at 3.02 ppm. The single "OFF" 68 ms sub-spectra was t-phased with respect to both the zero- and first-order phases. Spectral fitting in Advanced Method for Accurate, Robust, and Efficient Spectral Fitting (AMARES) was performed after manually defining the center frequency and line width of the creatine peak and modeling the creatine peak as a singlet. AMARES represents an enhanced technique to precisely and efficiently estimate the parameters of noisy magnetic resonance spectroscopy (MRS) signals in the time domain. We calculated ratios for GABA relative to creatine.

2.8.2. Spectral Quality Assessment

We calculated the variances from the peak areas and the standard deviations of the fit for GABA in each participant to assess the goodness of fit. Average line widths and signal-to-noise ratios (SNRs) were also examined. We assessed SNRs using the peak amplitudes of N-acetylaspartate (NAA) in the GABA OFF spectrum compared with the peak amplitude of the noise from a signal-free section of the spectrum of approximately 10 ppm in each participant.

2.8.3. Data Analysis

We calculated means and standard deviations for NRS, VAS, and GABA/creatine ratios. Paired sample t-tests were used to examine alterations in pain intensity and GABA/creatine ratios measured before and after the VRWalk intervention. Significant correlations between pain and neurochemical data were examined through Pearson correlations. SPSS version 26.0 (IBM SPSS Statistics) was used to perform the statistical analyses. A significance level of $p < 0.05$ was used across this study.

3. Results

3.1. Pain Intensity

The demographics and pain characteristics of the sample are shown in Table 1. Although the time since injury varied, all participants had a complete thoracic spinal cord injury. Participants showed a significant decrease in NRS ratings of average pain collected prior to and following the intervention (mean NRS $\pm$ SD PRE Intervention: 5.6 ± 2.4; mean NRS $\pm$ SD POST Intervention: 3.4 ± 1.7; t = -0.037, df = 6, $p = 0.023$; Figure 3, individual NRS values are represented in Table 2). Participants also showed a significant decrease in VAS ratings of pain collected prior to and after the intervention (mean VAS $\pm$ SD PRE Intervention: 52 ± 31; mean VAS $\pm$ SD POST Intervention: 22 ± 19; t = 3.648, df = 6, $p = 0.011$; Figure 3, individual VAS values are represented in Table 2). There was a decrease in NPS ratings of pain severity from pre- to post-intervention that approached significance (mean PDI PRE Intervention: 19 ± 10; mean PDI POST Intervention $\pm$ SD POST Intervention: 21 ± 20; t = -0.486, df = 6, $p = 0.644$; mean Pain Interference PRE Intervention: 2.1 ± 2.3; mean Pain Interference POST Intervention $\pm$ SD POST Intervention: 0.6 ± 0.8; t = 3.161, df = 6, $p = 0.052$). Participants showed a marginal trend toward a significant decrease in NPS ratings of pain severity collected prior to and following the intervention (mean NPS $\pm$ SD PRE Intervention: 40.6 ± 15; mean NRS $\pm$ SD POST Intervention: 25.0 ± 16; t = 2.408, df = 6, $p = 0.053$; Figure 3, individual NPS values are represented in Table 2). None of the seven participants reported any adverse effects related to the VRWalk intervention.

Table 1. Participant Demographic and Pain Characteristics.

Code	Sex	Age	ASIA ISNCSCI Grade	Level of Injury	Years Since Injury	Pain Duration (Years)	Pain Location	Pain Level	Pain Medication
1	M	23	A	T7	5	5	Bilateral back, feet	Below	None
2	M	35	A	T7	15	15	Bilateral feet, shins	Below	None
3	M	36	A	T12	10	10	Left buttocks, left lower back	Below	None
4	M	48	A	T12	6	6	Bilateral toes	Below	Baclofen, gabapentin
5	M	48	A	T1	14	14	Bilateral buttocks, feet	Below	None
6	M	56	A	T10	11	11	Bilateral toes, upper legs	Below	Baclofen, gabapentin
7	M	70	A	T11–12	4	4	Bilateral abdomen, legs	Below	None

Note. M = male; ASIA ISNCSCI = International Standards for Neurological Classification of Spinal Cord Injury American Spinal Injury Association; Neurological level: T = thoracic level.

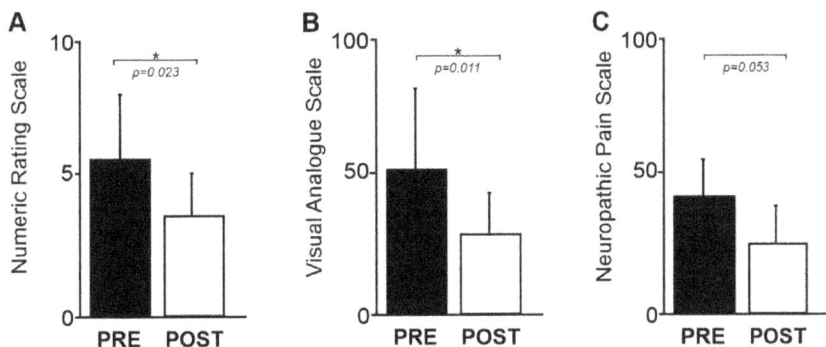

Figure 3. (**A**) A plot of the mean (±SD) numeric rating scale (NRS) rating over the preceding week before the VRWalk intervention as well as approximately one week following the completion of the 10 day intervention. (**B**) A plot of the mean (±SD) visual analog scale (VAS) values of current pain intensity of participants prior to and after 10 days of VRWalk intervention. (**C**) A plot of the mean (±SD) neuropathic pain scale (NPS) ratings of pain severity prior to and after 10 days of VRWalk intervention.

Table 2. Individual GABA/creatine ratios, numeric rating scale (NRS), and visual analog Scale (VAS) values.

Code	Pain Duration (Years)	GABA/Cr (ppm) PRE Therapy	GABA/Cr (ppm) POST Therapy	NRS PRE Therapy	NRS POST Therapy	VAS PRE Therapy	VAS POST Therapy	NPS PRE Therapy	NPS POST Therapy
1	5	0.25	0.31	6	2	30	8	24	11
2	15	0.21	0.27	9	6	85	48	63	15
3	10	0.24	0.36	8	5	80	13	55	56
4	6	0.28	0.26	3	3	77	50	27	10
5	14	0.21	0.27	6	3	55	15	46	21
6	11	0.24	0.29	4	1	3	1	36	28
7	4	0.22	0.31	3	4	32	21	33	34
Mean (±SD)	9.3 ± 4.4	0.24 ± 0.022	0.30 ± 0.034	5.6 ± 2.4	3.4 ± 1.7	52 ± 31	22 ± 19	40.6 ± 15	25 ± 16

Note. Cr = Creatine; NRS = Numeric Rating Scale; VAS = Visual Analogue Scale; ppm = ppm: parts per million; GABA = gamma-aminobutyric acid; NPS = Neuropathic Pain Scale.

3.2. GABA-Edited MEGA-PRESS Spectroscopy

Participants showed a significant decrease in mean GABA/creatine ratios from pre- to post-VRWalk intervention (mean GABA/creatine ratio ± SD PRE Intervention: 0.24 ± 0.022; mean GABA/creatine ratio ± SD POST Intervention: 0.3 ± 0.034; t = −3.825, df = 6, p = 0.009; Figure 1, individual GABA/creatine ratios are represented in Table 2). However, there was no significant linear relationship between the change in GABA/creatine ratios and the change in pain intensity from pre- to post-intervention (NRS: r = −0.282, p = 0.3; VAS: r = −0.417, p = 0.2, Table 3). There was also no significant linear correlation between pre-intervention GABA/creatine ratios and pre-intervention NRS ratings (r = −0.2, p = 0.3, Table 3) and pre-intervention GABA/creatine ratios and participants' pain duration (r = −0.4, p = 0.2, Table 3). Though the Pearson correlation coefficient was of moderate strength between pre-intervention GABA/creatine ratios and pre-intervention VAS ratings, it did not reach significance (r = 0.5, p = 0.1, Table 3). Similarly, there was a positive linear correlation between post-intervention GABA/creatine ratios and post-intervention NRS ratings; this relationship did not reach the statistical threshold for significance (r = 0.6, p = 0.1, Table 3). Lastly, there was no significant relationship between post-intervention GABA/creatine ratios and post-intervention VAS ratings (r = −0.2, p = 0.3, Table 3).

Table 3. Correlations.

Variable 1	Variable 2	Correlation Coefficient (r)	Significance Level (p)
Change in GABA/creatine ratios from pre- to post-intervention	Change in pain intensity (NRS) from pre- to post-intervention	−0.282	0.3
Change in GABA/creatine ratios from pre- to post-intervention	Change in pain intensity (VAS) from pre- to post-intervention	0.417	0.2
Pre-intervention GABA/creatine ratios	Pre-intervention NRS ratings	−0.2	0.3
Pre-intervention GABA/creatine ratios	Pain duration	−0.04	0.2
Pre-intervention GABA/creatine ratios	Pre-intervention VAS ratings	0.5	0.1
Post-intervention GABA/creatine ratios	Post-intervention NRS ratings	0.6	0.1
Post-intervention GABA/creatine ratios	Post-intervention NRS ratings	−0.2	0.3

Note. Cr = NRS = Numeric Rating Scale; VAS = Visual Analogue Scale; GABA = gamma-aminobutyric acid.

Two of the seven participants were treated with baclofen and gabapentin (Table 1). Both participants' medication regimens were constant across the intervention. When both participants were excluded from the paired t-test analysis, the results still showed a significant decrease in mean GABA/creatine ratios from pre- to post-VRWalk intervention (mean GABA/creatine ratio ± SD PRE Intervention: 0.23 ± 0.016; mean GABA/creatine ratio ± SD POST Intervention: 0.3 ± 0.032; t = −7.364, df = 4, p = 0.002).

3.3. Spectral Quality Assessment

Line widths, SNRs, and variances of GABA and creatine were all well within acceptable limits for data quality according to the consensus on clinical MRS of the brain [40,41]. Line widths for all spectra were <10 Hz after manual shimming. Furthermore, there was no significant difference in the mean-variance of GABA (%) between pre- and post-intervention (GABA variance mean ± SD: PRE Intervention: 17.4 ± 4.5% (minimum 13.12; maximum 26.17); POST Intervention: 18.1 ± 4.1% (minimum 13.0; maximum 23.06); t = −0.305, df = 6, p = 0.77). There was also no significant difference in the mean-variance (%) of creatine between pre- and post-intervention (creatine variance mean ± SD: PRE Intervention:

5.0 ± 0.67% (minimum 4.18; maximum 5.26); POST Intervention: 5.00 ± 0.61% (minimum 4.40; maximum 5.95); t = −0.037, df = 6, p = 0.97). Finally, there was no significant difference in mean SNR ratios between before and after intervention (SNR ratios mean GABA spectra: PRE Intervention ± SD: 11.0 ± 2.2 (minimum 8.83; maximum 13.25); POST Intervention: 11.4 ± 3.7 (minimum 3.28; maximum 13.3); t = −0.339, df = 6, p = 0.75).

4. Discussion

This study demonstrated that individuals with SCI NP have a significant change in thalamic GABA content pre- compared with post-VWalk treatment. That is, individuals with SCI NP have significantly increased GABA/creatine ratios following a 10 day immersive, interactive virtual walking therapy compared with pre-intervention. Participants also reported a significant decline in SCI NP intensity following VRWalk treatment [13], though there was no significant correlation between GABA/creatine ratios and SCI NP intensity as well as pain duration, as evidenced by the present pilot results. Nevertheless, these results indicate an association between SCI NP and neurotransmitter dysregulation in the thalamus, consistent with similar dysregulation observed in other central nervous system regions, such as the medial prefrontal cortex in SCI NP [42,43].

While speculative in the context of the current finding, this plausibly aligns with a cortical model of disinhibition in which the cortical inability to suppress pain potentially underlies the experience of SCI NP [44]. In line with this model, we suggested that a decrease in the inhibitory neurotransmitter GABA in the thalamic reticular nucleus (TRN) results in an altered thalamocortical connection between the TRN and the sensorimotor cortex [22]. The disruption of TRN—sensorimotor cortex connection may lead to functional changes within the sensorimotor cortex. For instance, individuals experiencing SCI NP have shown reorganization in the primary somatosensory (S1) cortex, leading to a diminution of activity in regions related to innervating the legs and a rearrangement of cortical representation for other body regions (i.e., the little finger and thumb) toward regions normally associated with innervating the legs [23]. Additionally, individuals with SCI NP exhibit functional alterations in the primary motor cortex (M1) when engaging with imagery of lower extremity movement, resulting in modulation of SCI NP through neural processes or neuromodulation [21]. Notably, the extent of these sensorimotor functional changes significantly relates to SCI NP intensity [21,23], making these functional alterations a potential target for intervention. Indeed, evidence suggests visual feedback interventions may activate sensorimotor areas in the brain, resulting in decreased SCI NP [1,14–17,30]. Thus, visual illusion modalities, such as virtual walking, may activate the sensorimotor cortex in an adaptive manner with the consequence that SCI NP is reduced. Moreover, incorporating a first-person perspective to such modalities, as was performed in the VRWalk intervention, may engage cortical motor networks to a greater extent than third-person perspectives [18,19]. These effects could potentially be amplified by the heightened presence and immersion achieved from a first-person perspective [45], which are characteristics of VR paradigms previously associated with increased reductions in pain [46–48].

Although preliminary, the results of the current study indicate that creating a completely immersive experience of walking in a normal gait, as achieved in the VRWalk intervention, could potentially activate cortical regions associated with sensorimotor execution and control (i.e., S1 and M1). This, in turn, might positively influence the corticothalamic circuit, resulting in the stabilization of neurotransmitter dysregulation associated with pain, as evident in the elevated thalamic GABA content. Although we did not measure S1 and M1 activation in this study, participants reported a sensation of performing and sensing a walking motion [13], providing anecdotal evidence that both S1 and M1 might have been activated in an adaptive manner. In line with this argument, evidence shows that both real and illusory sensorimotor stimulation results in a decrease in neuropathic pain by targeting the sensorimotor cortex, which has been previously found to functionally reorganize following SCI and amputation [14,16,49].

The specific cortical mechanisms underlying pain relief of illusory sensorimotor stimulation remain unclear. For example, any temporal causal relationship that exists between illusory sensorimotor cortex stimulation via the immersive VRWalk intervention and sensorimotor cortex activation, thalamocortical connection, and thalamic GABA concentration is not evident from this study. Nonetheless, this preliminary study indicates that further investigation of changes in thalamic GABA concentrations and its role in normalizing inhibitory function is potentially a fruitful line of future research. Specifically, future studies with larger samples are needed to determine the potential mediating role of changes in thalamic GABA on SCI NP reductions following the VRWalk intervention, as well as its role in reversing maladaptive sensorimotor cortex reorganization associated with chronic pain.

5. Limitations

The current study was pilot in nature, and while it provides direction for future research, it lacks a sufficient sample size to infer true population effects from these results alone. The small sample size also prevented the control of individual differences in medication types (i.e., two out of seven participants were treated with baclofen and gabapentin), even though participants' medication regimens remained constant during the intervention. Despite this, the results still demonstrated a significant decrease in mean GABA/creatine ratios from pre- to post-VWalk intervention, even after excluding the two participants on pain medications. Nevertheless, it is important to consider that certain SCI NP medications, such as anticonvulsants, may impact GABAergic systems [50]. Future research investigating neurotransmitter mechanisms underlying pain reduction should take this into account. Furthermore, since all seven participants were exposed to the interactive VRWalk intervention, there is no comparator group to definitively rule out any effect of time on changes in thalamic GABA concentrations and pain intensity or to account for other potential confounding factors. Thus, we cannot fully determine whether the observed reduction in GABA content and pain intensity was due to the intervention or other factors. This study also lacks an able-bodied control or non-SCI chronic pain comparator group, which would clarify whether changes in GABA/creatine ratios following VRWalk intervention are unique to those with SCI-NP. Due to the lack of follow-up scanning sessions, we were not able to determine if both the decrease in pain intensity and the increase in GABA content persisted over time. Future studies should incorporate follow-up measurements to investigate whether the effects of 10 days of interactive VRWalk treatment on pain intensity and GABA content extend beyond the intervention period.

6. Conclusions

The current study advances existing research on illusory walking treatment for SCI NP by providing first hints about the action of immersive virtual reality treatment on the human brain. While caution should be used when interpreting these preliminary results, they nonetheless suggest that immersive virtual walking may alleviate SCI NP through the normalization of thalamic neurotransmitter dysregulation. Future studies are called for to better understand and confirm causal mechanisms. GABAergic changes may play a role in a larger model of cortical change associated with virtual reality walking that involves activating the sensorimotor cortex. Neuromodulative interventions aimed at increasing thalamic inhibitory function may provide more effective pain relief than currently available treatments.

Author Contributions: S.M.G., M.B. and Z.T. designed the work that led to the submission. All authors played an important role in interpreting the results. S.M.G. and E.R. drafted the manuscript. All authors revised the manuscript for important intellectual content and approved the final version. All authors agreed to be accountable for all aspects of the work in ensuring that questions related to the accuracy or integrity of any part of the work are appropriately investigated and resolved. All authors have read and agreed to the published version of the manuscript.

Funding: This work was supported by the Craig H. Neilsen Foundation (Spinal Cord Injury on the Translational Spectrum [SCIRTS] Pilot Grant), International Association for the Study of Pain ([IASP] Collaborative International Grant), the Congressionally Designated Medical Research Program ([CDMRP SCIRP] Spinal Cord Injury Research Development Grant), University of Alabama at Birmingham (UAB) Department of Radiology and the Rebecca L. Cooper Medical Research Foundation.

Institutional Review Board Statement: The study was conducted in accordance with the Declaration of Helsinki, and approved by the University of Alabama at Birmingham (UAB) Institutional Review Board (IRB-300001463, approved on 3 May 2019).

Informed Consent Statement: Informed consent was obtained from all subjects involved in the study.

Data Availability Statement: The datasets generated and/or analyzed during the current study are available from the corresponding author upon reasonable request.

Conflicts of Interest: The authors declare no competing interests.

References

1. Moseley, G.L. Using visual illusion to reduce at-level neuropathic pain in paraplegia. *Pain* **2007**, *130*, 294–298. [PubMed]
2. Finnerup, N.B. Pain in patients with spinal cord injury. *PAIN®* **2013**, *154*, S71–S76. [PubMed]
3. Siddall, P. Management of neuropathic pain following spinal cord injury: Now and in the future. *Spinal Cord* **2009**, *47*, 352–359.
4. Finnerup, N.B.; Attal, N.; Haroutounian, S.; McNicol, E.; Baron, R.; Dworkin, R.H.; Gilron, I.; Haanpää, M.; Hansson, P.; Jensen, T.S.; et al. Pharmacotherapy for neuropathic pain in adults: A systematic review and meta-analysis. *Lancet Neurol.* **2015**, *14*, 162–173. [CrossRef]
5. Baastrup, C.; Finnerup, N.B. Pharmacological management of neuropathic pain following spinal cord injury. *CNS Drugs* **2008**, *22*, 455–475. [PubMed]
6. Mehta, S.; McIntyre, A.; Janzen, S.; Loh, E.; Teasell, R.; Spinal Cord Injury Rehabilitation Evidence Team. Systematic review of pharmacologic treatments of pain after spinal cord injury: An update. *Arch. Phys. Med. Rehabil.* **2016**, *97*, 1381–1391.e1.
7. Snedecor, S.; Sudharshan, L.; Cappelleri, J.C.; Sadosky, A.; Desai, P.; Jalundhwala, Y.J.; Botteman, M. Systematic review and comparison of pharmacologic therapies for neuropathic pain associated with spinal cord injury. *J. Pain Res.* **2013**, *6*, 539. [PubMed]
8. Finnerup, N.B.; Haroutounian, S.; Baron, R.; Dworkin, R.H.; Gilron, I.; Haanpaa, M.; Jensen, T.S.; Kamerman, P.R.; McNicol, E.; Moore, A.; et al. Neuropathic pain clinical trials: Factors associated with decreases in estimated drug efficacy. *Pain* **2018**, *159*, 2339–2346. [CrossRef]
9. Hagen, E.M.; Rekand, T. Management of neuropathic pain associated with spinal cord injury. *Pain Ther.* **2015**, *4*, 51–65.
10. Ahn, S.-H.; Park, H.-W.; Lee, B.-S.; Moon, H.-W.; Jang, S.-H.; Sakong, J.; Bae, J.-H. Gabapentin effect on neuropathic pain compared among patients with spinal cord injury and different durations of symptoms. *Spine* **2003**, *28*, 341–346.
11. Cardenas, D.D.; Nieshoff, E.C.; Suda, K.; Goto, S.; Sanin, L.; Kaneko, T.; Sporn, J.; Parsons, B.; Soulsby, M.; Yang, R.; et al. A randomized trial of pregabalin in patients with neuropathic pain due to spinal cord injury. *Neurology* **2013**, *80*, 533–539. [CrossRef]
12. Boldt, I.; Eriks-Hoogland, I.; Brinkhof, M.W.; de Bie, R.; Joggi, D.; von Elm, E. Non-pharmacological interventions for chronic pain in people with spinal cord injury. *Cochrane Database Syst. Rev.* **2014**, CD009177. [CrossRef]
13. Trost, Z.; Anam, M.; Seward, J.; Shum, C.; Rumble, D.; Sturgeon, J.; Mark, V.; Chen, Y.Y.; Mitchell, L.; Cowan, R.; et al. Immersive Interactive Virtual Walking Reduces Neuropathic Pain in Spinal Cord Injury: Findings from a Preliminary Investigation of Feasibility and Clinical Efficacy. *Pain* **2022**, *163*, 350–361.
14. Eick, J.; Richardson, E.J. Cortical activation during visual illusory walking in persons with spinal cord injury: A pilot study. *Arch. Phys. Med. Rehabil.* **2015**, *96*, 750–753.
15. Jordan, M.; Richardson, E.J. Effects of Virtual Walking Treatment on Spinal Cord Injury–Related Neuropathic Pain: Pilot Results and Trends Related to Location of Pain and at-level Neuronal Hypersensitivity. *Am. J. Phys. Med. Rehabil.* **2016**, *95*, 390–396.
16. Soler, M.D.; Kumru, H.; Pelayo, R.; Vidal, J.; Tormos, J.M.; Fregni, F.; Navarro, X.; Pascual-Leone, A. Effectiveness of transcranial direct current stimulation and visual illusion on neuropathic pain in spinal cord injury. *Brain* **2010**, *133*, 2565–2577. [PubMed]
17. Richardson, E.J.; McKinley, E.C.; Rahman, A.; Klebine, P.; Redden, D.T.; Richards, J.S. Effects of virtual walking on spinal cord injury-related neuropathic pain: A randomized, controlled trial. *Rehabil. Psychol.* **2019**, *64*, 13. [PubMed]
18. Kobashi, N.; Holper, L.; Scholkmann, F.; Kiper, D.; Eng, K. Enhancement of motor imagery-related cortical activation during first-person observation measured by functional near-infrared spectroscopy. *Eur. J. Neurosci.* **2012**, *35*, 1513–1521. [PubMed]
19. Jackson, P.L.; Meltzoff, A.N.; Decety, J. Neural circuits involved in imitation and perspective-taking. *Neuroimage* **2006**, *31*, 429–439. [PubMed]
20. Gustin, S.; Wrigley, P.; Siddall, P.; Henderson, L. Brain anatomy changes associated with persistent neuropathic pain following spinal cord injury. *Cereb. Cortex* **2010**, *20*, 1409–1419.
21. Gustin, S.M.; Wrigley, P.J.; Henderson, L.A.; Siddall, P.J. Brain circuitry underlying pain in response to imagined movement in people with spinal cord injury. *PAIN®* **2010**, *148*, 438–445.

22. Gustin, S.M.; Wrigley, P.J.; Youssef, A.M.; McIndoe, L.; Wilcox, S.L.; Rae, C.D.; Edden, R.; Siddall, P.J.; Henderson, L.A. Thalamic activity and biochemical changes in individuals with neuropathic pain after spinal cord injury. *PAIN®* **2014**, *155*, 1027–1036. [CrossRef]
23. Wrigley, P.J.; Press, S.R.; Gustin, S.M.; Macefield, V.G.; Gandevia, S.C.; Cousins, M.J.; Middleton, J.W.; Henderson, L.A.; Siddall, P. Neuropathic pain and primary somatosensory cortex reorganization following spinal cord injury. *PAIN®* **2009**, *141*, 52–59. [CrossRef]
24. Kramer, P.R.; Stinson, C.; Umorin, M.; Deng, M.; Rao, M.; Bellinger, L.L.; Yee, M.B.; Kinchington, P.R. Lateral thalamic control of nociceptive response after whisker pad injection of varicella zoster virus. *Neuroscience* **2017**, *356*, 207–216. [CrossRef] [PubMed]
25. Zhang, C.; Chen, R.-X.; Zhang, Y.; Wang, J.; Liu, F.-Y.; Cai, J.; Liao, F.-F.; Xu, F.-Q.; Yi, M.; Wan, Y. Reduced GABAergic transmission in the ventrobasal thalamus contributes to thermal hyperalgesia in chronic inflammatory pain. *Sci. Rep.* **2017**, *7*, 41439. [CrossRef]
26. Wang, C.; Hao, H.; He, K.; An, Y.; Pu, Z.; Gamper, N.; Zhang, H.; Du, X. Neuropathic Injury–Induced Plasticity of GABAergic System in Peripheral Sensory Ganglia. *Front. Pharmacol.* **2021**, *12*, 702218. [CrossRef] [PubMed]
27. Bryce, T.N.; Budh, C.N.; Cardenas, D.D.; Dijkers, M.; Felix, E.R.; Finnerup, N.B.; Kennedy, P.; Lundeberg, T.; Richards, J.S.; Rintala, D.H. Pain after spinal cord injury: An evidence-based review for clinical practice and research: Report of the National Institute on Disability and Rehabilitation Research Spinal Cord Injury Measures meeting. *J. Spinal Cord Med.* **2007**, *30*, 421–440. [CrossRef] [PubMed]
28. Karcioglu, O.; Topacoglu, H.; Dikme, O.; Dikme, O. A systematic review of the pain scales in adults: Which to use? *Am. J. Emerg. Med.* **2018**, *36*, 707–714. [CrossRef]
29. Williamson, A.; Hoggart, B. Pain: A review of three commonly used pain rating scales. *J. Clin. Nurs.* **2005**, *14*, 798–804. [CrossRef]
30. Acerra, N.; Souvlis, T.; Moseley, G. Does mirror-box therapy improve sensory and motor changes in the early post-stroke population? A randomised controlled trial. *Aust. J. Physiother.* **2005**, *51*, S7.
31. Biering-Sørensen, F.; Alai, S.; Anderson, K.; Charlifue, S.; Chen, Y.; DeVivo, M.; Flanders, A.E.; Jones, L.; Kleitman, N.; Lans, A. Common data elements for spinal cord injury clinical research: A National Institute for Neurological Disorders and Stroke project. *Spinal Cord* **2015**, *53*, 265–277. [CrossRef]
32. Ferreira-Valente, M.A.; Pais-Ribeiro, J.L.; Jensen, M.P. Validity of four pain intensity rating scales. *Pain* **2011**, *152*, 2399–2404. [CrossRef] [PubMed]
33. Widerström-Noga, E.; Biering-Sørensen, F.; Bryce, T.; Cardenas, D.; Finnerup, N.; Jensen, M.; Richards, J.; Siddall, P. The international spinal cord injury pain basic data set (version 2.0). *Spinal Cord* **2014**, *52*, 282–286. [CrossRef] [PubMed]
34. Dworkin, S.F. Research diagnostic criteria for temporomandibular disorders: Review, criteria, examinations and specifications, critique. *J. Craniomandib. Disord.* **1992**, *6*, 301–355.
35. Collins, S.L.; Moore, A.R.; McQuay, H.J. The visual analogue pain intensity scale: What is moderate pain in millimetres? *Pain* **1997**, *72*, 95–97. [CrossRef] [PubMed]
36. Tait, R.; Pollard, C.A.; Margolis, R.; Duckro, P.N.; Krause, S.J. The Pain Disability Index: Psychometric and validity data. *Arch. Phys. Med. Rehabil.* **1987**, *68*, 438–441. [PubMed]
37. Amtmann, D.; Cook, K.F.; Jensen, M.P.; Chen, W.H.; Choi, S.; Revicki, D.; Cella, D.; Rothrock, N.; Keefe, F.; Callahan, L.; et al. Development of a PROMIS item bank to measure pain interference. *Pain* **2010**, *150*, 173–182. [CrossRef]
38. Galer, B.S.; Jensen, M.P. Development and preliminary validation of a pain measure specific to neuropathic pain: The Neuropathic Pain Scale. *Neurology* **1997**, *48*, 332–338. [CrossRef] [PubMed]
39. Spreafico, R.; Frassoni, C.; Arcelli, P.; De Biasi, S. GABAergic interneurons in the somatosensory thalamus of the guinea-pig: A light and ultrastructural immunocytochemical investigation. *Neuroscience* **1994**, *59*, 961–973. [CrossRef]
40. Choi, I.Y.; Andronesi, O.C.; Barker, P.; Bogner, W.; Edden, R.A.; Kaiser, L.G.; Lee, P.; Marjańska, M.; Terpstra, M.; de Graaf, R.A. Spectral editing in 1H magnetic resonance spectroscopy: Experts' consensus recommendations. *NMR Biomed.* **2020**, *34*, e4411. [CrossRef]
41. Wilson, M.; Andronesi, O.; Barker, P.B.; Bartha, R.; Bizzi, A.; Bolan, P.J.; Brindle, K.M.; Choi, I.Y.; Cudalbu, C.; Dydak, U. Methodological consensus on clinical proton MRS of the brain: Review and recommendations. *Magn. Reson. Med.* **2019**, *82*, 527–550. [CrossRef]
42. Kang, D.; Hesam-Shariati, N.; McAuley, J.H.; Alam, M.; Trost, Z.; Rae, C.D.; Gustin, S.M. Disruption to normal excitatory and inhibitory function within the medial prefrontal cortex in people with chronic pain. *Eur. J. Pain* **2021**, *25*, 2242–2256. [CrossRef]
43. Naylor, B.; Hesam-Shariati, N.; McAuley, J.H.; Boag, S.; Newton-John, T.; Rae, C.D.; Gustin, S.M. Reduced glutamate in the medial prefrontal cortex is associated with emotional and cognitive dysregulation in people with chronic pain. *Front. Neurol.* **2019**, *10*, 1110. [CrossRef]
44. Henderson, L.A.; Peck, C.C.; Petersen, E.T.; Rae, C.D.; Youssef, A.M.; Reeves, J.M.; Wilcox, S.L.; Akhter, R.; Murray, G.M.; Gustin, S.M. Chronic pain: Lost inhibition? *J. Neurosci.* **2013**, *33*, 7574–7582. [CrossRef] [PubMed]
45. Trost, Z.; France, C.; Anam, M.; Shum, C. Virtual reality approaches to pain: Toward a state of the science. *Pain* **2021**, *162*, 325–331. [CrossRef] [PubMed]
46. Boesch, E.; Bellan, V.; Moseley, G.L.; Stanton, T.R. The effect of bodily illusions on clinical pain: A systematic review and meta-analysis. *Pain* **2016**, *157*, 516–529. [CrossRef] [PubMed]
47. Garrett, B.; Taverner, T.; Masinde, W.; Gromala, D.; Shaw, C.; Negraeff, M. A rapid evidence assessment of immersive virtual reality as an adjunct therapy in acute pain management in clinical practice. *Clin. J. Pain* **2014**, *30*, 1089–1098. [CrossRef] [PubMed]

48. Thieme, H.; Morkisch, N.; Rietz, C.; Dohle, C.; Borgetto, B. The efficacy of movement representation techniques for treatment of limb pain—A systematic review and meta-analysis. *J. Pain* **2016**, *17*, 167–180. [CrossRef]
49. Lotze, M.; Grodd, W.; Birbaumer, N.; Erb, M.; Huse, E.; Flor, H. Does use of a myoelectric prosthesis prevent cortical reorganization and phantom limb pain? *Nat. Neurosci.* **1999**, *2*, 501–502. [CrossRef]
50. Cai, K.; Nanga, R.P.; Lamprou, L.; Schinstine, C.; Elliott, M.; Hariharan, H.; Reddy, R.; Epperson, C.N. The impact of gabapentin administration on brain GABA and glutamate concentrations: A 7T 1 H-MRS study. *Neuropsychopharmacology* **2012**, *37*, 2764–2771. [CrossRef]

Disclaimer/Publisher's Note: The statements, opinions and data contained in all publications are solely those of the individual author(s) and contributor(s) and not of MDPI and/or the editor(s). MDPI and/or the editor(s) disclaim responsibility for any injury to people or property resulting from any ideas, methods, instructions or products referred to in the content.

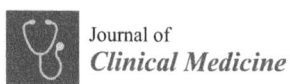

Case Report

A Case Study of Hypnosis Enhanced Cognitive Therapy for Pain in a Ventilator Dependent Patient during Inpatient Rehabilitation for Spinal Cord Injury

Amy J. Starosta [1,*], Katherine S. Wright [1], Charles H. Bombardier [1], Faran Kahlia [1], Jason Barber [2], Michelle C. Accardi-Ravid [3], Shelley A. Wiechman [1], Deborah A. Crane [1] and Mark P. Jensen [1]

[1] Department of Rehabilitation Medicine, University of Washington, Seattle, WA 98195, USA; wright6@uw.edu (K.S.W.); chb@uw.edu (C.H.B.); fkahlia@uw.edu (F.K.); wiechman@uw.edu (S.A.W.); dacrane@uw.edu (D.A.C.); mjensen@uw.edu (M.P.J.)
[2] Department of Neurological Surgery, University of Washington, Seattle, WA 98195, USA; barber@neurosurgery.washington.edu
[3] Department of Physical Medicine and Rehabilitation, University of Utah, Salt Lake City, UT 84132, USA; michelle.accardiravid@hsc.utah.edu
* Correspondence: starosta@uw.edu

Abstract: Early, acute pain following spinal cord injury (SCI) is common, can negatively impact SCI rehabilitation, and is frequently not responsive to biomedical treatment. Nonpharmacological interventions show promise in reducing pain for individuals with SCI. However, most psychological interventions rely heavily on verbal interaction between the individual being treated and the clinician, making them inaccessible for individuals with impaired verbal output due to mechanical ventilation. This case study aims to describe the adaptation and implementation of hypnotic cognitive therapy (HYP-CT) intervention for early SCI pain in the context of mechanical ventilation dependence and weaning. The participant was a 54-year-old male with C2 AIS A SCI requiring mechanical ventilation. Four sessions of HYP-CT were provided during inpatient rehabilitation with assessment prior to intervention, after the intervention sessions, and prior to discharge. The participant reported immediate reductions in pain intensity following each intervention session. Overall, he reported increases in self-efficacy and pain acceptance. He did not report any negative treatment effects and thought the intervention provided support during mechanical ventilation weaning. During treatment, he discontinued opioid pain medications and reported actively using intervention strategies. Our results support the potential for early, hypnotic cognitive therapy for individuals with SCI experiencing pain or distress while dependent on mechanical ventilation.

Keywords: pain; spinal cord injury; case study

1. Introduction

Chronic pain is a common issue following spinal cord injury (SCI), with reviews estimating that 40% to 80% of individuals with SCI report chronic pain [1] and that this pain is severe in 32% to 53% of those with SCI [2]. People with SCI can experience multiple types of pain simultaneously, including musculoskeletal, neuropathic, and visceral pain [3]. Nociceptive pain is pain that results from activation of (otherwise healthy) nociceptors related to tissue damage or the risk for tissue damage (e.g., muscle overuse) that can happen in any population. In contrast, neuropathic pain is associated with damage to neurons in the central nervous system (CNS: brain or spinal cord) or periphery that continues after the injury heals. In individuals with SCI, such pain is often experienced at or below the level of the SCI [3]. Both types of pain are common following SCI. A 2021 meta-analysis of SCI pain prevalence reported that 58% of people with SCI have neuropathic pain and 45% have nociceptive pain [4].

For many people with SCI, pain starts early following injury and adversely affects SCI rehabilitation. Siddall et al. found that at two weeks post-injury, 90% of people report pain [5]. Those with greater acute pain receive less time in therapy sessions during inpatient rehabilitation and need more modifications to therapy activities [6]. In many cases, more intense acute SCI pain predicts greater chronic pain [5,7]. When pain becomes chronic it is associated with negative outcomes such as depression, sleep disturbance, poorer physical, psychological, social, and occupational function, as well as lower quality of life in people with SCI [8–10].

Although longitudinal studies demonstrate the high prevalence of both early and chronic SCI pain, less is known about the factors that contribute to the development of pain after injury. Thus far, most pain prediction research has used a biomedical framework and has therefore focused on biomedical predictors. Although a number of biological predictors of SCI-related pain have been identified, such as sensory hypersensitivity [11], chronological age and sensory and motor preservation [12], and injuries due to gunshot wounds [13], these factors do not fully explain chronic pain intensity or interference. One reason that biological variables alone do not fully explain the development of chronic pain is that all chronic pain, including SCI-related pain, is influenced by psychological and social factors [14]. Dating back to at least the 1960s, pain clinicians and researchers have recognized that pain has multiple components including cognitive/evaluative and affective/emotional, as well as sensory/nociceptive elements [15]. Additionally, biological, psychological, and social factors influence chronic pain and pain behaviors [14]. The biopsychosocial model has been advanced as the way to understand and treat SCI-related pain by leading SCI pain researchers [7,9,16–19].

Despite the call to conceptualize pain and pain treatment from a biopsychosocial model, management of SCI-related pain continues to be primarily pharmacological. Unfortunately, SCI-related pain is often not responsive to pharmacological intervention. Optimal pharmacological treatment (often involving a combination of anticonvulsants, antidepressants, opioids, or antispasmodics) typically results in only about one third of people experiencing at least a 50% reduction in their pain [9]. Not only do medications have limited efficacy, commonly used pain medications, such as opioids, have negative side effects [8,20], For years, experts have called for research on nonpharmacological treatments for acute SCI-related pain to lessen the development of chronic pain and improve the quality of life [7,21]. In comparison to pharmacological interventions, nonpharmacological interventions have very few negative side effects, and have been found to reduce chronic pain in non-SCI populations [14].

One factor that has consistently been associated with pain intensity for individuals with chronic pain, including individuals with SCI-related chronic pain, is a tendency to focus on negative automatic thoughts about pain, also referred to as pain catastrophizing [22]. Individuals who have this tendency are more likely to experience increased pain intensity, and to have higher levels of physical disability, psychological distress [23], depression [24], and sleep disruption [25]. This issue is particularly relevant for SCI-related pain, as individuals with SCI may experience more pain catastrophizing than other chronic pain populations [26]. A tendency to catastrophize about pain may develop early following SCI and is related to long-term pain intensity and unpleasantness [27], suggesting that these cognitive appraisals about pain are potentially an important intervention target for any chronic SCI pain treatment.

The most common clinical approach for addressing pain catastrophizing is cognitive restructuring (also known as cognitive therapy; CT). This strategy focuses on teaching individuals to become aware of their thoughts about pain, evaluate the impact of those thoughts on their mood and behaviors, and—for those thoughts deemed to have negative effects—develop alternative thoughts that support improved mood or increased engagement with valued activities. Recent reviews recommend the use of CT strategies to manage SCI-related pain mostly based on evidence that CT can reduce pain interference, especially in the areas of sleep and mood [28–30]. Taken together, CT has a strong theoretical basis, evidence of some positive effects in SCI pain management, and merits further research.

Another promising nonpharmacological treatment for chronic pain is clinical hypnosis, defined as, "A state of consciousness involving focused attention and reduced peripheral awareness characterized by an enhanced capacity for response to suggestion" (p. 32) [31]. Clinical hypnosis usually involves two steps. First, a hypnotic "induction", which is designed to enhance responses to clinical suggestions. This is then followed by clinical suggestions, which are provided to engender changes in sensations, mood, or behavior. These suggestions differentiate hypnotic interventions from interventions including relaxation or clinical meditation, which also may be promising interventions for reducing pain interference for individuals with SCI [32]. Traditionally, the clinical suggestions for pain management focus on decreased pain, increased comfort, and improved ability to ignore or be distracted from pain, and/or changing the quality of pain. The last suggestion provided usually involves a "post-hypnotic" suggestion that the benefits experienced by the individual will last beyond the session. Individuals who receive hypnosis treatment may be given recordings of the treatment sessions in order to practice hypnosis on their own between treatment sessions, and also to perform self-hypnosis following a basic self-induction procedure and giving themselves helpful hypnotic suggestions. A recent meta-analysis found that for non-headache pain, hypnosis had a moderate beneficial effect on pain intensity compared to control conditions [33]. There is also evidence that hypnosis might be particularly effective in treating neuropathic pain, which is common among people with SCI [34].

In addition to hypnosis being an effective stand-alone treatment, there is substantial evidence that, when combined with other evidence based cognitive and behavioral therapies, hypnosis enhances the benefits of these treatments. Two meta-analyses—one published in 1985 and a second updated analysis published more recently—of studies that added hypnosis to cognitive and behavioral therapies for pain, insomnia, obesity, or hypertension concluded that the average effect size for the combined treatment was in the large range (e.g., Cohen's d = 1.36) [35,36]. Building on these findings, a hypnosis-enhanced cognitive therapy intervention (HYP-CT) was developed to target negative thoughts about chronic pain for people with disabilities and chronic pain. Initial pilot studies and follow-up clinical trials have consistently found HYP-CT to be effective, resulting in a marked reduction in pain intensity compared to pain education, CT, or hypnosis alone [37–39].

These psychological interventions rely heavily on collaboration with the individual receiving the treatment, which can be more difficult for those individuals who are unable to voice due to mechanical ventilation needs. As many as two thirds of individuals with new cervical-level SCI will experience respiratory complications during the acute phase of their injury, often requiring mechanical ventilation [40]. Patients requiring ventilation are a uniquely vulnerable group, as respiratory dysfunction is a major cause of both mortality and morbidity in SCI [40]. Anxiety is very common among those requiring mechanical ventilation [41], and prolonged anxiety and distress may predispose these individuals to more long-term negative psychological outcomes, including depression and posttraumatic stress disorder [42].

Despite the high need for psychological support and intervention for patients requiring mechanical ventilation, there is limited information on how effective psychological interventions are for this population. One case study reported positive results from HYP-CT for an individual with a high-level SCI who was dependent on mechanical ventilation in an outpatient setting [43]. After eight sessions, this individual showed clinically meaningful improvements in sleep quality and pain acceptance, and reductions in pain intensity, interference, and catastrophizing; these improvements were maintained for over a year.

All of the available evidence in individuals with SCI is from interventions offered on an outpatient basis after chronic pain has already developed. However, as previously discussed, studies have found that chronic pain often begins early in the course of SCI [6,44,45].

There is untapped clinical potential to reduce the negative impact of pain in this uniquely vulnerable population by intervening early in rehabilitation.

In order to provide early nonpharmacological SCI pain treatment, the previously evaluated CT and hypnosis intervention (HYP-CT) was adapted to be administered during inpatient rehabilitation following SCI. During the recruitment for this feasibility trial, an individual requiring mechanical ventilation was interested in participating in the intervention. This patient met all eligibility requirements, but due to the need to adjust the intervention to meet the patient's communication needs, he was not enrolled in the primary pilot project. Rather, the aim of this case study is to describe the process of adapting and implementing HYP-CT for early SCI pain in the context of mechanical ventilation-dependence and weaning.

2. Case Study

The participant is a 54-year-old Filipino man who was initially admitted to the intensive care unit (ICU) after an unwitnessed fall down a flight of stairs. He presented with polytrauma, including multiple facial fractures, wrist fractures, and a new onset spinal cord injury. The initial exam using the International Standards for Neurological Classification of SCI (ISNCSCI) on the day after his injury and surgery showed complete sensorimotor tetraplegia, C2, American Spinal Injury Association (ASIA) Impairment Scale (AIS) grade A, although 3 weeks later when he was being admitted to inpatient rehabilitation, his SCI was graded as C1 AIS B SCI. His spine injuries were treated with C2-5 posterior spinal instrumentation and fusion (PSIF) and C3-4 laminectomies. He required mechanical ventilation due to the level of his SCI. Both a tracheostomy and percutaneous endoscopic gastrostomy (PEG) tube were placed on hospital day 6. His course was complicated by ventilator-associated pneumonia. After 16 days of ICU management, the participant was medically stable and ready for an inpatient rehabilitation program.

Upon transfer to the inpatient rehabilitation unit on hospital day 17, the participant required total assistance for all aspects of self-care and functional mobility. During inpatient rehabilitation, he was actively engaged with therapy teams. He received 15 h of therapy per week, and his therapist rated his participation as "good" to "very good" on the Pittsburgh Rehabilitation Participation Scale (PRPS). On hospital day 13, he began weaning from mechanical ventilation via T-piece spontaneous breathing trials (SBTs) prior to his admission to inpatient rehabilitation and continued SBTs on inpatient rehabilitation. When the cuff was inflated, he communicated by mouthing words, using head nods/shakes, and occasional use of an eye-gaze board. He made steady positive progress and was independent from the ventilator for a full 24 h on hospital day 29. Post-wean progress was complicated by a lower lobe collapse on day 31 but was successfully managed with chest physiotherapy. During the weaning process, the participant continued to be mostly unable to voice due to cuff inflation. As the weaning protocol progressed, he was able to communicate at the 2–3-word level. He was decannulated on hospital day 52, at which point he was able to communicate fully with mild voice impairments mostly due to poor respiratory support. The participant was discharged home with his family 69 days after his injury and admission to the ICU.

The participant was followed by the Rehabilitation Psychology team throughout hospitalization, first by a clinical psychologist on the acute care consult service, and then by one of the authors (KSW), who is a clinical psychologist on inpatient rehabilitation. The participant denied any history of mental health diagnoses or treatment prior to this hospitalization. He noted that he was a generally positive person and had great support from family and friends. His significant other (SO) and adult son described him as "happy, loving, good humored, funny", and the "type of person who will do anything for anyone". Unfortunately, due to the hospital policy for COVID restrictions at the time, the participant was unable to have regular visitors at bedside initially. However, in preparation for discharge, his SO and his son were able to be with him in person to learn about his care and to participate in hands-on training, which the participant reported was very helpful for his mood.

At baseline assessment, the participant reported significant pain in his neck, chest, and throughout his back (average intensity = 4/10, worst intensity = 8/10). Upon initial presentation, pain was primarily musculoskeletal in nature. The participant reported that pain was often distressing to him and sometimes made it difficult for him to fall asleep. He reported that he felt the worst pain during turns with nursing staff, which occurred every two hours to protect his skin.

3. Methods

3.1. Intervention

The intervention was adapted from a standardized outpatient hypnotic cognitive therapy (HYP-CT) [38] protocol to fit into the busy schedule of the inpatient rehabilitation setting. Full descriptions of the intervention and pilot have been published elsewhere [46]. In brief, the intervention utilizes focused attention and perceived automaticity resulting from hypnosis to enhance the efficacy and extend the duration of the positive effects of CT. The primary goals of HYP-CT are to (1) increase the individual's comfort with ambiguity about the meaning of pain in order to reduce pain catastrophizing, (2) encourage the belief that the individual can gain control over pain and its impact, or self-efficacy, and (3) automatize the process of cognitive restructuring. The intervention sessions are described in Table 1.

Table 1. Intervention schedule.

Session	Hospital Day	Topics Reviewed (30–40 min)	Hypnotic Induction (~20 min) *
1	27	Psychoeducation on cognitive model of pain	Increasing tolerance of ambiguity regarding pain and its impact
2	40	Thought worksheets to identify negative and positive automatic thoughts	Automatization of the process of altering pain-related catastrophizing and any other alarming or maladaptive cognitions into more reassuring and realistic cognitions
3	47	Reviewing and adjusting negative and positive automatic thoughts	Continued automatization of reassuring or more realistic cognitions. Externalizing physical discomfort or unhelpful thoughts
4	55	Skill review. Use of Motivational Interviewing to promote continued practice	Age progression hypnosis strategy based on strategy described by Moshe Torem

* Every in-session hypnosis induction was audio recorded and provided to the patient.

3.2. Measures

The same outcome domains that were assessed in the pilot trial were administered (see Table 2) prior to the start of the intervention (baseline), at each intervention session, and prior to discharge (follow-up). A shortened post-discharge assessment was conducted during an outpatient Rehabilitation Medicine appointment 5.5 months after discharge (post-discharge). Full descriptions of all measures collected are published elsewhere [46], while a brief description of the measures relevant to the present case are provided below.

Table 2. Assessment schedule.

Measures		Timepoints			
Domain	Measure	Baseline	Intervention	Follow-Up	Post-Discharge
Pain intensity	Numerical Rating Scale (NRS) ranging from 0 (No pain) to 10 (Pain as bad as you can imagine)	X	X	X	X

Table 2. *Cont.*

Measures		Timepoints			
Domain	Measure	Baseline	Intervention	Follow-Up	Post-Discharge
Pain interference	Patient-Reported Outcomes Measurement Information System (PROMIS) Pain Interference (PI) Short Form	X		X	
	Single Pain Interference Item from Short Form Survey (SF-36)				X
Pain type	Spinal Cord Injury Pain Instrument (SCIPI)	X		X	X
Pain catastrophizing	University of Washington Concerns about Pain (UW-CAP)	X		X	
Pain self-efficacy	University of Washington Pain Related Self-Efficacy Scale (PRSE)	X		X	
Pain acceptance	Chronic Pain Acceptance Questionnaire-Revised (CPAQ-R)	X		X	
Depression	Patient Health Questionnaire-9 (PHQ-9)	X		X	
Sleep quality	PROMIS Sleep Disturbance Short Form	X		X	
Analgesic use	Medical chart review			X	X
Patient impression of change	Patient Global Impression of Change (PGIC)			X	X
Perceived benefit and satisfaction	Benefit, Satisfaction, and Willingness to Continue Treatment (BSW)			X	X
Skills practice	Patient report of number of times listening to recording or practicing self-hypnosis as well as amount of time spent on each practice		X	X	X
Relief during hypnosis	NRS ranging from 0 (No relief) to 10 (Complete relief)		X		

3.2.1. Demographic and Descriptive Measures

Demographic variables: Demographic information was collected using self-report including sex, race, ethnicity, education, employment status, and marital status.

Pain type: The pain type was classified as neuropathic or nociceptive based on the participants' responses to the Spinal Cord Injury Pain Instrument (SCIPI) [47]. The 4-item SCIPI short form is a screening tool that assesses the quality and features of the individual's worst pain in the past 7 days. Evidence supports its sensitivity and specificity for classifying neuropathic versus nociceptive pain types [47].

Pain locations: Information about each pain location was collected at baseline using Version 2.0 of the International SCI Pain Data Set [48]. The participants were asked to rank their three worst pain locations and provide information about each pain. The location, type of pain, intensity, duration, and treatment was collected for each of the three unique pain problems. The average pain intensity in the past week for each pain problem was rated on a 0–10 NRS from 0 = "No pain" to 10 = "Pain as bad as you can imagine".

3.2.2. Patient-Reported Outcome Measures

Treatment satisfaction: The Benefit, Satisfaction, and Willingness to Continue (BSW) scale was used to assess treatment satisfaction at discharge. The BSW is a patient-reported outcome that reflects the individuals' perception of the experience and effects of treatment. The question format for each of the 3 items was similar, with a yes/no question asked first; for example question 1 is "Did you receive any benefit from this treatment?" followed up with a question that rates the degree of benefit, satisfaction, or willingness to continue, for example "If yes, have you had little benefit or much benefit?" The BSW measure has shown validity for other symptom-based conditions including overactive bladder [49].

Global improvement: The Patient Global Impression of Change (PGIC) was used to assess perceived global improvement at discharge. The PGIC is a 7-point Likert scale on which participants describe how much better or worse they are now compared to the beginning of the intervention. The patients were asked to rate their overall status from the start of the study using the following scale: (1) very much improved; (2) much improved; (3) minimally improved; (4) no change; (5) minimally worse; (6) much worse; (7) very much worse. The PGIC is a standardized outcome measure for SCI clinical research and is often used as a secondary outcome measure [50].

Adverse events: At the beginning and end of intervention sessions, the study clinician asked participants if they experienced any adverse events between or during sessions. Adverse effects were also assessed at discharge by the research assistant.

Average and worst pain intensity: The average and worst pain intensity were assessed at baseline and discharge using the 0–10 Numerical Rating Scale (NRS). The participants were asked to rate their worst and average pain intensity in the past week from 0 "No pain" to 10 "Pain as bad as you can imagine". The NRS is recommended as a core outcome measure in pain studies [51] and has demonstrated validity as a measure of pain intensity through its strong association with other pain measures as well as its ability to detect changes in pain with treatment [52].

Immediate effects of the treatment sessions on pain: Prior to the start of each of the four intervention sessions, the current pain intensity was assessed on a 0–10 NRS, and reassessed at the end of the intervention session. In addition, the participants were asked to rate how much relief they experience during the session on a 0–10 scale, with 0 indicating "No relief" and 10 indicating "Complete relief".

Pain interference: The PROMIS Pain Interference Short Form (PROMIS PI) assesses the impact of pain with questions relevant to people during hospitalization for a traumatic injury [53]. The PROMIS PI has demonstrated validity in diverse clinical populations [54]. Higher scores indicate more pain interference. In order to reduce the assessment burden at post-discharge follow-up, a single pain interference from the Medical Outcomes Study SF-36 [55] was used. This item assesses pain interference on a 1–5 scale, with response options of "not at all", "a little bit", "moderately", "quite a bit", and "extremely". Responses can be transformed to a 0–100 score; however, to reduce direct comparisons to PROMIS PI scores, we elected to leave response in categorical format.

Pain catastrophizing: The Concerns about Pain (CAP) scale was used to assess pain catastrophizing at baseline and discharge. It was developed using item-response theory as well as expert and patient feedback [56] and has strong psychometric properties [57]. It is specifically designed to assess negative cognitive responses to anticipated or current pain [57]. The participants were asked how often they had each thought about pain using a response set rated from 1 "Never" to 5 "Always". Higher scores indicate more pain catastrophizing.

Pain self-efficacy: The 2-item short form of the Pain Related Self-Efficacy (PRSE) scale was administered at baseline and discharge [53]. It is an item-response theory measure designed to assess an individual's belief in their ability to accomplish tasks and activities despite their pain. Participants were prompted to rate their confidence about each item on a scale from 1 "not at all" to 5 "very much". Higher scores indicate more self-efficacy.

Pain acceptance: The Chronic Pain Acceptance Questionnaire-Revised (CPAQ-R) is a 20-item questionnaire that measures pain acceptance through two distinct factors: activity engagement and pain willingness [58]. Participants were asked to rate the truth of each of the twenty statements as it applied to them on a 7-point scale from 0 "never true" to 6 "always true". Items are summed for a total score, with higher scores indicating higher levels of acceptance.

Sleep disturbance: Sleep disturbance was assessed at baseline and discharge using the PROMIS sleep disturbance short form [59] which consists of 8 items assessing problems related to sleep quality over the past 7 days. The individual is prompted to rate each item on a 5-point scale of 1 "never" to 5 "always". Higher scores indicate more sleep disturbance.

4. Findings
4.1. Changes in Study Outcome Variables
4.1.1. Pre- to Post-Session Effects

Pain intensity was assessed before and after each session. For all four sessions, the participant reported stable or reduced pain intensity from before to after hypnosis (see Table 3). It is important to highlight that these improvements are considered clinically significant, as they all exceed the suggested 1.6 point clinically significant cut off [60]. Additionally, the participant consistently reported positive responses to the hypnosis, and experiencing "complete relief" during two of the sessions. The participant denied any negative effects associated with the hypnosis treatment throughout the intervention time period.

Table 3. Response to sessions.

	Pre-Session		Post-Session	
	Avg. Pain 24 h	Current Pain	Current Pain	Relief in Session
Session 1	8	8	6	4
Session 2	8	5	5	10
Session 3	6	6	3	10
Session 4	8	8	6	6

Prior to the start of intervention, the participant was receiving an average 8.5 mg of oxycodone daily. He began to use his prescribed 5 mg PRN dose of oxycodone less and less frequently over a 3-week period and had self-weaned from opioids completely by session 3 (see Table 4). The patient continued to utilize acetaminophen and topical lidocaine for pain management throughout his inpatient rehabilitation admission.

Table 4. Opioid use.

	Mean Daily Oxycodone (Range)
Prior to session 1	8.50 mg (15–5 mg)
Session 1–2	4.62 mg (15–0 mg)
Session 2–3	0.71 mg (5–0 mg)
Session 3–4	0.00 mg
Post Session 4	0.00 mg

4.1.2. Pre- to Post-Intervention Effects

The participant reported increased average pain intensity during his hospitalization (Table 5). While the pain was initially musculoskeletal, over time it became more neuropathic. The participant noted an electrical shock quality to the pain in his neck and reported having painful spasms. He also reported increased pain interference as his pain increased. While pain intensity and interference increased, pain catastrophizing decreased, indicating that the participant had fewer negative automatic thoughts about his pain. Additionally, the participant's willingness to engage in activities even when he experienced significant pain, as measured by pain acceptance, also increased. His sleep worsened significantly during his hospitalization.

Table 5. Assessment outcomes.

Variable Name	Measure	Baseline	Follow-Up	Post-Discharge
Average pain Intensity	NRS	4	6	8.5
Worst pain intensity	NRS	8	8	9
Pain interference	PROMIS	59.9	67.4	4/5 "quite a bit"
Pain catastrophizing	CAP	35.9	31.3	35.9
Depression	PHQ9	5.63	6	--
Pain acceptance	CPAQ-R Activity Engagement	36	41.8	--
	CPAQ-R Pain Willingness	29	29.3	--
Pain self-efficacy	PRSE	52.7	52.7	69.2
Sleep disturbance	PROMIS	33.1	60.4	28.9

4.1.3. Clinical Presentation at Post-Intervention

Over his 53-day stay on the inpatient rehabilitation unit, the participant also received the standard of care Rehabilitation Psychology support. His psychologist (KSW), who was aware of his participation in the study, had a total of five visits with the participant, most of which occurred in the second half of the patient's admission. Frequency of visits was tailored to meet the participant's needs. Emotionally, the participant reported normative grief and worries about his prognosis, but he did not experience clinically significant symptoms of depression or acute stress disorder. He also did not experience symptoms of generalized anxiety disorder. However, over time the participant reported increased anxiety related to apneic events occurring more frequently during the night. Concurrently, he was evaluated by the Sleep Medicine consult service and was diagnosed with severe sleep apnea. The participant utilized nasal pillows and a CPAP machine during hospitalization. During these apneic events, he felt a sense of panic that was amplified by his memories of two frightening instances before he was fully weaned from the ventilator when he needed assistance managing secretions, but his call light malfunctioned.

The participant engaged well with psychological interventions and was successful in using pursed lip breathing to slow the breathing rate and count breaths. Once calm enough, he was able to initiate the self-hypnosis he learned in HYP-CT, which helped to further manage anxiety.

4.1.4. Post-Discharge Follow-Up

After discharge from the hospital, the participant reported increased pain intensity. His pain transitioned from musculoskeletal to neuropathic pain, and he reported that pain experience was primarily neuropathic at post-discharge follow-up. He stated that he continued to experience painful spasms on a daily basis. He stated that pain interfered with his daily activities "quite a bit". However, he reported increased self-efficacy in managing his pain during daily activities. His sleep quality also improved significantly. He reported he no longer used CPAP, but rather slept with his head elevated, which improved sleep quality. While not assessed formally, he continued to deny symptoms of depression, stating, "I think about the positive". Unfortunately, he did not have access to the audio recordings to engage in hypnosis practice at home. However, he stated that at least once per week, he would "think about the elevator" (i.e., a visualization of deepening during hypnosis induction) as a strategy to help build relaxation when he was experiencing pain. At a later follow-up, he reported using the image of the elevator every time he needed to transfer using the lift, a painful experience that occurred approximately four times daily.

4.2. Perception of Change and Treatment Satisfaction

On the PGIC, the participant reported that he was "much improved" since the start of the study on both post-intervention and post-discharge assessments. On the BSW, he rated that he received "much benefit" from the intervention and was "very satisfied". Additionally, he stated that he would be "very willing" to continue the therapy. In fact, at post-discharge follow-up, the participant inquired about initiating outpatient rehabilitation psychology treatment in order to receive further HYP-CT to address chronic pain. Additionally, he requested that audio recordings be sent again to his email address so he could restart home practice. Upon learning of the participant's inability to access hypnosis recordings, the study team again sent the hypnosis recordings to patient's primary caregiver in order to facilitate access.

The participant reported that the hypnosis inductions "gave me peace of mind". He reported "[the intervention] helped me a lot". He particularly noted that he liked the sense of relaxation that he got from hypnosis inductions. He noted that the skill of self-hypnosis was something that he used regularly, stating, "I have that information, and I can always use it".

5. Discussion

The results of this case study provide additional support for the promise of early, hypnotic cognitive therapy for individuals with SCI experiencing pain or distress while dependent on mechanical ventilation. Although average pain intensity and pain interference did not improve for this patient, he reported increases in self-efficacy and pain acceptance, both important factors in the experience of pain. He did not experience any negative effects and thought that the intervention provided helpful support during his weaning from mechanical ventilation. Additionally, he discontinued opioid pain medications and reported actively using the strategies taught in the intervention. Upon discharge to home, the participant most commonly used his self-hypnosis practice in preparation for transfers with his lift, one of the most painful parts of his care. Over time, it appeared that the lift had become a naturally occurring cue that induced the hypnotic response. Finally, this early introduction to HYP-CT prompted the participant to re-engage with listening to the recording of the hypnosis induction for continued management of his chronic pain at home.

5.1. Challenges during the Intervention

Standard application of this intervention involves significant verbal collaboration with the person receiving the treatment to identify both helpful and unhelpful thoughts, feedback on hypnosis sessions, practice planning, and evaluating barriers to utilizing learned skills. For the first two sessions, the participant was unable to phonate due to mechanical ventilation, which limited his ability to engage in this collaborative process. Communication style was adjusted based on the patient's needs. The provider offered lip reading and use of a communication board. Open-ended questions were rephrased to yes/no or multiple-choice format when needed. By the third session, the participant was able to voice two to three words at a time, and by the fourth session, he was able to communicate more freely.

Due to the high level of care and therapy needs, the participant was only available to meet with the study provider approximately once per week. Several attempts had to be made each week before a suitable time for a treatment session was found. Despite these scheduling challenges, the participant received four intervention sessions within five weeks.

5.2. Practice

The participant reported significant barriers to self-hypnosis practice, noting that he was very busy throughout his day and rarely had uninterrupted time to listen to recordings. Additionally, because of COVID-related hospital visitor restrictions, the participant did not have visitors at bedside during most of his hospitalization and did not have regular help accessing his phone or other audio devices.

While the participant stated that he was unable to utilize the audio recordings due to access issues, he reported that he was able to, and did, practice self-hypnosis regularly without the recording. He noted that he often used this strategy to prepare himself before staff offered turns in bed, which was a time when he reported experiencing the most pain. By Session 4, the participant reported that it was getting easier to allow himself to be hypnotized. He stated that as he listed to the psychologist start the induction, he would focus on her voice and "the next thing you know, I'm so relaxed". Additionally, he was able to access this self-created relaxation during turns, even without a full hypnotic induction. He reports that he would take a deep breath, feel more relaxation and comfort and the "pain [during turns] is not as bad as it was before".

5.3. Conclusions

This case report, as well as our initial pilot study [46], confirms that it is practical to teach HYP-CT techniques to individuals with SCI during inpatient rehabilitation, even if those individuals are limited in their ability to engage in verbal exchanges due to mechanical ventilation needs. Offering psychological pain treatment during inpatient rehabilitation could serve as an avenue to increase accessibility to effective treatment that may reduce the negative impacts of pain, ultimately improving quality of life over the long-term for individuals with SCI. Development of interventions to address pain in SCI is a critical unmet need for this population, as SCI pain has generally been refractory to pain treatments [61–63]. As strictly biological interventions, such as pharmacology, continue to be limited, it is important to continue to develop and evaluate interventions from a biopsychosocial conceptualization of SCI pain. Future research should continue to evaluate the effectiveness of intervention on pain intensity, but should also include interventions to address other factors of pain, including cognitive/evaluative, affective/emotional, and behavioral elements as well as other conditions that can be related to pain following SCI, such as spasticity. We will continue to evaluate HYP-CT in an ongoing RCT focusing on effectiveness, mechanisms of change, and long-term impact of this intervention on pain and pain interference. Particularly for those individuals utilizing mechanical ventilation, it may be important to examine how HYP-CT impacts factors related to their respiratory function, such as respiratory rate or breathing quality. However, anecdotal reports such as this case study suggest HYP-CT has strong potential as a nonpharmacological treatment for early SCI-related pain.

Author Contributions: Conceptualization, A.J.S., C.H.B. and M.P.J.; Formal Analysis, J.B.; Data Curation, F.K. and J.B.; Writing—Original Draft Preparation, A.J.S. and K.S.W.; Writing—Review and Editing, C.H.B., S.A.W., C.H.B., D.A.C., M.P.J. and M.C.A.-R.; Funding Acquisition, A.J.S. All authors have read and agreed to the published version of the manuscript.

Funding: This project is funded by the Craig H. Nielsen Foundation (#646809).

Institutional Review Board Statement: Individual Institutional Review Board approval was received from the University of Washington (STUDY00009601). We certify that all applicable institutional and governmental regulations concerning the ethical use of human volunteers were followed during this research. Written informed consent was obtained from participant and verbal consent was given to publish this paper.

Data Availability Statement: The datasets generated during and/or analyzed during the current study are available from the corresponding author on reasonable request.

Acknowledgments: This case report was written with express permission from the participant receiving the treatment. The participant was also given the opportunity to review this report to ensure that it was an accurate description of his response to the treatment. The authors would like to express their appreciation to the participant for both his willingness to participate and share his experience. This study was supported and financed by the Craig H. Nielsen Foundation (#646809).

Conflicts of Interest: The authors declare no conflict of interest.

References

1. Van Gorp, S.; Kessels, A.; Joosten, E.; Van Kleef, M.; Patijn, J. Pain prevalence and its determinants after spinal cord injury: A systematic review. *Eur. J. Pain* **2015**, *19*, 5–14. [CrossRef]
2. Ehde, D.M.; Jensen, M.P.; Engel, J.M.; Turner, J.A.; Hoffman, A.J.; Cardenas, D.D. Chronic pain secondary to disability: A review. *Clin. J. Pain* **2003**, *19*, 3–17. [CrossRef] [PubMed]

3. Bryce, T.N.; Biering-Sørensen, F.; Finnerup, N.B.; Cardenas, D.D.; Defrin, R.; Lundeberg, T.; Norrbrink, C.; Richards, J.S.; Siddall, P.; Stripling, T.; et al. International spinal cord injury pain classification: Part I. Background and description. *Spinal cord.* **2012**, *50*, 413. [CrossRef] [PubMed]
4. Hunt, C.; Moman, R.; Peterson, A.; Wilson, R.; Covington, S.; Mustafa, R.; Murad, M.H.; Hooten, W.M. Prevalence of chronic pain after spinal cord injury: A systematic review and meta-analysis. *Reg. Anesth. Pain Med.* **2021**, *46*, 328–336. [CrossRef] [PubMed]
5. Siddall, P.J.; McClelland, J.M.; Rutkowski, S.B.; Cousins, M.J. A longitudinal study of the prevalence and characteristics of pain in the first 5 years following spinal cord injury. *Pain* **2003**, *103*, 249–257. [CrossRef]
6. Zanca, J.M.; Dijkers, M.P.; Hammond, F.M.; Horn, S.D. Pain and its impact on inpatient rehabilitation for acute traumatic spinal cord injury: Analysis of observational data collected in the SCIRehab study. *Arch. Phys. Med. Rehabil.* **2013**, *94*, S137–S144. [CrossRef]
7. Finnerup, N.B.; Jensen, M.P.; Norrbrink, C.; Trok, K.; Johannesen, I.L.; Jensen, T.S.; Werhagen, L. A prospective study of pain and psychological functioning following traumatic spinal cord injury. *Spinal Cord.* **2016**, *54*, 816–821. [CrossRef]
8. Bloemen-Vrencken, J.H.; Post, M.W.; Hendriks, J.M.; De Reus, E.C.; De Witte, L.P. Health problems of persons with spinal cord injury living in the Netherlands. *Disabil. Rehabil.* **2005**, *27*, 1381–1389. [CrossRef]
9. Siddall, P.J. Management of neuropathic pain following spinal cord injury: Now and in the future. *Spinal Cord.* **2009**, *47*, 352–359. [CrossRef]
10. Widerstrom-Noga, E.G.; Felipe-Cuervo, E.; Yezierski, R.P. Chronic pain after spinal injury: Interference with sleep and daily activities. *Arch. Phys. Med. Rehabil.* **2001**, *82*, 1571–1577. [CrossRef]
11. Finnerup, N.B.; Norrbrink, C.; Trok, K.; Piehl, F.; Johannesen, I.L.; Sørensen, J.C.; Jensen, T.S.; Werhagen, L. Phenotypes and predictors of pain following traumatic spinal cord injury: A prospective study. *J. Pain* **2014**, *15*, 40–48. [CrossRef] [PubMed]
12. Warner, F.M.; Cragg, J.J.; Jutzeler, C.R.; Finnerup, N.B.; Werhagen, L.; Weidner, N.; Maier, D.; Kalke, Y.-B.; Curt, A.; Kramer, J.L. Progression of Neuropathic Pain after Acute Spinal Cord Injury: A Meta-Analysis and Framework for Clinical Trials. *J. Neurotrauma* **2019**, *36*, 1461–1468. [CrossRef] [PubMed]
13. Margot-Duclot, A.; Tournebise, H.; Ventura, M.; Fattal, C. What are the risk factors of occurence and chronicity of neuropathic pain in spinal cord injury patients? *Ann. Phys. Rehabil. Med.* **2009**, *52*, 111–123. [CrossRef]
14. Jensen, M.P.; Turk, D.C. Contributions of psychology to the understanding and treatment of people with chronic pain: Why it matters to ALL psychologists. *Am. Psychol.* **2014**, *69*, 105–118. [CrossRef] [PubMed]
15. Melzack, R.; Casey, K. Sensory, Motivational, and Central Control Determinants of Pain. In *The Skin Senses*; Kenshalo, D.R., Ed.; Charles C Thomas: Springfield, IL, USA, 1968; pp. 423–439.
16. Siddall, P.J.; Middleton, J.W. A proposed algorithm for the management of pain following spinal cord injury. *Spinal Cord.* **2006**, *44*, 67–77. [CrossRef]
17. Widerstrom-Noga, E.G.; Finnerup, N.B.; Siddall, P.J. Biopsychosocial perspective on a mechanisms-based approach to assessment and treatment of pain following spinal cord injury. *J. Rehabil. Res. Dev.* **2009**, *46*, 1–12. [CrossRef]
18. Jensen, M.P.; Hoffman, A.J.; Cardenas, D.D. Chronic pain in individuals with spinal cord injury: A survey and longitudinal study. *Spinal Cord.* **2005**, *43*, 704–712. [CrossRef]
19. Jensen, M.P.; Kuehn, C.M.; Amtmann, D.; Cardenas, D.D. Symptom burden in persons with spinal cord injury. *Arch. Phys. Med. Rehabil.* **2007**, *88*, 638–645. [CrossRef] [PubMed]
20. Stampas, A.; Pedroza, C.; Bush, J.N.; Ferguson, A.R.; Kramer, J.L.K.; Hook, M. The first 24 h: Opioid administration in people with spinal cord injury and neurologic recovery. *Spinal Cord.* **2020**, *58*, 1080–1089. [CrossRef]
21. Nicholson Perry, K.; Nicholas, M.K.; Middleton, J. Spinal cord injury-related pain in rehabilitation: A cross-sectional study of relationships with cognitions, mood and physical function. *Eur. J. Pain* **2009**, *13*, 511–517. [CrossRef]
22. Hanley, M.A.; Raichle, K.; Jensen, M.; Cardenas, D.D. Pain catastrophizing and beliefs predict changes in pain interference and psychological functioning in persons with spinal cord injury. *J. Pain* **2008**, *9*, 863–871. [CrossRef] [PubMed]
23. Turner, J.A.; Jensen, M.P.; Warms, C.A.; Cardenas, D.D. Catastrophizing is associated with pain intensity, psychological distress, and pain-related disability among individuals with chronic pain after spinal cord injury. *Pain* **2002**, *98*, 127–134. [CrossRef] [PubMed]
24. Craig, A.; Guest, R.; Tran, Y.; Perry, K.N.; Middleton, J. Pain catastrophizing and negative mood states after spinal cord injury: Transitioning from inpatient rehabilitation into the community. *J. Pain* **2017**, *18*, 800–810. [CrossRef]
25. Craig, A.; Tran, Y.; Guest, R.; Middleton, J. Excessive daytime sleepiness in adults with spinal cord injury and associations with pain catastrophizing and pain intensity. *Spinal Cord.* **2020**, *58*, 831–839. [CrossRef] [PubMed]
26. Gruener, H.; Zeilig, G.; Laufer, Y.; Blumen, N.; Defrin, R. Increased psychological distress among individuals with spinal cord injury is associated with central neuropathic pain rather than the injury characteristics. *Spinal Cord.* **2018**, *56*, 176–184. [CrossRef] [PubMed]
27. Taylor, J.; Huelbes, S.; Albu, S.; Gomez-Soriano, J.; Penacoba, C.; Poole, H.M. Neuropathic pain intensity, unpleasantness, coping strategies, and psychosocial factors after spinal cord injury: An exploratory longitudinal study during the first year. *Pain Med.* **2012**, *13*, 1457–1468. [CrossRef] [PubMed]
28. Ehde, D.M.; Jensen, M.P. Feasibility of a cognitive restructuring intervention for treatment of chronic pain in persons with disabilities. *Rehabil Psychol.* **2004**, *49*, 254–258. [CrossRef]

29. Loh, E.; Mirkowski, M.; Roa Agudelo, A.; Allison, D.J.; Benton, B.; Bryce, T.N.; Guilcher, S.; Jeji, T.; Kras Dupis, A.; Kreutzwiser, D.; et al. The CanPain SCI clinical practice guidelines for rehabiliation managemetn of neuropathic pain after spinal cord injury: 2021 update. *Spinal Cord.* **2022**, *60*, 548–566. [CrossRef]
30. Eller, O.C.; Willits, A.B.; Young, E.E.; Baumbauer, K.M. Pharmacological and non-pharmacological therapeutic interventions for the treatment of spinal cord injury-induced pain. *Front. Pain Res.* **2022**, *3*, 991736. [CrossRef]
31. Elkins, G.R.; Barabasz, A.F.; Council, J.R.; Spiegel, D. Advancing research and practice: The revised APA Division 30 definition of hypnosis. *Int. J. Clin. Exp. Hypn.* **2015**, *63*, 1–9. [CrossRef]
32. Zanca, J.M.; Gilchrist, C.; Ortiz, C.E.; Dyson-Hudson, T.A. Pilot clinical trial of a clinical meditation and imagery intervention for chronic pain after spinal cord injury. *J. Spinal Cord. Med.* **2022**, *45*, 339–353. [CrossRef] [PubMed]
33. Adachi, T.; Fujino, H.; Nakae, A.; Mashimo, T.; Sasaki, J. A meta-analysis of hypnosis for chronic pain problems: A comparison between hypnosis, standard care, and other psychological interventions. *Int. J. Clin. Exp. Hypn.* **2014**, *62*, 1–28. [CrossRef] [PubMed]
34. Stoelb, B.L.; Molton, I.R.; Jensen, M.P.; Patterson, D.R. The Efficacy of Hypnotic Analgesia in Adults: A Review of the Literature. *Contemp. Hypn.* **2009**, *26*, 24–39. [CrossRef] [PubMed]
35. Heutink, M.; Post, M.W.; Bongers-Janssen, H.M.; Dijkstra, C.A.; Snoek, G.J.; Spijkerman, D.C.; Lindeman, E. The CONECSI trial: Results of a randomized controlled trial of a multidisciplinary cognitive behavioral program for coping with chronic neuropathic pain after spinal cord injury. *Pain* **2012**, *153*, 120–128. [CrossRef]
36. Kirsch, I.; Montgomery, G.; Sapirstein, G. Hypnosis as an adjunct to cognitive-behavioral psychotherapy: A meta-analysis. *J. Consult. Clin. Psychol.* **1995**, *63*, 214–220. [CrossRef]
37. Jensen, M.P.; Ehde, D.M.; Gertz, K.J.; Stoelb, B.L.; Dillworth, T.M.; Hirsh, A.T.; Molton, I.R.; Kraft, G.H. Effects of self-hypnosis training and cognitive restructuring on daily pain intensity and catastrophizing in individuals with multiple sclerosis and chronic pain. *Int. J. Clin. Exp. Hypn.* **2011**, *59*, 45–63. [CrossRef]
38. Jensen, M.P.; Mendoza, M.E.; Ehde, D.M.; Patterson, D.R.; Molton, I.R.; Dillworth, T.M.; Gertz, K.J.; Chan, J.; Hakimian, S.; Battalio, S.L.; et al. Effects of hypnosis, cognitive therapy, hypnotic cognitive therapy, and pain education in adults with chronic pain: A randomized clinical trial. *Pain* **2020**, *161*, 2284–2298. [CrossRef]
39. Hesam-Shariati, N.; Newton-John, T.; Singh, A.K.; Cortes, C.A.T.; Do, T.-T.N.; Craig, A.; Middleton, J.W.; Jensen, M.P.; Trost, Z.; Lin, C.-T.; et al. Evaluation of the Effectiveness of a Novel Brain-Computer Interface Neuromodulative Intervention to Relieve Neuropathic Pain Following Spinal Cord Injury: Protocol for a Single-Case Experimental Design with Multiple Baselines. *JMIR Res. Protoc.* **2020**, *9*, e20979. [CrossRef]
40. Brown, R.; DiMarco, A.F.; Hoit, J.D.; Garshick, E. Respiratory dysfunction and management in spinal cord injury. *Respir. Care* **2006**, *51*, 853–870.
41. Tate, J.A.; Devito Dabbs, A.; Hoffman, L.A.; Milbrandt, E.; Happ, M.B. Anxiety and agitation in mechanically ventilated patients. *Qual. Health Res.* **2012**, *22*, 157–173. [CrossRef]
42. Jones, C.; Bäckman, C.; Capuzzo, M.; Flaatten, H.; Rylander, C.; Griffiths, R. Precipitants of post-traumatic stress disorder following intensive care: A hypothesis generating study of diversity in care. *Intensive Care Med.* **2007**, *33*, 978–985. [CrossRef]
43. de la Vega, R.; Mendoza, M.E.; Chan, J.F.; Jensen, M.P. Case study: Cognitive restructuring hypnosis for chronic pain in a quadriplegic patient. *Am. J. Clin. Hypn.* **2019**, *61*, 394–408. [CrossRef] [PubMed]
44. New, P.; Lim, T.; Hill, S.; Brown, D. A survey of pain during rehabilitation after acute spinal cord injury. *Spinal Cord.* **1997**, *35*, 658. [CrossRef] [PubMed]
45. Lamid, S.; Chia, J.; Kohli, A.; Cid, E. Chronic pain in spinal cord injury: Comparison between inpatients and outpatients. *Arch. Phys. Med. Rehabil.* **1985**, *66*, 777–778. [PubMed]
46. Starosta, A.J.; Bombardier, C.H.; Kahlia, F.; Barber, J.; Accardi-Ravid, M.C.; Wiechman, S.A.; Crane, D.A.; Jensen, M.P. Feasibility of brief, hypnotic enhanced cognitive therapy for SCI-related pain during inpatient rehabilitation. *Arch. Phys. Med. Rehabil.* **2023**, *online ahead of publication*.
47. Bryce, T.N.; Richards, J.S.; Bombardier, C.H.; Dijkers, M.; Fann, J.R.; Brooks, L.J.; Chiodo, A.E.; Tate, D.G.; Forchheimer, M. Screening for neuropathic pain after spinal cord injury with the spinal cord injury pain instrument (SCIPI): A preliminary validation study. *Spinal Cord.* **2014**, *52*, 407–412. [CrossRef] [PubMed]
48. Widerström-Noga, E.; Biering-Sørensen, F.; Bryce, T.N.; Cardenas, D.D.; Finnerup, N.B.; Jensen, M.P.; Richards, J.S.; Siddall, P.J. The international spinal cord injury pain basic data set (version 2.0). *Spinal Cord.* **2014**, *52*, 282–286. [CrossRef] [PubMed]
49. Pleil, A.M.; Coyne, K.S.; Reese, P.R.; Jumadilova, Z.; Rovner, E.S.; Kelleher, C.J. The validation of patient-rated global assessments of treatment benefit, satisfaction, and willingness to continue—The BSW. *Value Health* **2005**, *8*, S25–S34. [CrossRef]
50. Bryce, T.N.; Budh, C.N.; Cardenas, D.D.; Dijkers, M.; Felix, E.R.; Finnerup, N.B.; Kennedy, P.; Lundeberg, T.; Richards, J.S.; Rintala, D.H.; et al. Pain after spinal cord injury: An evidence-based review for clinical practice and research: Report of the National Institute on Disability and Rehabilitation Research Spinal Cord Injury Measures meeting. *J. Spinal Cord Med.* **2007**, *30*, 421–440. [CrossRef]
51. Dworkin, R.H.; Turk, D.C.; Farrar, J.T.; Haythornthwaite, J.A.; Jensen, M.P.; Katz, N.P.; Kerns, R.D.; Stucki, G.; Allen, R.R.; Bellamy, N.; et al. Core outcome measures for chronic pain clinical trials: IMMPACT recommendations. *Pain* **2005**, *113*, 9–19. [CrossRef]
52. Jensen, M.P.; Widerström-Noga, E.; Richards, J.S.; Finnerup, N.B.; Biering-Sørensen, F.; Cardenas, D.D. Reliability and validity of the International Spinal Cord Injury Basic Pain Data Set items as self-report measures. *Spinal Cord.* **2010**, *48*, 230–238. [CrossRef]

53. Amtmann, D.; Cook, K.F.; Jensen, M.P.; Chen, W.-H.; Choi, S.; Revicki, D.; Cella, D.; Rothrock, N.; Keefe, F.; Callahan, L.; et al. development of a PROMIS item bank to measure pain interference. *Pain* **2010**, *150*, 173–182. [CrossRef] [PubMed]
54. Askew, R.L.; Cook, K.F.; Revicki, D.A.; Cella, D.; Amtmann, D. Evidence from diverse clinical populations supported clinical validity of PROMIS pain interference and pain behavior. *J. Clin. Epidemiol.* **2016**, *73*, 103–111. [CrossRef]
55. Kean, J.; Monahan, P.; Kroenke, K.; Wu, J.; Yu, Z.; Stump, T.; Krebs, E.E. Comparative responsiveness of the PROMIS Pain Interference short forms, Brief Pain Inventory, PEG, and SF-36 Bodily Pain subscale. *Med. Care* **2016**, *54*, 414–421. [CrossRef] [PubMed]
56. Amtmann, D.; Liljenquist, K.; Bamer, A.; Bocell, F.; Jensen, M.; Wilson, R.; Turk, D. Measuring pain catastrophizing and pain-related self-efficacy: Expert panels, focus groups, and cognitive interviews. *Patient-Patient-Centered Outcomes Res.* **2018**, *11*, 107–117. [CrossRef]
57. Amtmann, D.; Bamer, A.M.; Liljenquist, K.S.; Cowan, P.; Salem, R.; Turk, D.C.; Jensen, M.P. The Concerns About Pain (CAP) Scale: A Patient-Reported Outcome Measure of Pain Catastrophizing. *J. Pain* **2020**, *21*, 1198–1211. [CrossRef]
58. McCracken, L.M.; Vowles, K.E.; Eccleston, C. Acceptance of chronic pain: Component analysis and a revised assessment method. *Pain* **2004**, *107*, 159–166. [CrossRef]
59. Buysse, D.J.; Yu, L.; Moul, D.E.; Germain, A.; Stover, A.; Dodds, N.E.; Johnston, K.L.; Shablesky-Cade, M.A.; Pilkonis, P.A. Development and validation of patient-reported outcome measures for sleep disturbance and sleep-related impairments. *Sleep* **2010**, *33*, 781–792. [CrossRef]
60. Sobreira, M.; Almeida, M.P.; Gomes, A.; Lucas, M.; Oliveira, A.; Marques, A. Minimal clinically important differences for measures of pain, lung function, fatigue, and functionality in spinal cord injury. *Phys. Ther.* **2021**, *101*, pzaa210. [CrossRef]
61. Burke, D.; Fullen, B.M.; Stokes, D.; Lennon, O. Neuropathic pain prevalence following spinal cord injury: A systematic review and meta-analysis. *Eur. J. Pain* **2017**, *21*, 29–44. [CrossRef] [PubMed]
62. Boldt, I.; Eriks-Hoogland, I.; Brinkhof, M.W.; de Bie, R.; Joggi, D.; von Elm, E. Non-pharmacological interventions for chronic pain in people with spinal cord injury. *Cochrane Database Syst. Rev.* **2014**, *28*, CD009177. [CrossRef] [PubMed]
63. Gibbs, K.; Beaufort, A.; Stein, A.; Leung, T.M.; Sison, C.; Bloom, O. Assessment of pain symptoms and quality of life using the International Spinal Cord Injury Data Sets in persons with chronic spinal cord injury. *Spinal Cord. Ser. Cases* **2019**, *5*, 32. [CrossRef] [PubMed]

Disclaimer/Publisher's Note: The statements, opinions and data contained in all publications are solely those of the individual author(s) and contributor(s) and not of MDPI and/or the editor(s). MDPI and/or the editor(s) disclaim responsibility for any injury to people or property resulting from any ideas, methods, instructions or products referred to in the content.

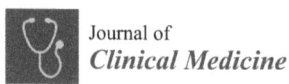

Article

Spinal Cord Stimulation Prevents Autonomic Dysreflexia in Individuals with Spinal Cord Injury: A Case Series

Soshi Samejima [1,2], Claire Shackleton [1,2], Raza N. Malik [1,2], Kawami Cao [1,2], Anibal Bohorquez [2,3], Tom E. Nightingale [1,4,5], Rahul Sachdeva [1,2] and Andrei V. Krassioukov [1,2,3,*]

1 International Collaboration on Repair Discoveries, Faculty of Medicine, University of British Columbia, Vancouver, BC V5Z 1M9, Canada
2 Division of Physical Medicine and Rehabilitation, Department of Medicine, University of British Columbia, Vancouver, BC V5Z 2G9, Canada
3 Spinal Cord Program, GF Strong Rehabilitation Centre, Vancouver Coastal Health, Vancouver, BC V5Z 2G9, Canada
4 School of Sport, Exercise and Rehabilitation Sciences, University of Birmingham, Edgbaston, Birmingham B15 2TT, UK
5 Centre for Trauma Sciences Research, University of Birmingham, Edgbaston, Birmingham B15 2TT, UK
* Correspondence: andrei.krassioukov@vch.ca; Tel.: +1-604-675-8810

Abstract: Spinal cord injury (SCI) results in severe cardiovascular dysfunction due to the disruption of supraspinal control. Autonomic dysreflexia (AD), an uncontrolled rise in blood pressure in response to peripheral stimuli including common bowel routine, digital anorectal stimulation (DARS), reduces the quality of life, and increases morbidity and mortality. Recently, spinal cord stimulation (SCS) has emerged as a potential intervention to mitigate unstable blood pressure following SCI. The objective of this case series was to test the real-time effect of epidural SCS (eSCS) at the lumbosacral spinal cord, the most common implant location, on mitigating AD in individuals with SCI. We recruited three individuals with cervical and upper thoracic motor-complete SCI who have an implanted epidural stimulator. We demonstrated that eSCS can reduce the elevation in blood pressure and prevent DARS-induced AD. The blood pressure variability analysis indicated that eSCS potentially reduced vascular sympathetic nervous system activity during DARS, compared to without eSCS. This case series provides evidence to support the use of eSCS to prevent AD episodes during routine bowel procedures, improving the quality of life for individuals with SCI and potentially reducing cardiovascular risks.

Keywords: spinal cord injury; spinal cord stimulation; autonomic dysreflexia; cardiovascular function; epidural stimulation

1. Introduction

Spinal cord injury (SCI) results in a disconnect between the supraspinal autonomic control center and the spinal autonomic circuits below the injury [1]. The disrupted autonomic pathways lead to impaired cardiovascular control following SCI, especially with injuries at or above the sixth thoracic spinal cord segment (T6) [2]. Cardiovascular dysfunction not only disturbs activities of daily living and detrimentally impacts the health-related quality of life for individuals with SCI, but also contributes to the deterioration of vascular health, increasing the risk of cerebro- and cardio-vascular diseases [3–6].

These cardiovascular impairments include episodes of uncontrolled blood pressure (BP) elevation in response to afferent inputs below the injury, a condition known as autonomic dysreflexia (AD) [7,8]. The severity of AD is associated with the completeness of SCI, and 91% of people with cervical SCI present with AD signs [9]. In addition to the loss of supraspinal inhibitory inputs to sympathetic preganglionic neurons (SPNs) below the lesion [10], the neuroplastic changes of SPNs [11–15], changes within propriospinal neurons [16], as well as aberrant plasticity within afferent fibers [17] increase the excitability of the spinal cord in response to peripheral stimulation [18]. AD is commonly caused by bowel routines following SCI, including the regularly used procedure of digital anorectal stimulation (DARS) [19]. DARS can also cause increased sympathetic activity and the development of AD [19]. Inadequate interventions for AD lead to severe cardiovascular conditions, stroke and even death [4,20]. Preventing AD is one of the key health priorities for recovery identified by individuals with cervical and thoracic SCI [21,22]. Current options for managing AD, including non-pharmacological and pharmacological agents [23], frequently have limited effects or significant side effects and a delayed onset of action [24,25]. For instance, some antihypertensive agents (e.g., Nifedipine) can decrease arterial BP below the desired levels, which is sustained for hours, and requires further monitoring and management [24,25]. Alternative options for the management of AD, without significant adverse effects, are needed to improve care for individuals with SCI.

Spinal cord stimulation (SCS) has been used clinically to treat pain since 1967 [26,27]. There is a growing body of evidence indicating that epidural SCS (eSCS), an FDA-approved means to treat pain, potentially modulates spinal circuits via primary afferent inputs, resulting in motor [28–31] and autonomic [32–38] recovery following SCI. These studies indicate that the most common positioning of epidural implants is on the lumbosacral spinal cord to target direct innervation of lower extremity muscles and pelvic organs. Furthermore, early work investigating eSCS at the lumbosacral spinal segment demonstrated the long-term effect of stimulation on mitigating AD in four out of five individuals with SCI [39]. However, this study only reported anecdotal evidence (e.g., frequency of AD), without systematic BP measurements, and did not test any real-time effects of eSCS on AD.

Therefore, this study aimed to assess the real-time impact of clinically approved eSCS on preventing DARS-induced AD in three individuals with cervical and upper thoracic motor-complete SCI. We also evaluated the impact of eSCS on vasculature sympathetic nervous system activity during DARS. It was hypothesized that real-time eSCS at the lumbosacral spinal segments could prevent AD during DARS by preventing the increase in sympathetic nervous system activity.

2. Methods

This study was approved by the University of British Columbia Clinical Ethics Board (UBC CREB H19-00932) and was conducted in accordance with the Declaration of Helsinki. The participants provided written informed consent prior to their participation.

We recruited individuals with sensorimotor-complete or motor-complete SCI (American Spinal Injury Association impairment scale (AIS) AIS A and B) at T6 or above, who presented with documented AD signs and received the epidural stimulator implantation. We included consecutive participants under the criteria. The participants included two males with traumatic cervical SCI, and one female with traumatic thoracic SCI. All participants underwent implantation of a 16-electrode array (Restore-ADVANCED neurostimulator, Specify 5-6-5, Medtronic, Minneapolis, MN, USA) between T10 and T12 vertebral levels (i.e., the lumbosacral spinal segments) prior to the study. Each individual's neurological level of injury (NLI) and AIS were determined according to the International Standards for Neurological Classification of Spinal Cord Injury (ISNCSCI) [40].

2.1. Study Design and Assessments

A summary of participant demographics and injury characteristics are presented in Figure 1. Following screening and informed consent, participants attended their first visit in which their severity of neurological impairment and autonomic cardiovascular dysfunction was assessed using the ISNCSCI exam and 24 h Ambulatory BP Monitoring (ABPM) (Meditech Ltd., Budapest, Hungary) [41], respectively. Prior to the 24 h ABPM, baseline resting BP and heart rate (HR) values were established as the average of three measurements. The ABPM device was applied with appropriate cuff sizes to the non-dominant arm and preprogrammed to record systolic BP (SBP), diastolic BP (DBP) and HR. Cardiovascular parameters were recorded automatically every 15 min during the daytime and every 60 min during the nighttime, based on the individual's usual sleeping routines.

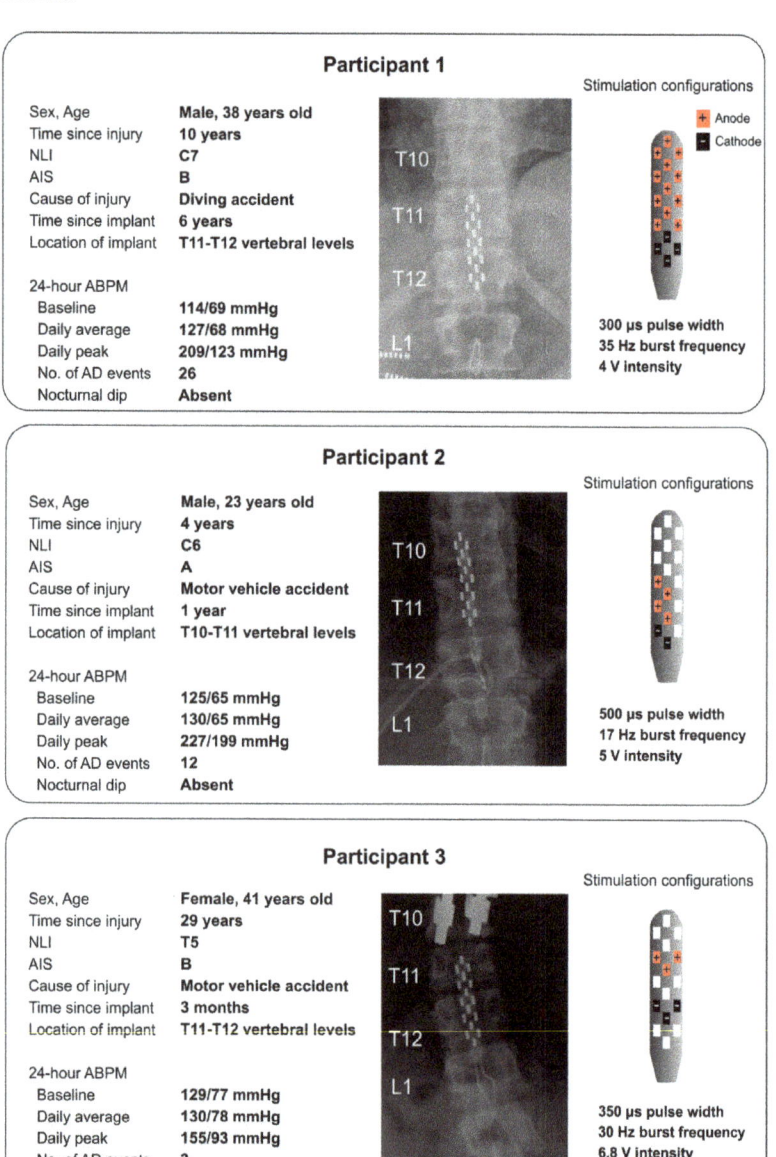

Figure 1. Demographics, blood pressure responses, epidural implant location and stimulation configuration, including active anodic and cathodic electrodes on the implants in three individuals with SCI. Anatomical placement of the 16-electrode array: conventional radiography of the thoracic and lumbar spines displays the position of the 16-electrode array. Stimulation configurations: red identifies anodes and black identifies cathodes. Cathodes were the caudal electrodes in all participants. Abbreviations: ABPM, ambulatory blood pressure monitoring; AD, autonomic dysreflexia; AIS, American Spinal Injury Association Impairment Scale; BP, blood pressure; C, cervical; DBP, diastolic blood pressure; Hz: hertz; SBP, systolic blood pressure; us, microseconds; V, volts.

The second visit involved the DARS procedure with continuous BP monitoring. DARS is a routine procedure to initiate a bowel evacuation and has previously been employed to trigger controlled elevation in arterial BP in individuals with SCI [19,42]. The participants were requested to complete a bowel routine 24 h prior to the assessment. Participants were positioned in the left lateral decubital position and baseline hemodynamics were recorded. Next, an experienced clinician (AVK) delivered DARS in accordance with published recommendations [43]. The index finger was inserted into the rectum and gentle pressure was applied for 30 s. Throughout the assessment, continuous hemodynamic data were recorded to monitor cardiovascular safety and report on the severity of AD experienced by the participants. Beat-by-beat BP and HR were continuously recorded via finger photoplethysmography and five-lead electrocardiography (ECG) using Finapres NOVA (Finapres Medical Systems, Amsterdam, Netherlands), respectively, and brachial BP recorded every minute (Dinamap PRO, GE Healthcare, Chicago, IL, USA). Beat-by-beat BP and HR were sampled at 1000 Hz via an analog-to-digital converter (Powerlab 16/35 System, ADInstruments, Colorado Springs, CO, USA). DARS was performed twice without eSCS and twice with eSCS in a randomized order. Both the clinician and participants remained blinded to the selected eSCS program and BP responses during the DARS procedure. eSCS was selected to target the lumbosacral area involved in bowel control, based on the program in which the cathode electrodes were caudally positioned within the array (Figure 1). To determine the ability of eSCS in preventing an episode of AD, eSCS was initiated 60 s prior to DARS and was sustained for an additional 60 s after DARS was completed.

2.2. Data Processing and Analysis

The ABPM data were downloaded for offline analysis using the CardioVisions 1.13.0 software (Meditech Ltd., Budapest, Hungary). Furthermore, participants diarized the time and type of event (e.g., bowel routine initiation) that could have resulted in BP fluctuations and described any potential AD signs and symptoms experienced during the 24 h ABPM period. Based on the clinical definition of AD, in which SBP rises more than 20 mmHg from the baseline resting SBP, all episodes of daily AD were identified for the 24 h period [44].

Offline hemodynamic data analyses of the digitized Finapres signals were performed at a temporal resolution of one millisecond using MATLAB R2021b (Mathworks, Natick, MA, USA). Time series of successive beats were extracted for SBP, DBP and HR. Occasional ectopic beats were corrected by linear interpolation of adjacent normal beats. Baseline BP and HR with and without eSCS were collected for 60 s in the absence of DARS. The magnitude of change in SBP, DBP and HR in response to DARS were calculated as the differences between the average baseline measurements prior to a DARS application and the peak values obtained during DARS. The calculated changes were averaged across two trials per participant under each stimulation condition (eSCS OFF and eSCS ON).

The periodic content of BP variability was assessed using validated wavelet decomposition [45]. This analysis was implemented using the continuous wavelet transform (cwt) function from the MATLAB Wavelet Toolbox, using the default settings with the analytic Morse wavelet. A scalogram was generated to represent the time and frequency domains of BP variability and the amplitude of the frequency power was shown by the intensity of that point using color. By taking the integral of the wavelet power over the selected frequency range, the total power of the scalogram was determined, which is an index of BP variability. The magnitude of the change in lower frequency (LF) power of BP variability was extracted as the difference between the average LF power of the 40 s baseline prior to DARS and the average LF power of the 40 s measurement from the finger insertion. The data period was selected to account for the time from finger insertion (5–10 s) to the completion of DARS (30 s). Specific LF components (i.e., 0.05–0.15 Hz) of BP variability were assessed to estimate vasculature sympathetic activity [46,47]. All data were reported as the mean ± standard deviation.

3. Results

All participants experienced episodes of AD during a daily 24 h period (Figure 1). In addition to the frequent episodes of AD, Participants 1 and 2 had no nocturnal dipping, indicative of severe cardiovascular dysfunction. The effect of eSCS on resting cardiovascular parameters showed that there were minimal changes in resting SBP, DBP and HR between the stimulation conditions in all participants (Table 1). Subsequently, we evaluated the cardiovascular responses to DARS with and without eSCS. DARS without eSCS induced an elevation in SBP of greater than 20 mmHg (Participant 1: change of (Δ)SBP 31 ± 14 mmHg, Participant 2: ΔSBP 22 ± 1 mmHg, Participant 3: ΔSBP 26 ± 2 mmHg) and a simultaneous reduction in HR (Table 1), indicative of AD. Active eSCS during DARS prevented AD, as evidenced by a marginal elevation in SBP of less than the 20 mmHg threshold for AD diagnosis (Participant 1: ΔSBP 16 ± 0.2 mmHg, Participant 2: ΔSBP 13 ± 3 mmHg, Participant 3: ΔSBP 8 ± 5 mmHg) and a minimal reduction in HR (Table 1, Figure 2a,b).

Table 1. Cardiovascular responses at rest (supine) and in response to DARS, with and without eSCS in individuals with SCI.

	Participant 1		Participant 2		Participant 3	
	Without eSCS	With eSCS	Without eSCS	With eSCS	Without eSCS	With eSCS
Baseline SBP (mmHg)	110 ± 10	118 ± 12	102 ± 2	96 ± 1	134 ± 1	137 ± 4
Baseline DBP (mmHg)	63 ± 7	66 ± 10	62 ± 3	53 ± 2	93 ± 5	91 ± 1
Baseline HR (bpm)	71 ± 8	71 ± 14	47 ± 1	46 ± 1	69 ± 0.1	70 ± 1
Baseline LF wavelet power (a.u.)	0.0047 ± 0.0030	0.0051 ± 0.0015	0.0050 ± 0.0044	0.0050 ± 0.0013	0.0058 ± 0.0014	0.0052 ± 0.0003
Δ SBP during DARS (mmHg)	31 ± 14	16 ± 0.2	22 ± 1	13 ± 3	26 ± 2	8 ± 5
Δ DBP during DARS (mmHg)	13 ± 6	4 ± 2	14 ± 2	7 ± 1	7 ± 0.2	−1 ± 2
Δ HR during DARS (bpm)	−20 ± 8	−9 ± 3	−5 ± 1	−3 ± 0.2	−8 ± 2	−2 ± 2
Δ LF wavelet power during DARS (a.u.)	0.0021 ± 0.0006	−0.0001 ± 0.0011	0.0015 ± 0.0003	−0.0002 ± 0.0002	0.0029 ± 0.0001	0.0007 ± 0.0003

Abbreviations: a.u., arbitrary unit; bpm, beats per minute; DARS, digital anorectal stimulation; DBP, diastolic blood pressure; eSCS, epidural spinal cord stimulation; HR, heart rate; LF, low frequency; mmHg, millimeter of mercury; SBP, systolic blood pressure; SCI, spinal cord injury; Δ, change. Data are represented as the mean of two measurements ± standard deviation.

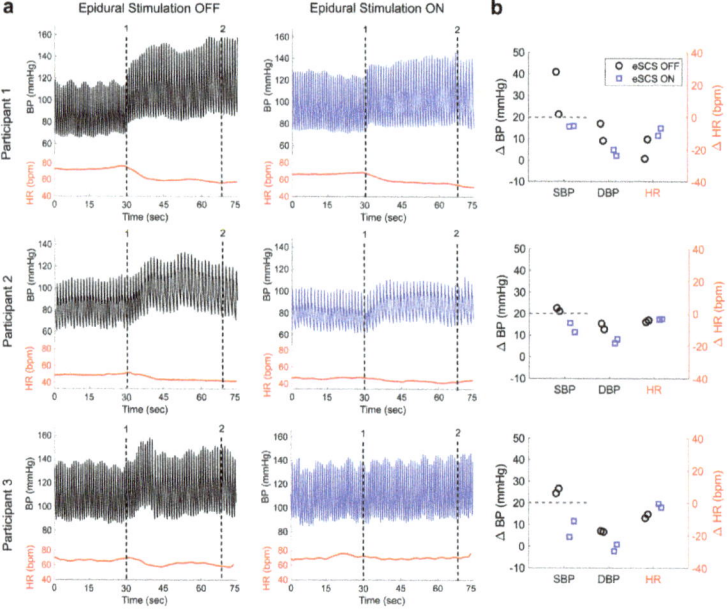

Figure 2. Cont.

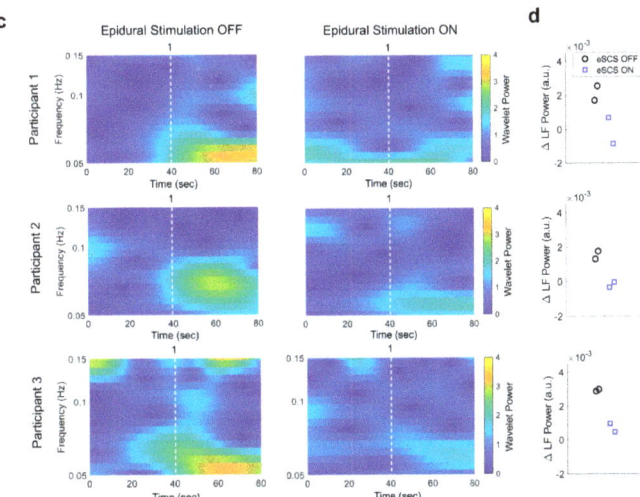

Figure 2. Effect of eSCS on AD during DARS in three individuals with SCI. (**a**) Cardiovascular responses during DARS with eSCS OFF (grey shading) and eSCS ON (blue shading). The first vertical black dotted line (1) shows the start of DARS (i.e., insertion of index finger into the rectum), and the second vertical black dotted line (2) shows the completion of DARS (i.e., removal of finger). (**b**) Changes in SBP, DBP and HR during DARS with (blue symbols) and without (black symbols) eSCS in each participant. During DARS without eSCS, all participants showed an elevation in SBP greater than the 20-mmHg threshold for AD diagnosis (gray dotted lines). However, DARS with eSCS consistently reduced changes in SBP, keeping it below the threshold for AD diagnosis (grey dotted lines). (**c**) Scalogram showing wavelet power (yellow color) at low frequencies (0.05–0.15 Hz, y-axis) over time (x-axis). Wavelet power scalogram shows increased low frequency power during DARS without eSCS. However, with eSCS, all participants showed a decrease in wavelet power following the start of DARS (white dotted vertical line 1). (**d**) The elevation in low frequency power following DARS was prevented with eSCS ON compared to eSCS OFF in all participants. Abbreviations: a.u., arbitrary unit; BPM, beats per minute; DARS, digital anorectal stimulation; DBP, diastolic blood pressure; eSCS, epidural spinal cord stimulation; HR, heart rate; Hz, hertz; LF, low frequency; mmHg, millimeter of mercury; SBP, systolic blood pressure; Δ, change.

Wavelet decomposition analysis of BP variability, in the absence of eSCS, showed a higher LF wavelet power concomitant with the elevation of SBP during DARS (Table 1). However, real-time eSCS resulted in decreased LF wavelet power (Participant 1: 0.0021 ± 0.0006 vs. -0.0001 ± 0.0011, Participant 2: 0.0015 ± 0.0003 vs. -0.0002 ± 0.0002, Participant 2: 0.0029 ± 0.0001 vs. -0.0007 ± 0.0003), concomitant with the mitigation of AD during DARS (Figure 2c,d).

4. Discussion

Severe AD symptoms during bowel management (e.g., DARS) are associated with a lower quality of life following SCI [48–50]. In addition, the labile BP is the leading cause of cardiovascular morbidity and mortality after SCI [6,51–53]. Despite the risk of potentially life-threatening episodes of AD associated with DARS, it is still a commonly used method for bowel evacuation following SCI. In this case series, we demonstrated the effect of real-time eSCS on preventing AD during DARS in three individuals with cervical and upper thoracic motor-complete SCI. Our results show that real-time eSCS during DARS decreased the elevation of LF wavelet power in BP variability, indicating reduced vasculature sympathetic nerve activity [46,47]. Therefore, clinically available lumbosacral eSCS is potentially a fast-acting and effective alternative to pharmacological management of AD, which could reduce cardiovascular risk and improve the health-related quality of life.

Previous neurostimulation studies have shown that by targeting the SPNs directly, SCS can mitigate AD [42]. In this study, we used eSCS programs where the active electrodes (i.e., cathode) stimulated the caudal lumbosacral spinal segments. Therefore, we show that eSCS delivered at the lumbosacral region (i.e., outside the T1–L2 segments that contain SPNs) can similarly effectively mitigate AD. These results suggest that SCS over the caudal lumbosacral spinal segments can impact the SPNs potentially via propriospinal neurons [32]. This contrasts previous studies which proposed eSCS at the lower thoracic spinal segments as a "hemodynamic hot spot" for BP control [33,54]. Thus, it is possible that eSCS at the lumbosacral spinal segments, which targets motor and pelvic organ function, could be repurposed for the recovery of cardiovascular control following SCI.

The most plausible mechanism for the effect of SCS on AD relies on the gate control theory [55]. This theory proposes that primary afferent inputs induce inhibitory mechanisms to close the gate to visceral or noxious inputs at the spinal cord level. Based on the gate control theory and the location of the active electrodes in this study, we propose that eSCS-induced primary afferent inputs at the sacral spinal segments likely inhibited the activation of excitatory interneurons (e.g., long propriospinal neurons) [16] in response to visceral inputs (i.e., DARS) via inhibitory interneurons [32]. These inhibitory interneurons (e.g., GABAergic interneurons) can be activated via large afferent fibers [56,57]. A previous study showed that DARS increased the vasculature sympathetic outflow, measured by norepinephrine, in individuals with SCI [19]. In our study, the smaller changes in LF wavelet power indicate that eSCS potentially inhibited the excitation of the vascular sympathetic nervous system activity in all participants. Based on our case series results, we hypothesize that eSCS prevented AD through inhibitory interneurons in the sacral spinal cord, potentially preventing the activation of maladapted sympathetic spinal circuits controlling hyperexcitable SPNs in T6–L2 spinal segments (Figure 3).

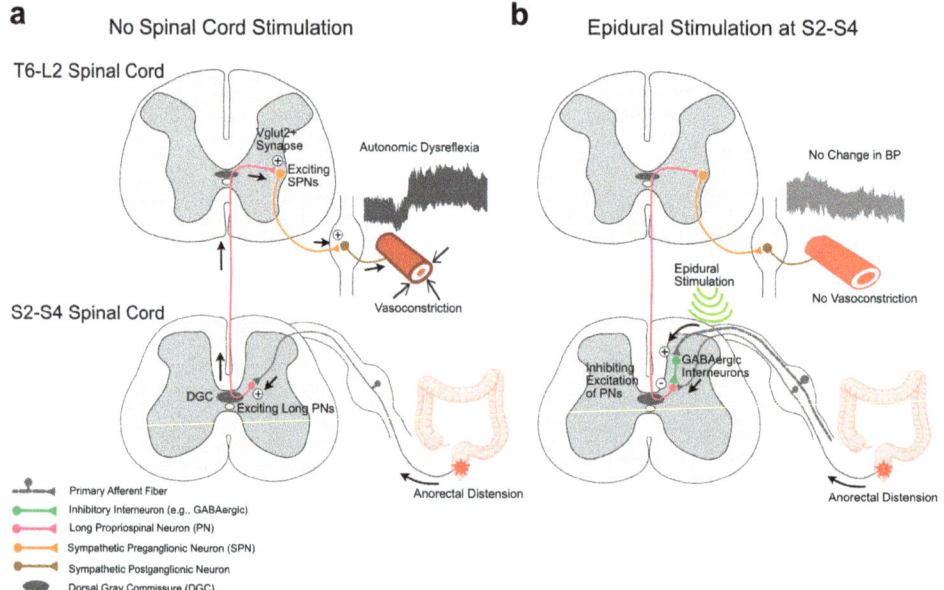

Figure 3. Potential mechanism of epidural spinal cord stimulation for mitigating autonomic dysreflexia. This figure shows the effect of eSCS at the caudal lumbosacral spinal segments (S2–S4) on visceral stimuli in the intact and injured spinal cord, at or above T6. (**a**) Without eSCS, visceral inputs by anorectal distention activate excitatory interneurons (red) through afferent fibers. The excitatory inputs polysynaptically ascend to thoracolumbar spinal segments (T6–L2), likely via long propriospinal neurons in the dorsal gray commissure (DGC) [16]. The ascending inputs activate

sympathetic preganglionic neurons (SPNs, orange) via glutamatergic synapses (e.g., vesicular–glutamate transporter positive (Vglut2+) synapses), increasing vasculature of the sympathetic nervous system activity, leading to autonomic dysreflexia [13,14]. (**b**) With eSCS, primary afferent inputs (gray with myelination) potentially activate inhibitory interneurons (e.g., GABAergic interneurons, green) [56,57]. The inhibitory interneurons may inhibit the activation of excitatory interneurons (red), which results in no excitation of SPNs to prevent vasoconstriction related to visceral inputs from S2 to S4.

There are several limitations to this study. First, we tested the effect of eSCS in only three participants. Consequently, investigations in a larger cohort, with more diverse injury and demographic characteristics are warranted to confirm the efficacy of eSCS for preventing AD in this population. Second, this study presents an experimental AD assessment in participants under a controlled laboratory manner to ensure cardiovascular safety. The preliminary findings of this study need to be translated into investigating the effect of eSCS on uncontrolled hypertensive episodes across various daily activities (e.g., bladder distension, catheterization, and sexual activity) or iatrogenic clinical procedures (e.g., urodynamics, penile vibrostimulation). Future studies also need to examine the long-term effect of eSCS on targeting the sacral spinal segments for mitigating AD. Third, although eSCS is approved by the FDA for pain management, the implantation of eSCS involve several risks, including surgical complications, cost and pulse generator battery life. The community needs to test whether a non-invasive means, such as tSCS which has not been approved by the FDA, can be an alternative therapy for mitigating AD [42]. Finally, this clinical study should be reverse-translated into rat SCI models to dissect activated and inhibited spinal neurons during the intervention, to better understand the precise mechanisms of action.

5. Conclusions

Lumbosacral eSCS prevented AD induced by DARS and decreased LF wavelet power in individuals with cervical and upper thoracic motor-complete SCI. More evidence is needed to clarify the underlying inhibitory mechanisms of eSCS and verify the best location of spinal cord stimulation to optimize the prevention of AD. eSCS could serve as a fast-acting therapeutic tool for mitigating uncontrolled BP fluctuations following SCI, leading to a decreased risk of associated cardiovascular consequences and an improved quality of life for individuals with SCI.

Author Contributions: A.V.K. and T.E.N. designed the case series. S.S., C.S., R.S. and A.V.K. contributed to conceptualizing the organizational structure, content, and scope of the manuscript. S.S. and A.V.K. were primarily responsible for writing the manuscript and creating the figures. All authors contributed to editing the entire document. All authors have read and agreed to the published version of the manuscript.

Funding: This case series study received no external funding.

Informed Consent Statement: Informed consent was obtained from all subjects involved in the study.

Data Availability Statement: The data that support the findings of this study can be available contacting the corresponding author via e-mail.

Acknowledgments: A.V.K. holds Endowed Chair in rehabilitation medicine, University of British Columbia, and his lab is supported by funds from the Canadian Institute for Health Research, Canadian Foundation for Innovation and BC Knowledge Development Fund, International Spinal Research Trust, Rick Hansen Foundation, PRAXIS Spinal Cord Institute, Wings for life Research Foundation and the US Department of Defense. S.S. is supported by Paralyzed Veterans of America Fellowship and Wings for Life Spinal Cord Research Foundation. C.S. and R.N.M are supported by Paralyzed Veterans of America Fellowship. R.S. is supported by Wings for Life Spinal Cord Research Foundation and the US Department of Defense. Lastly, we would like to thank Tiev Miller for the data collection support.

Conflicts of Interest: The authors declare no conflict of interest.

References

1. Krassioukov, A. Autonomic function following cervical spinal cord injury. *Respir. Physiol. Neurobiol.* **2009**, *169*, 157–164. [CrossRef] [PubMed]
2. Krassioukov, A.; Weaver, L. Physical medicine and rehabilitation: State of the Art reviews. In *Anatomy of the Autonomic Nervous System*; Teasell, R., Baskerville, V.B., Eds.; Hanley and Belfus, Inc.: Philadelphia, PA, USA, 1996; Volume 10, Chapter 1, pp. 1–14.
3. Wu, J.C.; Chen, Y.C.; Liu, L.; Chen, T.J.; Huang, W.C.; Cheng, H.; Tung-Ping, S. Increased risk of stroke after spinal cord injury: A nationwide 4-year follow-up cohort study. *Neurology* **2012**, *78*, 1051–1057. [CrossRef]
4. Wan, D.; Krassioukov, A.V. Life-threatening outcomes associated with autonomic dysreflexia: A clinical review. *J. Spinal Cord Med.* **2014**, *37*, 2–10. [CrossRef]
5. Forrest, G.P. Atrial fibrillation associated with autonomic dysreflexia in patients with tetraplegia. *Arch. Phys. Med. Rehabil.* **1991**, *72*, 592–594.
6. Cragg, J.J.; Noonan, V.K.; Krassioukov, A.; Borisoff, J. Cardiovascular disease and spinal cord injury: Results from a national population health survey. *Neurology* **2013**, *81*, 723–728. [CrossRef]
7. Guttmann, L.; Whitteridge, D. Effects of bladder distension on autonomic mechanisms after spinal cord injuries. *Brain J. Neurol.* **1947**, *70*, 361–404. [CrossRef] [PubMed]
8. Mathias, C.J.; Frankel, H.L. Cardiovascular control in spinal man. *Annu. Rev. Physiol.* **1988**, *50*, 577–592. [CrossRef]
9. Curt, A.; Nitsche, B.; Rodic, B.; Schurch, B.; Dietz, V. Assessment of autonomic dysreflexia in patients with spinal cord injury. *J. Neurol. Neurosurg. Psychiatry* **1997**, *62*, 473–477. [CrossRef] [PubMed]
10. Stjernberg, L.; Blumberg, H.; Wallin, B.G. Sympathetic activity in man after spinal cord injury. Outflow to muscle below the lesion. *Brain J. Neurol.* **1986**, *109 Pt 4*, 695–715. [CrossRef]
11. Krassioukov, A.V.; Weaver, L.C. Morphological changes in sympathetic preganglionic neurons after spinal cord injury in rats. *Neuroscience* **1996**, *70*, 211–225. [CrossRef] [PubMed]
12. Krenz, N.R.; Weaver, L.C. Changes in the morphology of sympathetic preganglionic neurons parallel the development of autonomic dysreflexia after spinal cord injury in rats. *Neurosci. Lett.* **1998**, *243*, 61–64. [CrossRef]
13. Maiorov, D.N.; Krenz, N.R.; Krassioukov, A.V.; Weaver, L.C. Role of spinal NMDA and AMPA receptors in episodic hypertension in conscious spinal rats. *Am. J. Physiol.* **1997**, *273*, H1266–H1274. [CrossRef] [PubMed]
14. Ueno, M.; Ueno-Nakamura, Y.; Niehaus, J.; Popovich, P.G.; Yoshida, Y. Silencing spinal interneurons inhibits immune suppressive autonomic reflexes caused by spinal cord injury. *Nat. Neurosci.* **2016**, *19*, 784–787. [CrossRef] [PubMed]
15. Sachdeva, R.; Hutton, G.; Marwaha, A.S.; Krassioukov, A.V. Morphological maladaptations in sympathetic preganglionic neurons following an experimental high-thoracic spinal cord injury. *Exp. Neurol.* **2020**, *327*, 113235. [CrossRef] [PubMed]
16. Hou, S.; Duale, H.; Cameron, A.A.; Abshire, S.M.; Lyttle, T.S.; Rabchevsky, A.G. Plasticity of lumbosacral propriospinal neurons is associated with the development of autonomic dysreflexia after thoracic spinal cord transection. *J. Comp. Neurol.* **2008**, *509*, 382–399. [CrossRef] [PubMed]
17. Krenz, N.R.; Weaver, L.C. Sprouting of primary afferent fibers after spinal cord transection in the rat. *Neuroscience* **1998**, *85*, 443–458. [CrossRef]
18. Krassioukov, A.V.; Johns, D.G.; Schramm, L.P. Sensitivity of sympathetically correlated spinal interneurons, renal sympathetic nerve activity, and arterial pressure to somatic and visceral stimuli after chronic spinal injury. *J. Neurotrauma* **2002**, *19*, 1521–1529. [CrossRef]
19. Faaborg, P.M.; Christensen, P.; Krassioukov, A.; Laurberg, S.; Frandsen, E.; Krogh, K. Autonomic dysreflexia during bowel evacuation procedures and bladder filling in subjects with spinal cord injury. *Spinal Cord* **2014**, *52*, 494–498. [CrossRef]
20. Pan, S.L.; Wang, Y.H.; Lin, H.L.; Chang, C.W.; Wu, T.Y.; Hsieh, E.T. Intracerebral hemorrhage secondary to autonomic dysreflexia in a young person with incomplete C8 tetraplegia: A case report. *Arch. Phys. Med. Rehabil.* **2005**, *86*, 591–593. [CrossRef]
21. Simpson, L.A.; Eng, J.J.; Hsieh, J.T.; Wolfe, D.L. The health and life priorities of individuals with spinal cord injury: A systematic review. *J. Neurotrauma* **2012**, *29*, 1548–1555. [CrossRef]
22. Anderson, K.D. Targeting recovery: Priorities of the spinal cord-injured population. *J. Neurotrauma* **2004**, *21*, 1371–1383. [CrossRef] [PubMed]
23. Krassioukov, A.; Warburton, D.E.; Teasell, R.; Eng, J.J. A systematic review of the management of autonomic dysreflexia after spinal cord injury. *Arch. Phys. Med. Rehabil.* **2009**, *90*, 682–695. [CrossRef] [PubMed]
24. Krassioukov, A.; Linsenmeyer, T.A.; Beck, L.A.; Elliott, S.; Gorman, P.; Kirshblum, S.; Vogel, L.; Wecht, J.; Clay, S. Evaluation and Management of Autonomic Dysreflexia and Other Autonomic Dysfunctions: Preventing the Highs and Lows: Management of Blood Pressure, Sweating, and Temperature Dysfunction. *Top. Spinal Cord Inj. Rehabil.* **2021**, *27*, 225–290. [CrossRef]
25. Grossman, E.; Messerli, F.H.; Grodzicki, T.; Kowey, P. Should a moratorium be placed on sublingual nifedipine capsules given for hypertensive emergencies and pseudoemergencies? *JAMA* **1996**, *276*, 1328–1331. [CrossRef]
26. Shealy, C.N.; Mortimer, J.T.; Reswick, J.B. Electrical inhibition of pain by stimulation of the dorsal columns: Preliminary clinical report. *Anesth. Analg.* **1967**, *46*, 489–491. [CrossRef] [PubMed]
27. Cameron, T. Safety and efficacy of spinal cord stimulation for the treatment of chronic pain: A 20-year literature review. *J. Neurosurg.* **2004**, *100*, 254–267. [CrossRef] [PubMed]
28. Samejima, S.; Henderson, R.; Pradarelli, J.; Mondello, S.E.; Moritz, C.T. Activity-dependent plasticity and spinal cord stimulation for motor recovery following spinal cord injury. *Exp. Neurol.* **2022**, *357*, 114178. [CrossRef]

29. Rowald, A.; Komi, S.; Demesmaeker, R.; Baaklini, E.; Hernandez-Charpak, S.D.; Paoles, E.; Montanaro, H.; Cassara, A.; Becce, F.; Lloyd, B.; et al. Activity-dependent spinal cord neuromodulation rapidly restores trunk and leg motor functions after complete paralysis. *Nat. Med.* **2022**, *28*, 260–271. [CrossRef]
30. Angeli, C.A.; Boakye, M.; Morton, R.A.; Vogt, J.; Benton, K.; Chen, Y.; Ferreira, C.K.; Harkema, S.J. Recovery of Over-Ground Walking after Chronic Motor Complete Spinal Cord Injury. *N. Engl. J. Med.* **2018**, *379*, 1244–1250. [CrossRef]
31. Gill, M.L.; Grahn, P.J.; Calvert, J.S.; Linde, M.B.; Lavrov, I.A.; Strommen, J.A.; Beck, L.A.; Sayenko, D.G.; Van Straaten, M.G.; Drubach, D.I.; et al. Neuromodulation of lumbosacral spinal networks enables independent stepping after complete paraplegia. *Nat. Med.* **2018**, *24*, 1677–1682. [CrossRef]
32. Samejima, S.; Shackleton, C.; Miller, T.; Moritz, C.T.; Kessler, T.M.; Krogh, K.; Sachdeva, R.; Krassioukov, A.V. Mapping the Iceberg of Autonomic Recovery: Mechanistic Underpinnings of Neuromodulation following Spinal Cord Injury. *Neurosci. Rev. J. Bringing Neurobiol. Neurol. Psychiatry* **2023**. [CrossRef] [PubMed]
33. Squair, J.W.; Gautier, M.; Mahe, L.; Soriano, J.E.; Rowald, A.; Bichat, A.; Cho, N.; Anderson, M.A.; James, N.D.; Gandar, J.; et al. Neuroprosthetic baroreflex controls haemodynamics after spinal cord injury. *Nature* **2021**, *590*, 308–314. [CrossRef]
34. Herrity, A.N.; Aslan, S.C.; Mesbah, S.; Siu, R.; Kalvakuri, K.; Ugiliweneza, B.; Mohamed, A.; Hubscher, C.H.; Harkema, S.J. Targeting bladder function with network-specific epidural stimulation after chronic spinal cord injury. *Sci. Rep.* **2022**, *12*, 11179. [CrossRef] [PubMed]
35. Harkema, S.J.; Ditterline, B.L.; Wang, S.; Aslan, S.; Angeli, C.A.; Ovechkin, A.; Hirsch, G.A. Epidural spinal cord stimulation training and sustained recovery of cardiovascular function in individuals with chronic cervical spinal cord injury. *JAMA Neurol.* **2018**, *75*, 1569–1571. [CrossRef]
36. Darrow, D.; Balser, D.; Netoff, T.I.; Krassioukov, A.; Phillips, A.; Parr, A.; Samadani, U. Epidural Spinal Cord Stimulation Facilitates Immediate Restoration of Dormant Motor and Autonomic Supraspinal Pathways after Chronic Neurologically Complete Spinal Cord Injury. *J. Neurotrauma* **2019**, *36*, 2325–2336. [CrossRef] [PubMed]
37. DiMarco, A.F.; Geertman, R.T.; Tabbaa, K.; Nemunaitis, G.A.; Kowalski, K.E. Effects of Lower Thoracic Spinal Cord Stimulation on Bowel Management in Individuals With Spinal Cord Injury. *Arch. Phys. Med. Rehabil.* **2021**, *102*, 1155–1164. [CrossRef]
38. Walter, M.; Lee, A.H.X.; Kavanagh, A.; Phillips, A.A.; Krassioukov, A.V. Epidural Spinal Cord Stimulation Acutely Modulates Lower Urinary Tract and Bowel Function Following Spinal Cord Injury: A Case Report. *Front. Physiol.* **2018**, *9*, 1816. [CrossRef]
39. Richardson, R.R.; Cerullo, L.J.; Meyer, P.R. Autonomic hyper-reflexia modulated by percutaneous epidural neurostimulation: A preliminary report. *Neurosurgery* **1979**, *4*, 517–520. [CrossRef] [PubMed]
40. Rupp, R.; Biering-Sørensen, F.; Burns, S.P.; Graves, D.E.; Guest, J.; Jones, L.; Read, M.S.; Rodriguez, G.M.; Schuld, C.; Tansey-Md, K.E.; et al. International Standards for Neurological Classification of Spinal Cord Injury: Revised 2019. *Top. Spinal Cord Inj. Rehabil.* **2021**, *27*, 1–22. [CrossRef]
41. Hubli, M.; Gee, C.M.; Krassioukov, A.V. Refined assessment of blood pressure instability after spinal cord injury. *Am. J. Hypertens.* **2015**, *28*, 173–181. [CrossRef]
42. Sachdeva, R.; Nightingale, T.E.; Pawar, K.; Kalimullina, T.; Mesa, A.; Marwaha, A.; Williams, A.M.M.; Lam, T.; Krassioukov, A.V. Noninvasive Neuroprosthesis Promotes Cardiovascular Recovery After Spinal Cord Injury. *Neurotherapeutics* **2021**, *18*, 1244–1256. [CrossRef] [PubMed]
43. Coggrave, M.J.; Norton, C. The need for manual evacuation and oral laxatives in the management of neurogenic bowel dysfunction after spinal cord injury: A randomized controlled trial of a stepwise protocol. *Spinal Cord* **2010**, *48*, 504–510. [CrossRef] [PubMed]
44. Wecht, J.M.; Krassioukov, A.V.; Alexander, M.; Handrakis, J.P.; McKenna, S.L.; Kennelly, M.; Trbovich, M.; Biering-Sorensen, F.; Burns, S.; Elliott, S.L.; et al. International Standards to document Autonomic Function following SCI (ISAFSCI): Second Edition. *Top. Spinal Cord Inj. Rehabil.* **2021**, *27*, 23–49. [CrossRef]
45. Ducla-Soares, J.L.; Santos-Bento, M.; Laranjo, S.; Andrade, A.; Ducla-Soares, E.; Boto, J.P.; Silva-Carvalho, L.; Rocha, I. Wavelet analysis of autonomic outflow of normal subjects on head-up tilt, cold pressor test, Valsalva manoeuvre and deep breathing. *Exp. Physiol.* **2007**, *92*, 677–686. [CrossRef] [PubMed]
46. Pagani, M.; Lombardi, F.; Guzzetti, S.; Rimoldi, O.; Furlan, R.; Pizzinelli, P.; Sandrone, G.; Malfatto, G.; Dell'Orto, S.; Piccaluga, E.; et al. Power spectral analysis of heart rate and arterial pressure variabilities as a marker of sympatho-vagal interaction in man and conscious dog. *Circ. Res.* **1986**, *59*, 178–193. [CrossRef]
47. Claydon, V.E.; Krassioukov, A.V. Clinical correlates of frequency analyses of cardiovascular control after spinal cord injury. *Am. J. Physiol. Heart Circ. Physiol.* **2008**, *294*, H668–H678. [CrossRef]
48. Inskip, J.A.; Lucci, V.M.; McGrath, M.S.; Willms, R.; Claydon, V.E. A Community Perspective on Bowel Management and Quality of Life after Spinal Cord Injury: The Influence of Autonomic Dysreflexia. *J. Neurotrauma* **2018**, *35*, 1091–1105. [CrossRef]
49. Pardee, C.; Bricker, D.; Rundquist, J.; MacRae, C.; Tebben, C. Characteristics of neurogenic bowel in spinal cord injury and perceived quality of life. *Rehabil. Nurs.* **2012**, *37*, 128–135. [CrossRef]
50. Coggrave, M.; Norton, C.; Wilson-Barnett, J. Management of neurogenic bowel dysfunction in the community after spinal cord injury: A postal survey in the United Kingdom. *Spinal Cord* **2009**, *47*, 323–333. [CrossRef] [PubMed]
51. Garshick, E.; Kelley, A.; Cohen, S.A.; Garrison, A.; Tun, C.G.; Gagnon, D.; Brown, R. A prospective assessment of mortality in chronic spinal cord injury. *Spinal Cord* **2005**, *43*, 408–416. [CrossRef] [PubMed]
52. DeVivo, M.J.; Krause, J.S.; Lammertse, D.P. Recent trends in mortality and causes of death among persons with spinal cord injury. *Arch. Phys. Med. Rehabil.* **1999**, *80*, 1411–1419. [CrossRef] [PubMed]

53. Myers, J.; Lee, M.; Kiratli, J. Cardiovascular disease in spinal cord injury: An overview of prevalence, risk, evaluation, and management. *Am. J. Phys. Med. Rehabil.* **2007**, *86*, 142–152. [CrossRef] [PubMed]
54. Soriano, J.E.; Hudelle, R.; Squair, J.W.; Anderson, M.A.; Gautier, M.; Mahe, L.; Tso, M.; Amir, S.; Courtine, G.; Phillips, A.A. Long-term neuroprosthetic hemotherapy treats autonomic dysreflexia after spinal cord injury. *FASEB J.* **2022**, *36*. [CrossRef]
55. Melzack, R.; Wall, P.D. Pain mechanisms: A new theory. *Science* **1965**, *150*, 971–979. [CrossRef] [PubMed]
56. Daniele, C.A.; MacDermott, A.B. Low-threshold primary afferent drive onto GABAergic interneurons in the superficial dorsal horn of the mouse. *J. Neurosci. Off. J. Soc. Neurosci.* **2009**, *29*, 686–695. [CrossRef]
57. Cui, J.G.; O'Connor, W.T.; Ungerstedt, U.; Linderoth, B.; Meyerson, B.A. Spinal cord stimulation attenuates augmented dorsal horn release of excitatory amino acids in mononeuropathy via a GABAergic mechanism. *Pain* **1997**, *73*, 87–95. [CrossRef]

Disclaimer/Publisher's Note: The statements, opinions and data contained in all publications are solely those of the individual author(s) and contributor(s) and not of MDPI and/or the editor(s). MDPI and/or the editor(s) disclaim responsibility for any injury to people or property resulting from any ideas, methods, instructions or products referred to in the content.